NEUROLOGY AND NEUROSURGERY ILLUSTRATED

NEUROLOGY AND NEUROSURGERY ILLUSTRATED

KENNETH W. LINDSAY PhD FRCS

Consultant Neurosurgeon, Royal Free Hospital;
Honorary Senior Lecturer, Royal Free Hospital School of Medicine,
University of London, London, UK

IAN BONE MRCP (UK) FRCP (G)

Consultant Neurologist, Institute of Neurological Sciences;
Honorary Clinical Lecturer, University of Glasgow,
Glasgow, UK

ROBIN CALLANDER FFPh FMAA AIMBI

Medical Illustrator

CHURCHILL LIVINGSTONE
EDINBURGH LONDON MELBOURNE AND NEW YORK 1986

CHURCHILL LIVINGSTONE
Medical Division of Longman Group UK Limited

Distributed in the United States of America by
Churchill Livingstone Inc., 1560 Broadway, New York,
N.Y. 10036, and by associated companies, branches and
representatives throughout the world.

First published 1986
  Reprinted 1988

ISBN 0-443-02945-8

British Library Cataloguing in Publication Data
Lindsay, Kenneth W.
  Neurology and neurosurgery illustrated.
  1. Nervous system — Diseases
  I. Title   II. Bone, Ian   III. Callander, Robin
  616.8   RC346

Produced by Longman Group (FE) Ltd
Printed in Hong Kong

PREFACE

Although neurology and neurosurgery are inevitably interlinked, sharing similar examination and investigative techniques, most postgraduate and undergraduate texts present each subject separately. In this book we adopt an integrated approach and take advantage of the highly visual nature of the subject by producing an illustrated text.

In the first part of the book, we place particular emphasis on the method of approaching clinical problems. We describe how clinical findings combined with a good knowledge of anatomy and physiology aid lesion localisation and guide the investigative approach towards a final diagnosis. The second part of the book concentrates on the clinical presentation and management of those neurological disorders occurring in specific sites and of those disorders involving multiple sites.

The text in small print is intended only as a source of reference for the undergraduate but provides more comprehensive coverage for the postgraduate reader. In some neurosurgical conditions we detail various operative approaches, but make no attempt to describe operative techniques.

We are indebted to numerous colleagues and friends in London, Glasgow and elsewhere who have taken the time and trouble to comment on and criticise parts of the text. Finally we would like to thank our wives and families for their continual encouragement and support.

1986

K. W. L.
I. B.
R. C.

CONTENTS

SECTION I

General Approach to History
and Examination

Nervous System — History

An accurate description of the patient's neurological symptoms is an important aid in establishing the diagnosis; but this must be taken in conjunction with information from other systems, previous medical history, family and social history and current medication. Often the patient's history requires confirmation from a relative or friend.

The following outline indicates the relevant information to obtain for each symptom, although some may require further clarification.

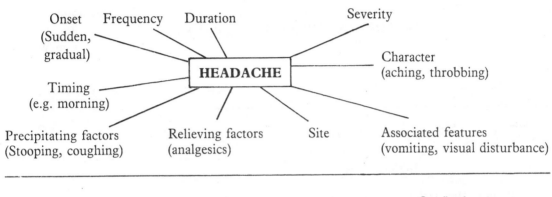

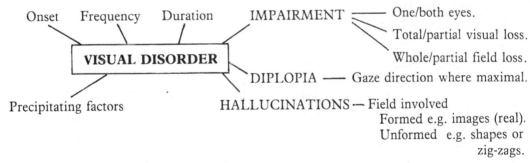

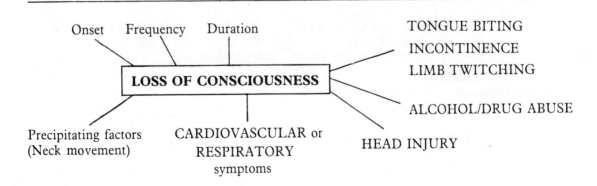

Nervous System — History

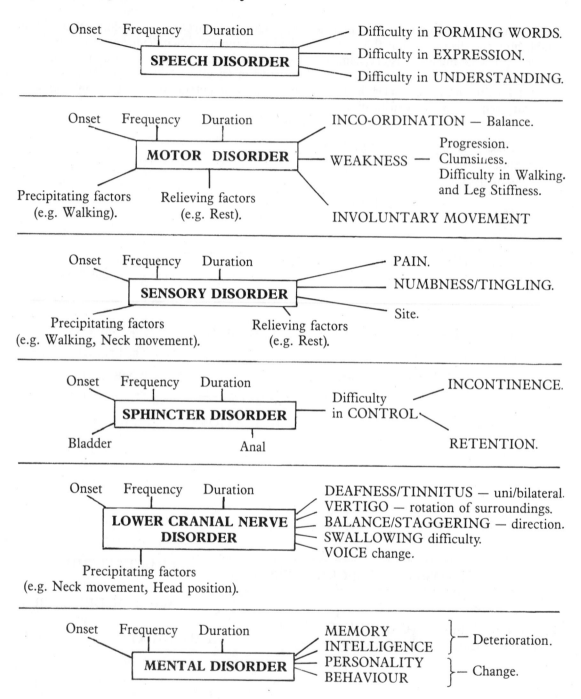

Onset Frequency Duration

SPEECH DISORDER

- Difficulty in FORMING WORDS.
- Difficulty in EXPRESSION.
- Difficulty in UNDERSTANDING.

Onset Frequency Duration

MOTOR DISORDER

Precipitating factors (e.g. Walking).

Relieving factors (e.g. Rest).

INCO-ORDINATION — Balance.

WEAKNESS — Progression. Clumsiness. Difficulty in Walking. and Leg Stiffness.

INVOLUNTARY MOVEMENT

Onset Frequency Duration

SENSORY DISORDER

Precipitating factors (e.g. Walking, Neck movement).

Relieving factors (e.g. Rest).

- PAIN.
- NUMBNESS/TINGLING.
- Site.

Onset Frequency Duration

SPHINCTER DISORDER

Bladder   Anal

Difficulty in CONTROL

INCONTINENCE.

RETENTION.

Onset Frequency Duration

LOWER CRANIAL NERVE DISORDER

Precipitating factors (e.g. Neck movement, Head position).

DEAFNESS/TINNITUS — uni/bilateral.
VERTIGO — rotation of surroundings.
BALANCE/STAGGERING — direction.
SWALLOWING difficulty.
VOICE change.

Onset Frequency Duration

MENTAL DISORDER

MEMORY
INTELLIGENCE } — Deterioration.
PERSONALITY
BEHAVIOUR } — Change.

Nervous System — Examination

Neurological disease may produce systemic signs and systemic disease may affect the nervous system. A complete general examination must therefore accompany that of the central nervous system. In particular, note the following:

Temperature.
Blood pressure.
Neck stiffness.
Pulse irregularity.
Carotid bruit.
Cardiac murmurs.
Cyanosis/Respiratory insufficiency.

Evidence of weight loss.
Breast lumps.
Lymphadenopathy.
Hepatic and splenic
    enlargement.
Prostatic irregularity.

Septic source e.g. teeth, ears.
Skin marks e.g. rashes,
    cafe-au-lait spots,
    angiomata.
Anterior fontanelle ⎫
Head circumference ⎭ in baby.

CNS examination is described systematically from the head downwards and includes:

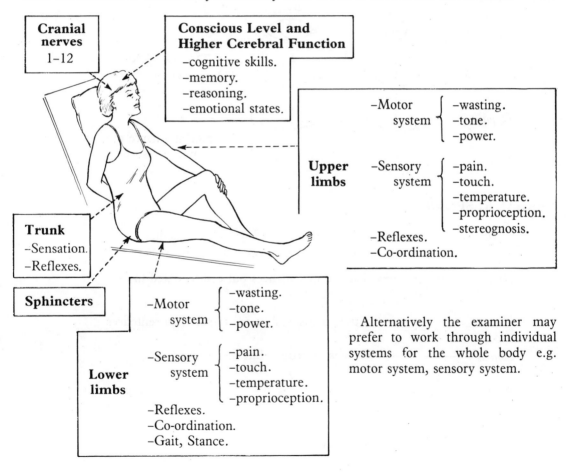

Cranial nerves 1–12

Conscious Level and Higher Cerebral Function
–cognitive skills.
–memory.
–reasoning.
–emotional states.

Upper limbs
–Motor system
  –wasting.
  –tone.
  –power.
–Sensory system
  –pain.
  –touch.
  –temperature.
  –proprioception.
  –stereognosis.
–Reflexes.
–Co-ordination.

Trunk
–Sensation.
–Reflexes.

Sphincters

Lower limbs
–Motor system
  –wasting.
  –tone.
  –power.
–Sensory system
  –pain.
  –touch.
  –temperature.
  –proprioception.
–Reflexes.
–Co-ordination.
–Gait, Stance.

Alternatively the examiner may prefer to work through individual systems for the whole body e.g. motor system, sensory system.

Examination — Conscious Level Assessment

A wide variety of systemic and intracranial problems produce depression of conscious level. Accurate assessment and recording are essential to determine deterioration or improvement in a patient's condition. In 1974 Teasdale and Jennett, in Glasgow, developed a system for conscious level assessment. They discarded vague terms such as stupor, semicoma and deep coma, and described conscious level in terms of EYE opening,
VERBAL response and
MOTOR response.

The Glasgow coma scale is now used widely in Britain and in many centres throughout the world. Recording is consistent irrespective of the status of the observer and can be carried out just as reliably by nurse as by neurosurgeon.

EYE OPENING

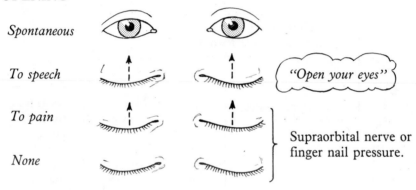

Spontaneous

To speech — "Open your eyes"

To pain

None — Supraorbital nerve or finger nail pressure.

VERBAL RESPONSE

Orientated ——————— Knows place, e.g. Royal Free Hospital and time e.g. day, month and year.

Confused ——————— Talking in sentences but disorientated in time and place.

Words ——————— Utters occasional words rather than sentences.

Sounds ——————— Groans or grunts, but no words.

None

Examination — Conscious Level Assessment

MOTOR RESPONSE

Obeys commands

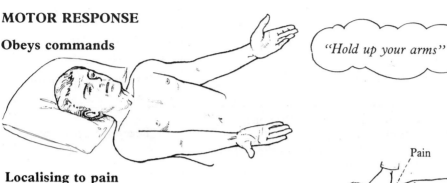

"Hold up your arms"

Localising to pain

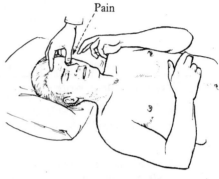

Apply a painful stimulus to the supraorbital nerve e.g. rub thumb nail in the supraorbital groove, increasing pressure until a response is obtained. If the patient responds by bringing the hand up beyond the chin = 'localising to pain'. (Pressure to nail beds or sternum at this stage may not differentiate 'localising' from 'flexing'.)

Flexing to pain

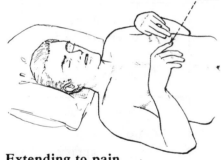

If the patient does not localise to supraorbital pressure, apply pressure with a pen or hard object to the nail bed. Record elbow flexion as 'flexing to pain'. Spastic wrist flexion may or may not accompany this response.

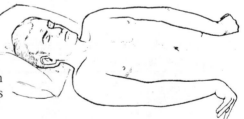

Extending to pain

If in response to the same stimulus elbow extension occurs, record as 'extending to pain'. This is always accompanied by spastic flexion of the wrist.

None   Before recording a patient at this level, ensure that the painful stimulus is adequate.

During examination the motor response may vary. Supraorbital pain may produce an extension response, whereas finger nail pressure produces flexion. Alternatively one arm may localise to pain; the other may flex. When this occurs record the *best* response during the period of examination (this correlates best with final outcome). For the purpose of conscious level assessment use only the *arm* response. Leg response to pain produces less consistent results and inappropriate spinal reflexes are more likely to occur.

7

Examination — Higher Cerebral Function

COGNITIVE SKILL

	Dominant Hemisphere Disorders
Listen to language pattern — hesitant — fluent.	Expressive dysphasia Receptive dysphasia
Does the patient understand simple/complex spoken commands? E.g. "Hold up both arms, touch the right ear with the left fifth finger."	Receptive dysphasia
Ask the patient to name objects.	Nominal dysphasia
Does the patient read correctly?	Dyslexia
Does the patient write correctly?	Dysgraphia
Ask the patient to perform a numerical calculation e.g. Serial 7 test, where 7 is subtracted serially from 100.	Dyscalculia
Can the patient recognise objects? E.g. ask patient to select an object from a group.	Agnosia

	Non-Dominant Hemisphere Disorders
Note patient's ability to find his way around the ward or his home.	Geographical agnosia
Can the patient dress himself?	Dressing apraxia
Note the patient's ability to copy a geometric pattern e.g. ask patient to form a star with matches or copy a drawing of a cube.	Constructional apraxia

Examination — Higher Cerebral Function

MEMORY Test

IMMEDIATE memory —— Digit span — ask patient to repeat a sequence of 5, 6 or 7 random numbers.

RECENT memory ——— Ask patient to describe present illness, duration of hospital stay or recent events in the news.

REMOTE memory ——— Ask about events and circumstances occurring more than 5 years previously.

VERBAL memory ——— Ask patient to remember a sentence or a short story and test after 15 minutes.

VISUAL memory ——— Ask patient to remember objects on a tray and test after 15 minutes.

Note: Memory cannot be tested in a confused or dysphasic patient.

REASONING and PROBLEM SOLVING

Test patient with two-step calculations e.g. "I wish to buy 12 articles at 7 pence each. How much change will I receive from £1?"

Ask patient to reverse 3 or 4 random numbers.

Ask patient to explain proverbs.

The examiner must compare patient's present reasoning ability with expected abilities based on job history and/or school work.

EMOTIONAL STATE

Note:
Anxiety or excitement.
Depression or apathy.
Emotional behaviour.
Uninhibited behaviour.
Slowness of movement or responses.

Cranial Nerve Examination

OLFACTORY NERVE (I)

Test using aromatic non-irritant materials e.g. soap, tobacco.

One nostril is closed while the patient sniffs with the other.

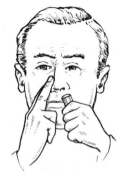

OPTIC NERVE (II)

Visual acuity
- *severe* deficit — Can patient see — light? — movement?
  - Can patient count fingers?
- *mild* deficit — Record reading acuity with wall or hand chart.

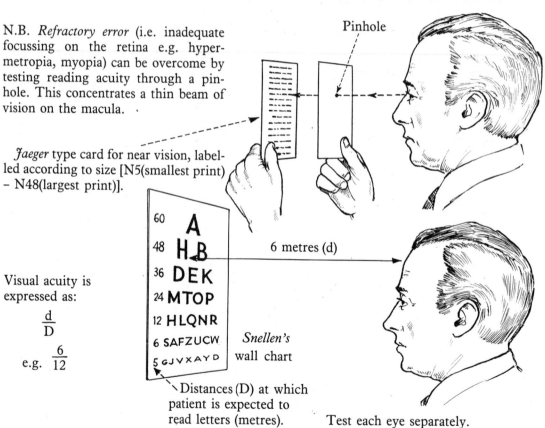

N.B. *Refractory error* (i.e. inadequate focussing on the retina e.g. hypermetropia, myopia) can be overcome by testing reading acuity through a pinhole. This concentrates a thin beam of vision on the macula.

Pinhole

Jaeger type card for near vision, labelled according to size [N5(smallest print) – N48(largest print)].

60 A
48 H B   6 metres (d)
36 DEK
24 MTOP
12 HLQNR
6 SAFZUCW   *Snellen's*
5 GJVXAYD   wall chart

Visual acuity is expressed as:

$$\frac{d}{D}$$

e.g. $\frac{6}{12}$

Distances (D) at which patient is expected to read letters (metres).

Test each eye separately.

Cranial Nerve Examination

The **Visual Fields**

1. Gross testing by CONFRONTATION.

Compare the patient's fields of vision by advancing a moving finger or, more accurately, a red 5mm pin from the extreme periphery towards the fixation point. This maps out 'cone' vision. A 2mm pin will define central field defects which may only manifest as a loss of colour perception.

In the temporal portion of the visual field the physiological blind spot may be detected. A 3mm object should disappear here.

The patient must fixate on the examiner's pupil.

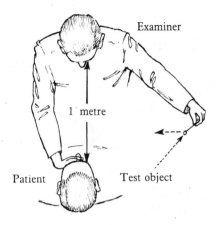

2. Peripheral visual fields are more sensitive to a *moving* target and are tested with a MECHANICAL PERIMETER.

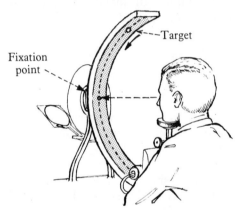

The patient fixates on a central point. A white target (3 – 10mm) is moved centrally around the arc of a perimeter from the extreme periphery until observed in the patient's peripheral field. The field charts thus obtained provide a permanent record with which comparisons can be made at a later date.

Record target diameter/distance of eye from fixation point e.g. 3/250.

3. The TANGENT SCREEN is a more accurate test of the central fields within 30° of the fixation point.

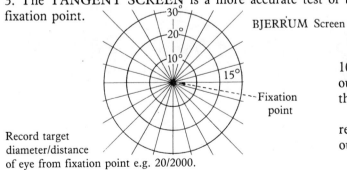

BJERRUM Screen

The screen is flat. A large white 10mm target is moved in from outside while the patient fixates on the centre.

By using smaller targets (e.g. 2mm red pin) the central field is mapped out.

Record target diameter/distance of eye from fixation point e.g. 20/2000.

Cranial Nerve Examination

Optic Fundus

Ask the patient to fixate on a distant object away from any bright light. Use the right eye to examine the patient's right eye and the left eye to examine the patient's left eye.

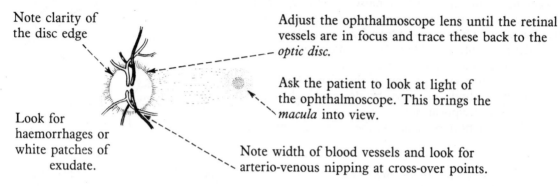

Note clarity of the disc edge

Adjust the ophthalmoscope lens until the retinal vessels are in focus and trace these back to the *optic disc.*

Ask the patient to look at light of the ophthalmoscope. This brings the *macula* into view.

Look for haemorrhages or white patches of exudate.

Note width of blood vessels and look for arterio-venous nipping at cross-over points.

If small pupil size prevents fundal examination, then dilate pupil with homatropine. This is contraindicated if either an acute expanding lesion or glaucoma is suspected.

Pupils   Note:
- size.
- shape.
- equality.
- reaction to light: both pupils constrict when light is shone in either eye.
- reaction to accommodation and convergence: pupil constriction occurs when gaze is transferred to a near point object.

A lesion of the *optic nerve* will abolish pupillary response to light on the same side as well as in the contralateral eye.

When light is shone in the *normal* eye, it and the contralateral pupil will constrict.

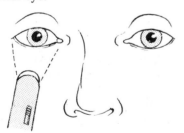

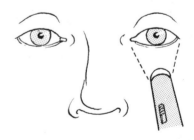

Cranial Nerve Examination

OCULOMOTOR(III), TROCHLEAR(IV) and ABDUCENS(VI) NERVES

A lesion of the III nerve produces impairment of eye and lid movement as well as disturbance of pupillary response.

Pupil: The pupil dilates and becomes 'fixed' to light.

Shine torch in *affected* eye - contra-lateral pupil constricts (its III nerve intact). Absent or impaired response in illuminated eye.

When light is shone into the *normal* eye, only the pupil on that side constricts.

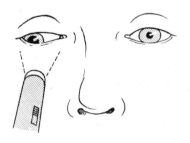
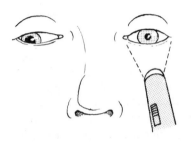

Ptosis: Ptosis is present if the eyelid droops over the pupil when the eyes are fully open.

Since the levator palpebrae muscle contains both skeletal and smooth muscle, ptosis signifies either a III nerve palsy or a sympathetic lesion.

Ocular Movement

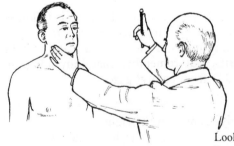

Steady the patient's head and ask him to follow an object held at arm's length. Observe the full range of horizontal and vertical movements.

Note any *malalignment or limitation of range.*

Examine eye movements in the six different directions of gaze representing maximal individual muscle strength.

```
                      Upward movement
                  Looking out        Looking in
                  Sup.rectus(III)   Inf.oblique(III)

     Lateral                                            Medial
     movement  ─────────┼─────────────┼──────────       movement
     Lat.rectus(VI)                                   Med.rectus(III)

                  Downward movement
                  Looking out        Looking in
                  Inf.rectus(III)   Sup.oblique(IV)
```

Cranial Nerve Examination

Question patient about *diplopia*; the patient is more likely to notice this before the examiner can detect impairment of eye movement. If present:

> – note the *direction of maximum displacement* of the images and determine the pair of muscles involved.
> – identify the source of the *outer image* (from the defective eye) using a transparent coloured lens.

e.g.

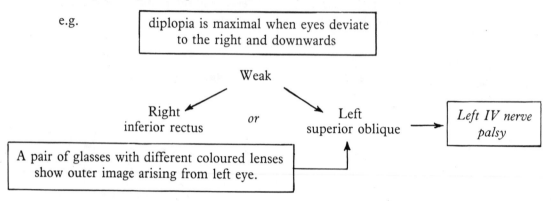

diplopia is maximal when eyes deviate to the right and downwards

Weak

Right inferior rectus   *or*   Left superior oblique → *Left IV nerve palsy*

A pair of glasses with different coloured lenses show outer image arising from left eye.

CONJUGATE MOVEMENT:

Note the ability of the eyes to move together (conjugately) in horizontal or vertical direction or tendency for gaze to fix in one particular direction.

NYSTAGMUS:

This is an upset in the normal balance of eye control. A slow drift in one direction is followed by a fast corrective movement. Nystagmus is maximal when the eyes are turned in the direction of the fast phase. Nystagmus 'direction' is usually described in terms of the fast phase and may be horizontal or vertical. Test as for other eye movements, but remember that 'physiological' nystagmus can occur when the eyes deviate more than 30° from central gaze.

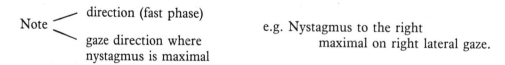

Note
- direction (fast phase)
- gaze direction where nystagmus is maximal

e.g. Nystagmus to the right
maximal on right lateral gaze.

Cranial Nerve Examination

TRIGEMINAL NERVE (V)

Test *pain* (pin prick) sensation
    temperature (cold object or
           hot/cold tubes)
    light touch
} over whole face

Compare each side.
Map out the sensory deficit,
testing from the abnormal
to the normal region.

Does distribution involve
         – a *root* pattern? ⟶
         – or a *brain stem*
            'onion skin' pattern?

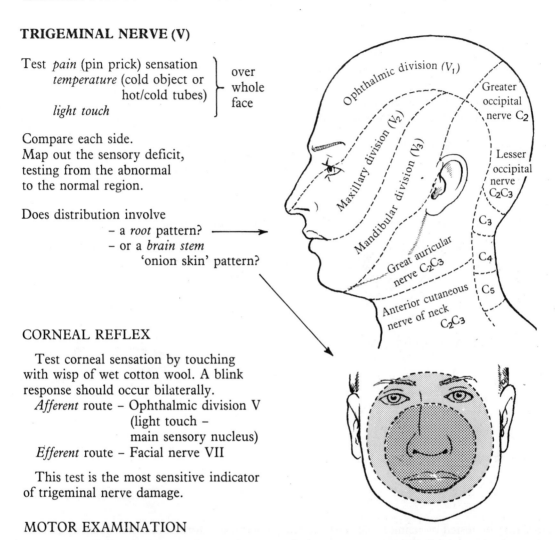

CORNEAL REFLEX

Test corneal sensation by touching
with wisp of wet cotton wool. A blink
response should occur bilaterally.
   Afferent route – Ophthalmic division V
         (light touch –
           main sensory nucleus)
   Efferent route – Facial nerve VII

This test is the most sensitive indicator
of trigeminal nerve damage.

MOTOR EXAMINATION

Observe for wasting and thinning of temporalis muscle – "hollowing out" the temporalis fossa.
Ask the patient to clamp jaws together. Feel temporalis and masseter muscles. Attempt to open patient's jaws by applying pressure to chin. Ask patient to open mouth. If pterygoid muscles are weak the jaw will deviate to the weak side, being pushed over by the unopposed pterygoid muscles of the good side.

JAW JERK

Ask patient to relax jaw. Place finger on the chin and tap with hammer. Slight or absent jerk – normal. Increased jerk – upper motor neurone lesion.

Cranial Nerve Examination

FACIAL NERVE (VII)

Observe patient as he talks and smiles, watching for:
- eye closure,
- asymmetrical elevation of one corner of mouth,
- flattening of naso-labial fold.

Patient is then instructed to

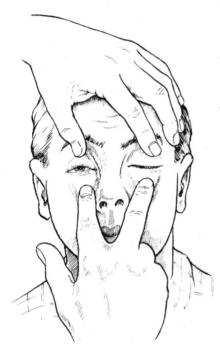

- wrinkle forehead
  (by looking upwards),

- close eyes while examiner
  attempts to open them,

- purse lips while examiner
  presses cheeks.

- show teeth,

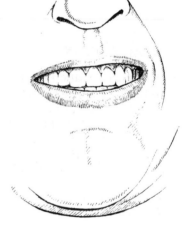

Taste may be tested by using sugar, tartaric acid or sodium chloride. A small quantity of each substance is placed on the appropriate side of the protruded tongue.

Cranial Nerve Examination

AUDITORY NERVE (VIII)

Cochlear Component:

Test by whispering numbers into one ear while masking hearing in the other ear by occluding and rubbing the external meatus. If hearing is impaired, examine external meatus and the tympanic membrane with auroscope to exclude wax or infection.

Differentiate conductive (middle ear) deafness from perceptive (nerve) deafness by:

1. WEBER's TEST

Hold base of tuning fork against the vertex. Ask patient if sound is heard more loudly in one ear.

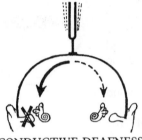 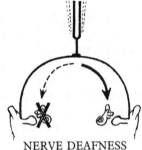

NORMAL hearing	CONDUCTIVE DEAFNESS	NERVE DEAFNESS
	Sound is louder in affected ear since distraction from external sounds is reduced in that ear.	Sound is louder in the normal ear

2. RINNE's TEST

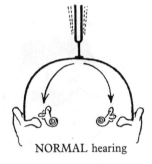

Hold the base of a vibrating tuning fork against the mastoid bone. Ask the patient if note is heard. When note disappears — hold tuning fork near the external meatus. Patient should hear sound again since air conduction via the ossicles is better than bone conduction.

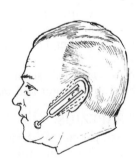

In *conductive deafness*, bone conduction is better than air conduction.
In *nerve deafness*, both bone and air conduction are impaired.

Further auditory testing and examination of the **vestibular component** requires specialised investigation (see pages 58–60).

Cranial Nerve Examination

GLOSSOPHARYNGEAL NERVE (IX):   VAGUS NERVE (X)

These nerves are considered jointly since they are examined together and their actions are seldom individually impaired.

Note patient's *voice* — if there is vocal cord paresis (X), voice may be high pitched. (Vocal cord examination is best left to an ENT specialist.)

Note any *swallowing* difficulty or nasal regurgitation of fluids.

Ask patient to open mouth and say *"Ah"*. Note any *asymmetry* of palatal movements (X nerve palsy).

GAG REFLEX

Depress patient's tongue and touch palate, pharynx or tonsil on one side until the patient 'gags'. Compare sensitivity on each side (*afferent* route — IX nerve) and observe symmetry of palatal contraction (*efferent* route — X nerve).

Absent gag reflex = loss of sensation and/or loss of motor power.

(Taste in the posterior $\frac{1}{3}$ of the tongue(IX) is impractical to test).

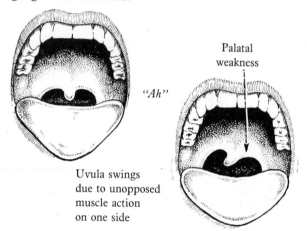

"Ah"

Palatal weakness

Uvula swings due to unopposed muscle action on one side

ACCESSORY NERVE (XI)

STERNOMASTOID

Ask patient to rotate head against resistance. Compare power and muscle bulk on each side. Also compare each side with the patient pulling head forward against resistance.

N.B. The left sternomastoid turns the head to the right and *vice versa*.

TRAPEZIUS

Ask patient to 'shrug' shoulders and to hold them in this position against resistance. Compare power on each side. Patient should manage to resist any effort to depress shoulders.

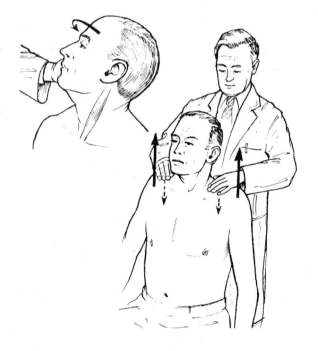

Cranial Nerve Examination

HYPOGLOSSAL NERVE (XII)

Ask patient to open mouth; inspect tongue.
Look for – evidence of atrophy (increased folds, wasting)
            – fasciculation (small wriggling movements).
Ask patient to protrude tongue.

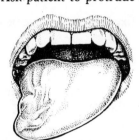

Note any difficulty or deviation
  (N.B. apparent deviation may occur with facial weakness
– if present, assess tongue in relation to teeth.)
Tongue deviates towards side of weakness.
Note any disturbance in patient's speech.

Examination – Upper Limbs

MOTOR SYSTEM

Appearance

Note:

  –any *asymmetry* or *deformity*

  –muscle *wasting* } If in doubt, measure circumference at fixed distance above/below
  –muscle *hypertrophy* } joint. Note muscle group involved.

  –muscle *fasciculation* — irregular, non-rhythmical contraction of muscle fascicles, increased after exercise and on smacking muscle surface.
  N.B. Fasciculation may occur in normal individuals. Distinguish from 'fibrillation' which is an E.M.G. finding

Tone

Ensure that the patient is relaxed, and assess tone by alternately flexing and extending the elbow or wrist.

Note:

  –decrease in tone

  –increase in tone {
  'Clasp-knife': the initial resistance to the movement is suddenly over-come (upper motor neurone lesion).
  'Lead-pipe': a steady increase in resistance throughout the movement (extrapyramidal lesion).
  'Cog-wheel': ratchet-like increase in resistance (extrapyramidal lesion).

Power

If a pyramidal weakness is suspect (i.e. a weakness arising from damage to the motor cortex or descending motor tracts (see pages 180–183) the following test is simple, quick yet sensitive.

Ask the patient to hold arms outstretched with the hands supinated for up to one minute. The eyes are closed (otherwise visual compensation occurs). The weak arm gradually pronates and drifts downwards.

With possible involvement at the spinal root or nerve level (lower motor neurone), it is essential to test individual muscle groups to help localise the lesion.

When testing muscle groups, think of *root* supply and *nerve* supply.

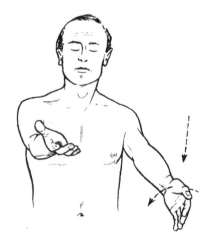

Examination – Upper Limbs

Shoulder Abduction

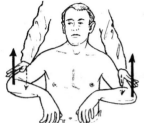

Deltoid: **C5**C6 roots. Axillary nerve.

Arm (at more than 15° from the vertical) abducts against resistance.

Shoulder Adduction

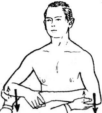

Pectoralis major: C5,**C6,7,8** roots. Lateral and med. pectoral nerves.
Latissimus dorsi: C6,**C7**,C8. Nerve to latissimus dorsi. Arm adducted against resistance.

Elbow Flexion

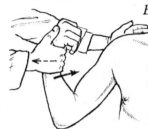

Biceps: **C5**,C6 roots. Musculocutaneous nerve.

Arm flexed against resistance with the hand fully supinated.

Elbow Extension

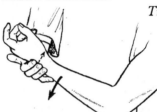

Triceps: **C7**,C8 roots. Radial nerve.

Patient extends arm against resistance.

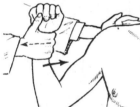

Brachioradialis: **C5,C6** roots. Radial nerve.

Arm flexed against resistance with hand in mid-position between pronation and supination.

Wrist Extension

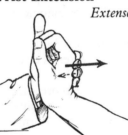

Extensor carpi radialis longus: C6,**C7** roots.
Extensor carpi ulnaris: **C7**,C8 roots. Radial nerve.

Wrist is extended against resistance.

Finger Flexion – terminal phalanx

Flexor digitorum profundus I and II: **C8**T1 roots. Median nerve.
Flexor digitorum profundus III and IV: **C8**,T1 roots. Ulnar nerve.

Examiner tries to extend patient's flexed terminal phalanges.

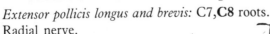

Thumb Extension – terminal phalanx

Extensor pollicis longus and brevis: C7,**C8** roots. Radial nerve.

Thumb is extended against resistance.

Examination – Upper Limbs

Thumb Opposition

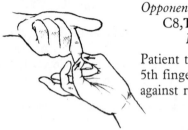

Opponens pollicis:
C8, **T1** roots.
Median nerve.

Patient tries to touch
5th finger with thumb
against resistance.

Finger Abduction

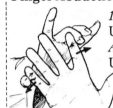

1st Dorsal interosseus: C8, **T1**
Ulnar nerve. roots.
Abductor digiti minimi: C8, **T1**
Ulnar nerve. roots.

Fingers abducted against
resistance.

[Note: Not all muscle groups are included in the foregoing, but only those required to identify and differentiate nerve and root lesions.]

SENSATION

Pain

Pin prick provides a simple method of testing this important modality. Firstly, check that the patient detects the pin as 'sharp' i.e. painful, then rapidly test each dermatome in turn.

Memorising the dermatome distribution is simplified by noting that 'C7' extends down the second finger.

If pin prick is impaired, then more carefully map out the extent of the abnormality, moving from the abnormal to the normal area.

Light Touch

This is tested in a similar manner, using a wisp of cotton wool.

Temperature

Temperature testing seldom provides any additional information. If required, use a cold object or hot and cold test tubes.

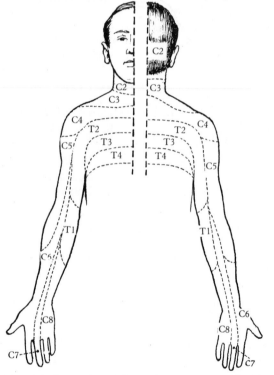

Examination – Upper Limbs

Joint Position Sense

Hold the sides of the patient's finger or thumb and demonstrate 'up and down' movements.

Repeat with the patient's eyes closed. Ask patient to specify the direction of movement.

Ask the patient, with eyes closed, to touch his nose with his forefinger or to bring forefingers together with the arms outstretched.

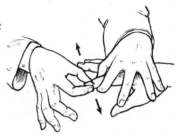

Vibration

Place a vibrating tuning fork (usually 128 c.p.s.) on a bony prominence e.g. radius. Ask the patient to indicate when the vibration, if felt, ceases. If impaired, move more proximally and repeat. Vibration testing is of value in the early detection of demyelinating disease and peripheral neuropathy, but otherwise is of limited benefit.

If the above modalities are normal and a cortical lesion is suspected, it is useful to test for the following:

Two Point Discrimination: the ability to discriminate two blunt points when simultaneously applied to the finger, 5mm apart. (Cf. 4cm in the legs.)

Blunt ends

5mm

Sensory Inattention (Perceptual Rivalry): the ability to detect stimuli (pin prick or touch) in both limbs, when applied to both limbs simultaneously.

Stereognosis: the ability to recognise objects placed in the hand.

Graphaesthesia: the ability to recognise numbers or letters traced out on the palm.

REFLEXES

Biceps Jerk   C5,C6 roots.
          Radial nerve.

Ensure patient's arm is relaxed and slightly flexed. Palpate the biceps tendon with the thumb and strike with tendon hammer. Look for elbow flexion and biceps contraction.

Supinator Jerk   C5,C6 roots.
          Radial nerve.

Strike the lower end of the radius with the hammer and watch for elbow and finger flexion.

23

Examination – Upper Limbs

Triceps Jerk

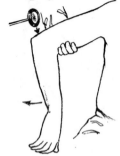

C7,C8 roots.
Radial nerve.

Strike the patient's elbow a few inches above the olecranon process. Look for elbow extension and triceps contraction.

Hoffman Reflex

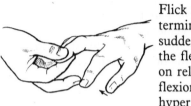

C7,C8,T1

Flick the patient's terminal phalanx, suddenly stretching the flexor tendon on release. Thumb flexion indicates hyperreflexia.

Reflex Enhancement

When reflexes are difficult to elicit, enhancement occurs if the patient is asked to 'clench the teeth'.

CO-ORDINATION

Inco-ordination (ataxia) and muscular hypotonicity are often prominent features of cerebellar disease (see page 169). Prior to testing, ensure that power and proprioception are normal.

Hypotonicity

Arm Bounce

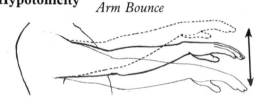

Downward pressure and sudden release of the patient's outstretched arm causes excessive swinging.

Rebound Phenomenon

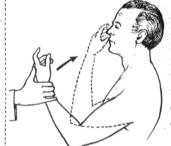

Ask the patient to flex elbow against resistance. Sudden release may cause the hand to strike the face due to delay in triceps contraction.

Inco-ordination

Finger-Nose Testing

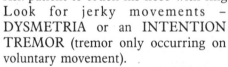

Ask patient to touch his nose with finger (eyes open). Look for jerky movements – DYSMETRIA or an INTENTION TREMOR (tremor only occurring on voluntary movement).
Ask patient to alternately touch his own nose then the examiner's finger as fast as he can. This may exaggerate the intention tremor and may demonstrate DYSDIADOCHOKINESIA – an inability to perform rapidly alternating movements.

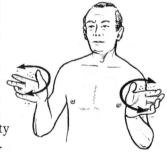

This may also be shown by asking the patient to rapidly supinate and pronate the forearms or to perform rapid and repeated tapping movements.

Examination – Trunk

SENSATION

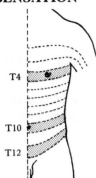

Test pin prick and light touch in dermatome distribution as for the upper limbs.

Levels to remember: T4 – at *nipple*
T10 – at *umbilicus*
T12 – at *inguinal ligament*

Abdominal Reflexes

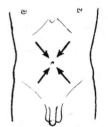

T7 – T12 roots.

Stroke or lightly scratch the skin towards the umbilicus in each quadrant in turn. Look for abdominal muscle contraction and note if absent or impaired. (N.B. Reflexes may be absent in obesity, after pregnancy or after abdominal operations.)

Cremasteric Reflex L1 root. Scratch inner thigh. Observe contraction of cremasteric muscle causing testicular elevation.

SPHINCTERS

Examine abdomen for distended bladder.

Note evidence of urinary or faecal incontinence.

Note tone of anal sphincter during rectal examination.

Anal Reflex S4,S5 roots.

A scratch on the skin beside the anus causes a reflex contraction of the anal sphincter.

Examination – Lower Limbs

MOTOR SYSTEM

Appearance   Note: – *asymmetry* or *deformity*.
– muscle *wasting*.
– muscle *hypertrophy*.
– muscle *fasciculation*.

} As in the upper limbs.

Tone

Try to relax the patient and alternately flex and extend the knee joint. Note the resistance.

Roll the patient's legs from side to side. Suddenly lift the thigh and note the response in the lower leg. With increased tone the leg kicks upwards.

Clonus

Ensure that the patient is relaxed. Apply sudden and sustained flexion to the ankle. A few oscillatory beats may occur in the normal subject, but when this persists it indicates increased tone.

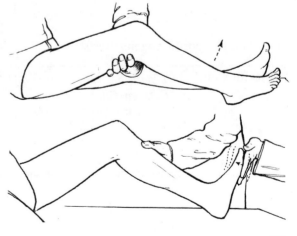

Examination – Lower Limbs

Power
When testing each muscle group, think of *root* and *nerve* supply.

Hip Flexion

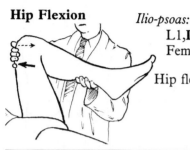

Ilio-psoas:
L1,L2,L3 roots.
Femoral nerve.

Hip flexed against
resistance.

Hip Extension

Glutei:
L4,L5,S1 roots.
Gluteal nerves.

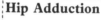

Patient attempts to keep heel on
bed against
resistance.

Hip Abduction

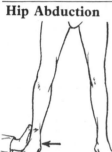

*Glutei and Tensor fascia
lata:* **L4,L5,S1** roots.
Superior gluteal nerve.

Patient lying on
back tries to abduct
the leg against
resistance.

Hip Adduction

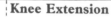

Adductors:
L2,L3,L4 roots.
Obturator nerve.

Patient lying on back
tries to pull knees
together against
resistance.

Knee Flexion

Hamstrings:
L4,L5,S1,S2 roots.
Sciatic nerve.

Patient pulls
heel towards
the buttock
and tries to
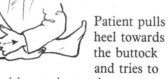
maintain this position against resistance.

Knee Extension

Quadriceps:
L2,L3,L4 roots.
Femoral nerve.

Patient tries
to maintain
knee extension.
Examiner with an arm under the patient's
thigh tries to flex the knee.

Dorsiflexion

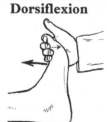

*Tibialis anterior,
Extensor hallucis longus,
Extensor digitorum longus:*
L4,L5,S1 roots.
Peroneal division of
Sciatic nerve.
Patient dorsiflexes the ankle
and toes against resistance.
May have difficulty in walking on heels.

Plantarflexion

*Gastrocnemius,
Tibialis posterior.*
S1,S2 roots.
Tibial division of
Sciatic nerve.
Patient plantarflexes the
ankle against resistance.
May have difficulty in walking on
toes before weakness can be directly detected.

Examination – Lower Limbs

Inversion

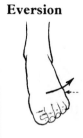

Tibialis anterior,
Tibialis posterior:

L4 root.

Peroneal and tibial
divisions of Sciatic nerve.

Patient inverts foot
against resistance.

Eversion

Peroneus longus and brevis:

L5,S1 roots.

Peroneal division
of Sciatic nerve.

Patient everts foot
against resistance.

SENSATION

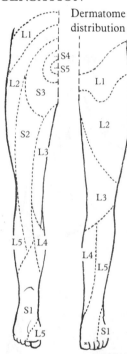

Dermatome
distribution

Test:
Pain
Light touch
(Temperature)
} Follow the dermatome
distribution as in the
upper limb.

Joint Position Sense

Firstly, demonstrate flexion
and extension movements of
the big toe. Then ask
patient to specify the
direction with the
eyes closed.
    If deficient, test ankle
joint sense in the same
way.

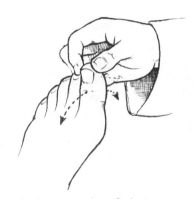

Vibration

Test vibration perception by placing a tuning fork
on the malleolus. If deficient, move up to the head of
the fibula or to the anterior superior iliac spine.

REFLEXES

Knee Jerk L2,L3,**L4** roots.

Ensure that the patient's leg is relaxed by
resting it over examiner's arm or by hanging
it over the edge of the bed. Tap the patellar
tendon with the hammer and observe quadriceps contraction. Note impairment or exaggeration.

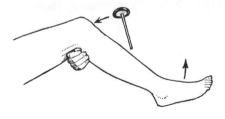

Examination – Lower Limbs

Ankle Jerk   **S1**, S2 roots.

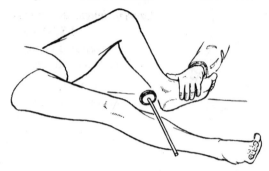

Externally rotate the patient's leg. Hold the foot in slight dorsiflexion. Ensure the foot is relaxed by palpating the tendon of tibialis anterior. If this is taut, then no ankle jerk will be elicited.

Tap the achilles tendon and watch for calf muscle contraction and plantarflexion.

Reflex Enhancement

When reflexes are difficult to elicit, they may be enhanced by asking the patient to clench the teeth or to try to pull clasped hands apart (Jendressik's manoeuvre).

Plantar Response

Check that the big toe is relaxed. Stroke the lateral aspect of the sole and across the ball of the foot. Watch for the first movement of the big toe.

Flexion should occur.

Extension (a 'Babinski' response) indicates an upper motor neurone lesion.

To avoid ambiguity do not touch the innermost aspect of the sole or the toes themselves.

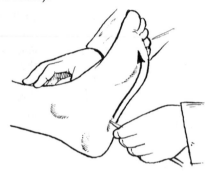

CO-ORDINATION

Ask patient to repeatedly run the heel from the opposite knee down the shin to the big toe. Look for ATAXIA (inco-ordination).   Ask patient to repeatedly tap the floor with the foot. Note any DYSDIADOCHOKINESIA (difficulty with rapidly alternating movement).

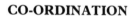

Examination – Posture and Gait

Romberg's Test

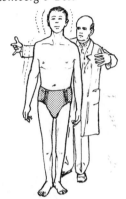

Ask patient to stand with the heels together, first with the eyes open, then with the eyes closed.

Note any excessive postural swaying or loss of balance.

Present when eyes open or closed = Cerebellar deficit (cerebellar ataxia)

Present only when eyes are closed = Proprioceptive deficit (sensory ataxia)

GAIT

Note:
- Length of step and width of base
- Abnormal leg movements (e.g. excessively high step)
- Instability (gait ataxia)
- Associated postural movements (e.g. pelvic swinging)

Normal

Abnormal

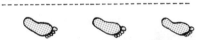

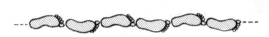

If normal, repeat with *tandem* walking i.e. heel to toe. This will exaggerate any instability.

Examination of the Unconscious Patient

HISTORY

Questioning relatives, friends or the ambulance team is an essential part of the assessment of the unconscious or the uncooperative patient.

- Has the patient sustained a head injury – leading to admission, or in the preceding weeks?
- Did the patient collapse suddenly?
- Did limb twitching occur?
- Have symptoms occurred in the preceding weeks?
- Has the patient suffered a previous illness?
- Does the patient take medication?

GENERAL EXAMINATION

Lack of patient cooperation does not limit general examination, and this may reveal important diagnostic signs. In addition to those features described on page 5, also look for signs of head injury, needle marks on the arm, and evidence of tongue biting. Also note the smell of alcohol, but beware of attributing the patient's clinical state solely to alcohol excess.

NEUROLOGICAL EXAMINATION

Conscious level: This assessment is of major importance. It not only serves as an immediate prognostic guide, but also provides a baseline with which future examinations may be compared.

Assess conscious level as described previously (page 6) in terms of:

Eye Opening		Verbal Response		Motor Response	
– Spontaneous	4	– Orientated	5	– Obeying commands	5
– To speech	3	– Confused	4	– Localising	4
– To pain	2	– Words	3	– Flexing	3
– None	1	– Sounds	2	– Extending	2
		– None	1	– None	1

A score may be applied to each category of the grading system and the total summed to give an overall value ranging from 3–14 e.g. no eye opening, no verbal response and extending to pain = 4.

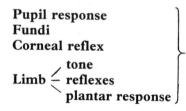

Pupil response
Fundi
Corneal reflex

Limb — tone / reflexes / plantar response

Lack of patient cooperation does not prevent objective assessment of these features described before, but other neurological features require a different approach.

Examination of the Unconscious Patient

Eye Movements
- observe any **spontaneous** eye movements.

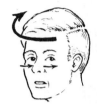

(Eyes held open by examiner)

- elicit the **oculocephalic (doll's eye) reflex.**
Rotation or flexion/extension of the head in a comatose patient produces transient eye movements in a direction opposite to the direction of movement.

Note whether the movements, if present, are *conjugate* (i.e. the eyes move in parallel) or *dysconjugate* (i.e. the eyes do not move in parallel).

- elicit the **oculovestibular reflex** (caloric testing – see page 60).

Visual fields
In the uncooperative patient, the examiner may detect a hemianopic field defect when 'menacing' from one side fails to produce a 'blink'.

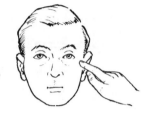

Facial weakness
Failure to 'grimace' on one side in response to bilateral supraorbital pain indicates a facial weakness.

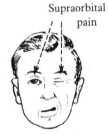

Supraorbital pain

Limb weakness
Detect by comparing the response in the limbs to painful stimuli. If pain produces an *asymmetric* response, then limb weakness is present.
[If the patient 'localises' with one arm, hold this down and retest to ensure that a similar response cannot be elicited from the other limb.]

e.g.

Supraorbital pain

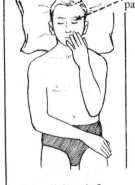

Localising left, flexing right.

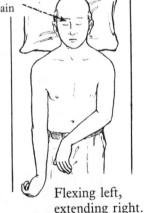

Flexing left, extending right.

Both patients are in coma; both have an asymmetric response to pain indicating a right arm weakness and focal brain damage.

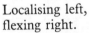

Pain stimulus applied to the toe nails or Achilles tendon similarly tests power in the lower limbs. Variation in tone, reflexes or plantar responses between each side also indicates a focal deficit. In practice, if the examiner fails to detect a difference in response to painful stimuli, these additional features seldom provide convincing evidence.

31

The Neurological Observation Chart

Despite major advances in intracranial investigative techniques, none have replaced clinical assessment for monitoring the patient's neurological state. The neurological observation chart produced by Jennett and Teasdale incorporates the most relevant clinical features viz. *coma scale (eye opening, verbal and motor response)*, *pupil size* and *reaction to light, limb responses* and *vital signs.* The frequency of observation (normally 2 hourly) depends on the individual patient's needs. The chart enables immediate evaluation of the trend in the patient's clinical state.

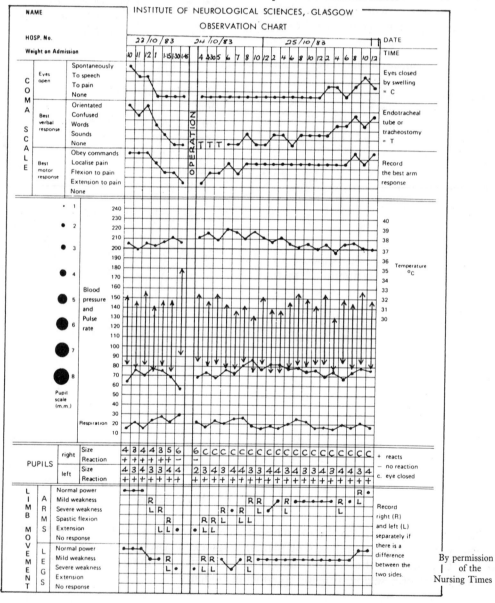

By permission of the Nursing Times

SECTION II

Investigations of the Central
and Peripheral Nervous Systems

Skull X-Ray

Despite the development of advanced radiological techniques, skull X-ray is still a useful preliminary investigation especially in head injured patients.

Standard views:
- Lateral
- Postero-anterior
- Towne's (fronto-occipital)

Learn to distinguish normal skull markings and sites of calcification (pineal and choroid plexus).

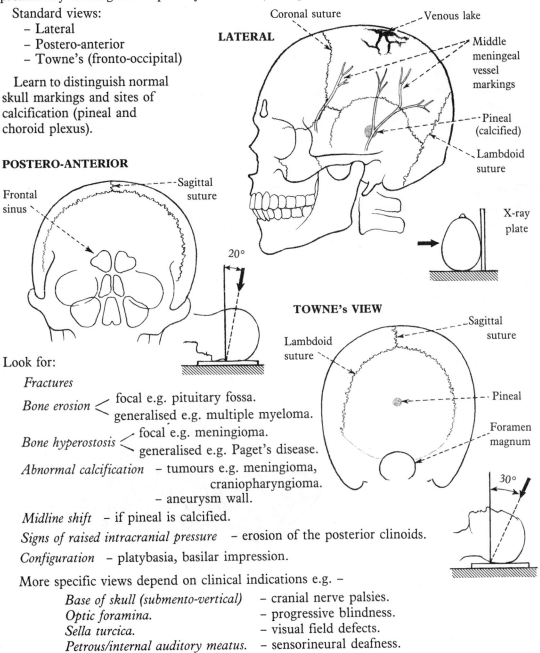

LATERAL

Coronal suture

Venous lake

Middle meningeal vessel markings

Pineal (calcified)

Lambdoid suture

X-ray plate

POSTERO-ANTERIOR

Sagittal suture

Frontal sinus

20°

TOWNE's VIEW

Lambdoid suture

Sagittal suture

Pineal

Foramen magnum

30°

Look for:

Fractures

Bone erosion < focal e.g. pituitary fossa.
generalised e.g. multiple myeloma.

Bone hyperostosis < focal e.g. meningioma.
generalised e.g. Paget's disease.

Abnormal calcification – tumours e.g. meningioma, craniopharyngioma.
– aneurysm wall.

Midline shift – if pineal is calcified.

Signs of raised intracranial pressure – erosion of the posterior clinoids.

Configuration – platybasia, basilar impression.

More specific views depend on clinical indications e.g. –

Base of skull (submento-vertical) – cranial nerve palsies.
Optic foramina. – progressive blindness.
Sella turcica. – visual field defects.
Petrous/internal auditory meatus. – sensorineural deafness.

Computerised Tomography (CT) Scanning

The development of this non-invasive technique in the 1970's, revolutionised the investigative approach to intracranial pathology.

A pencil beam of X-ray traverses the patient's head and a diametrically opposed detector measures the extent of its absorption. With the aid of computer processing, multiple beams and detectors rotating around the patient's head enable determination of absorption values for multiple small blocks of tissue (pixels). Reconstruction of these areas on a two dimensional display provides the characteristic CT scan appearance. For routine scanning, slices are 8–10mm wide. Slices of 2mm width provide even greater detail but these 'high attenuation' views take longer to acquire and process and this technique is usually reserved for examination of the orbit, the pituitary region and the posterior fossa.

An *intravenous contrast medium* is administered when the plain scan reveals an abnormality or if specific clinical indications exist e.g. suspected arterio-venous malformation, acoustic neurilemmoma or intracerebral abscess – with these lesions the plain scan may appear normal. Intravenous contrast shows areas with increased vascularity or with impairment of the blood brain barrier.

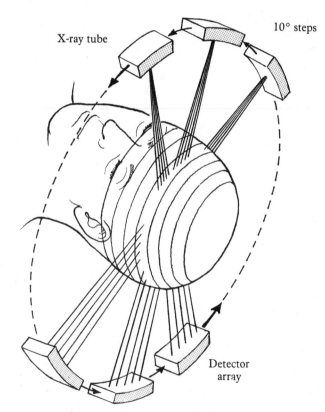

X-ray tube

10° steps

Detector array

Computerised Tomography (CT) Scanning

NORMAL SCAN

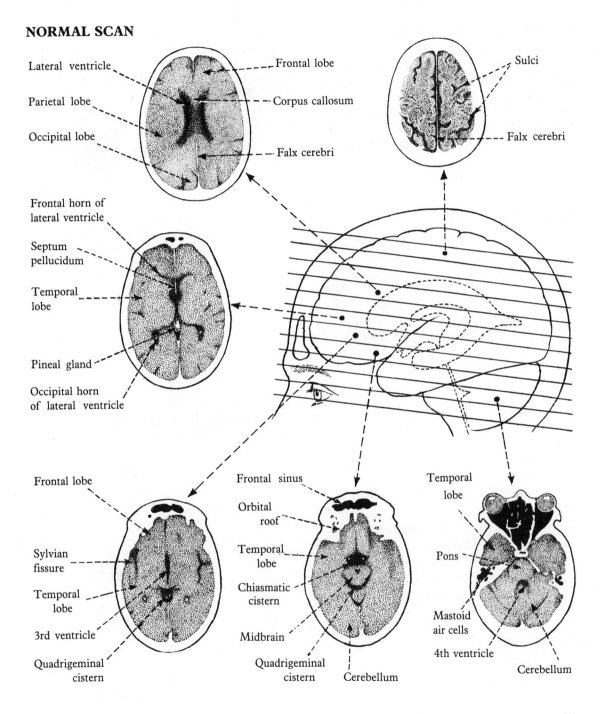

Lateral ventricle
Parietal lobe
Occipital lobe
Frontal lobe
Corpus callosum
Falx cerebri

Sulci
Falx cerebri

Frontal horn of lateral ventricle
Septum pellucidum
Temporal lobe
Pineal gland
Occipital horn of lateral ventricle

Frontal lobe
Sylvian fissure
Temporal lobe
3rd ventricle
Quadrigeminal cistern

Frontal sinus
Orbital roof
Temporal lobe
Chiasmatic cistern
Midbrain
Quadrigeminal cistern
Cerebellum

Temporal lobe
Pons
Mastoid air cells
4th ventricle
Cerebellum

37

Computerised Tomography (CT) Scanning

Coronal and Sagittal reconstruction

Computer reconstruction of images in the sagittal or coronal planes may occasionally provide more information, but requires CT slices of narrow width i.e. 2 mm. These are of particular value in demonstrating sellar and pineal region tumours and in lesions extending upwards from the skull base.

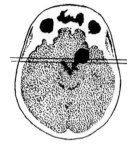

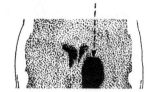

Coronal reconstruction showing relationships of an epidermoid cyst to the lateral ventricle.

Coronal CT scanning

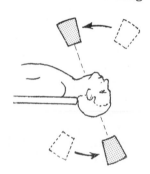

Coronal scan showing pneumocele arising from fracture in the orbital roof.

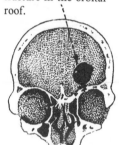

Full neck extension combined with maximal angulation of the CT gantry permits direct coronal scanning and may give greater definition than reconstructed views.

Orbital CT scanning

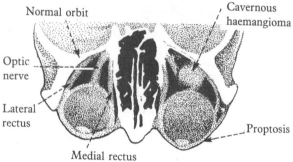

Normal orbit

Optic nerve

Lateral rectus

Medial rectus

Cavernous haemangioma

Proptosis

CT scanning clearly defines both normal and abnormal intraorbital contents and demonstrates any intracranial extension or bone destruction.

CT scanning with CSF contrast

CT scanning following the injection of metrizamide into the lumbar theca with head down tilt outlines filling defects within the basal cisterns. This aids early identification of small acoustic tumours and other cerebello-pontine angle lesions. When combined with coronal or sagittal reconstruction, the extent of any suprasellar extension is clearly shown. Occasionally this technique helps identify the exact site of a traumatic CSF fistula.

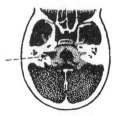

Small acoustic tumour outlined by contrast within the basal cisterns.

Computerised Tomography (CT) Scanning

Interpretation of the CT scan

Before contrast enhancement note:

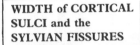

VENTRICULAR SYSTEM

- size
- position
- compression of
  one or more horns
  i.e. frontal, temporal
  or occipital

WIDTH of CORTICAL SULCI and the SYLVIAN FISSURES

SKULL BASE and VAULT

- hyperostosis
- osteolytic lesion
- remodelling
- depressed fracture

MULTIPLE LESIONS may result from:

- tumour – metastases
  – lymphoma
- abscesses
- granuloma
- infarction
- trauma

ABNORMAL TISSUE DENSITY

Identify the site, and whether the lesion lies within or without the brain substance.
Note the 'MASS EFFECT'
- midline shift
- ventricular compression
- obliteration of the basal cisterns

High density
- blood
- calcification
    - tumour
    - arterio-venous malformation/
                                    aneurysm
    - hamartoma
(Calcification of the pineal gland, choroid plexus, basal ganglia and falx may occur in normal scans.)

Low density
- infarction (arterial/venous)
- tumour
- abscess
- oedema
- encephalitis
- resolving haematoma

Mixed density
- tumour
- abscess
- arterio-venous malformation
- contusion
- haemorrhagic infarct

After contrast enhancement:
Look at the extent and pattern of contrast uptake in any abnormal region. Some lesions may only appear after contrast enhancement.

Radioisotope Scanning

The use of isotope brain scanning has diminished with the development of other imaging techniques, but this remains a sensitive detector of intracranial disease albeit limited in the recognition of the specific pathological process.

Following a blocking dose of potassium perchlorate (to prevent uptake in the choroid plexus and salivary glands), sodium pertechnetate, labelled with technetium^{99m}, is injected intravenously and its distribution within the brain detected with a gamma camera placed in the lateral, anterior or posterior positions.

Abnormalities of isotope distribution result from:

Lateral   **Antero-posterior**

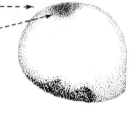 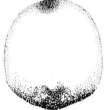

  – increased vascularity
    e.g. meningioma. - - - - - - - - - - - - →

Increased radioisotope - - - →
uptake over the
hemispheric convexity

  – abnormal presence of blood
    e.g. chronic subdural haematoma.

  – breakdown of the blood brain barrier
    e.g. herpes simplex encephalitis.

Scan timing after i.v. injection:

Vascular lesions e.g. arterio-venous malformation, — best detected *early*
                              meningioma.   i.e. 30 minutes after injection.

Less vascular lesions e.g. glioma — best detected *late* i.e. 2 hours after injection.

Limiting factors:

1. Degree of resolution – <2.5 cm.
2. Virtual inability in detecting posterior fossa lesions.

RADIOISOTOPE CISTERNOGRAPHY

Detection of radioisotope distributed throughout the cerebrospinal fluid (CSF) following injection into the lumbar theca, yields information about CSF flow. Reflux into the ventricular system, followed by slow clearance, suggests communicating or normal pressure hydrocephalus.

FUTURE APPLICATIONS

In the future, isotope scanning may resume an important role in *in vivo* localisation of radiolabelled monoclonal antibodies developed against specific tumour antigens, hormones and central nervous system receptors.

Electroencephalography (EEG)

Electroencephalography examines by means of scalp electrodes the spontaneous electrical activity of the brain. Tiny electrical potentials, which measure millionths of volts, are recorded, amplified and displayed on either 8 or 16 channels of a pen recorder. Low and high frequency filters remove unwanted signals such as muscle artefact and mains interference.

The system of electrode placement is referred to as the 10/20 system because the distance between bony points i.e. inion to nasion is divided into lengths of either 10 or 20% of the total, and the electrodes placed at each distance.

A switch changes recording from A (parasagittal) to B (transverse). Other electrode arrangements are also 'pre-set'. The numbering indicates the write out from top to bottom on an 8 channel record.

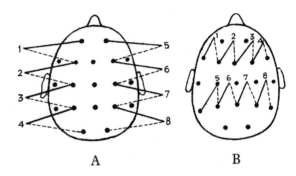

A   B

Normal rhythms

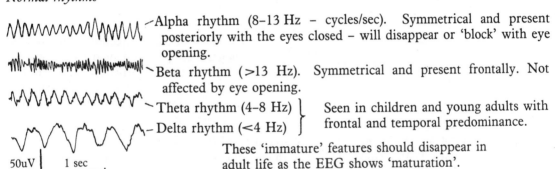

Alpha rhythm (8–13 Hz – cycles/sec). Symmetrical and present posteriorly with the eyes closed – will disappear or 'block' with eye opening.

Beta rhythm (>13 Hz). Symmetrical and present frontally. Not affected by eye opening.

Theta rhythm (4–8 Hz) ⎫ Seen in children and young adults with
Delta rhythm (<4 Hz) ⎭ frontal and temporal predominance.

These 'immature' features should disappear in adult life as the EEG shows 'maturation'.

50uV | 1 sec

As well as recording a resting EEG using various 'pre-set' electrode arrangements, stressing the patient by hyperventilation and photic stimulation (a flashing strobe light) may result in an electrical discharge supporting a diagnosis of epilepsy.

Less commonly drugs e.g. procyclidine, or fasting may be similarly employed.

The abnormal EEG

The EEG may reveal 3 types of abnormality:

1. A generalised excess of slow wave activity present in 'encephalopathy' of metabolic or infective aetiology.
2. A focal excess of slow wave activity indicative of a lateralised structural abnormality.
3. An abnormal electrical discharge of high voltage indicative of focal or generalised epilepsy.

Angiography

Many neurological and neurosurgical conditions require accurate delineation of both intra- and extra-cranial vessels. Angiography remains the standard technique although digital subtraction angiography (DSA) may become the optimal preliminary investigation in some conditions e.g. carotid stenosis, sagittal sinus thrombosis.

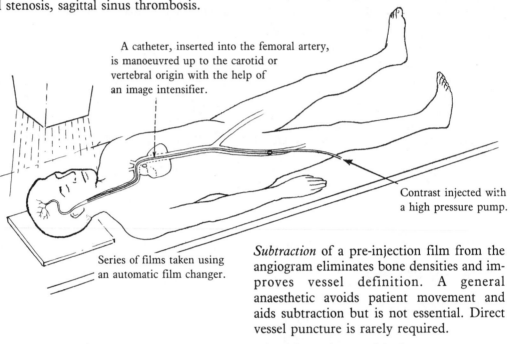

A catheter, inserted into the femoral artery, is manoeuvred up to the carotid or vertebral origin with the help of an image intensifier.

Contrast injected with a high pressure pump.

Series of films taken using an automatic film changer.

Subtraction of a pre-injection film from the angiogram eliminates bone densities and improves vessel definition. A general anaesthetic avoids patient movement and aids subtraction but is not essential. Direct vessel puncture is rarely required.

Phases   – arterial | Most information is now derived from the arterial phase.
         – capillary | Prior to the CT scan, the position of the cerebral veins helped localise
         – venous | intracranial structures.

CAROTID ANGIOGRAPHY

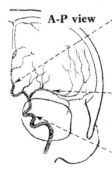

A-P view

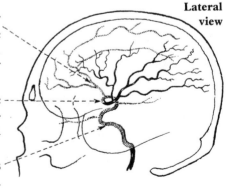

Lateral view

The *anterior cerebral arteries* run over the corpus callosum, supplying the medial aspects of the frontal lobes. Both anterior cerebral arteries may fill from each carotid injection.

The *middle cerebral artery* runs in the depth of the Sylvian fissure. Branches supply the frontal and temporal lobes.

The *internal carotid artery* bifurcates into the anterior and middle cerebral arteries.

Oblique views may aid identification of some lesions e.g. aneurysms.

Angiography

VERTEBRAL ANGIOGRAPHY

Towne's View

Lateral view

Posterior cerebral arteries supply the occipital lobes and parts of the parietal and temporal lobes.
Basilar artery: branches supply the brain stem and cerebellum.
Vertebral arteries: branches supply the spinal cord, brain stem and cerebellum.

Contrast medium

Compression of the contralateral vertebral artery in the neck during contrast injection produces retrograde flow and demonstrates both vessels with one injection.

Look for:

- vessel *occlusion, stenosis* or *plaque formation.*
- *aneurysms.*
- *arterio-venous malformations.*
- abnormal *tumour circulation.*
- vessel *displacement* or *compression.*

Although superceded by the CT scan in tumour detection angiography may give useful information about feeding vessels and the extent of vessel involvement with the tumour.

Complications:

The development of new contrast mediums e.g. iohexol, iopamidol, has considerably reduced the risk of complications during or following angiography; these seldom occur in the hands of experienced radiologists.

- *Cerebral ischaemia:* caused by emboli from an arteriosclerotic plaque broken off by the catheter tip, hypotension or vessel spasm following contrast injection.

- *Contrast sensitivity:* mild sensitivity to the contrast occasionally develops, but this rarely causes severe problems.

Digital Subtraction Angiography (DSA)

Digital subtraction angiography depends upon high speed digital computing. Exposures taken before and after the administration of contrast agents are instantly subtracted 'pixel by pixel'. Data manipulation allows enhancement of small differences of shading as well as magnification of specific areas of study.

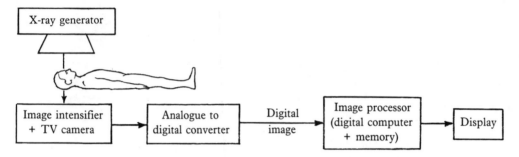

DSA results in improved contrast sensitivity, so much lower concentrations of contrast material are required –

Intravenous contrast administration provides good definition of extracranial vessels e.g. for investigation of transient ischaemic attacks.

Intraarterial contrast injection is required for intra-cranial vessel display e.g. for investigation of subarachnoid haemorrhage.

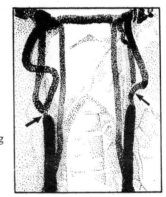

Computer enhancement of contrast showing moderate stenosis of both common carotid arteries with normal vertebral arteries.

Advantages of DSA over standard angiography
  - Fast, less costly technique
  - Less contrast required, therefore less risk (dose comparable to intravenous pyelogram).
  - Avoids intraarterial injection for extracranial vessels.

Problems with DSA
  - Superimposition of vessels may mask pathology.
  - Limited spacial resolution may prevent visualisation of small intracranial vessels – even with intraarterial injection.
  - Movement artefact (e.g. swallowing) may create image blurring.

Nuclear Magnetic Resonance (NMR)

For several years, NMR techniques have aided the chemical analysis of compounds in solution. The development of computerised imaging techniques (as in the CT scan) has extended its use to identification of *hydrogen atom densities* in vivo. These directly reflect *water content* and since this varies from tissue to tissue, NMR can provide a detailed image of both intra- and extracranial structures.

When a substance is placed in a magnetic field, the nuclei of the hydrogen atoms, i.e. single spinning protons, act like small magnets and align themselves with the magnetic field. A super-imposed electromagnetic pulse (radiowave) at a specific frequency displaces the protons causing them to 'resonate'. Since the protons act like magnets, a change in their position induces an e.m.f. in a surrounding coil. Various aspects of this signal (proton density and rate of proton realignment) provide information about surrounding nuclei (T1 'lattice') and interaction with other protons (T2). Computerised imaging is used to reconstruct the NMR scan.

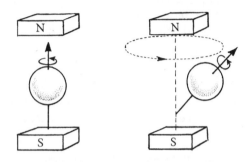

ADVANTAGES OVER CT SCANNING

- Hazards appear to be negligible (no ionising radiation).
- No bone artefact. Lesions around the skull base and in the posterior fossa are clearly identified.
- Small changes in tissue water content are detected prior to change on CT scan e.g. cerebral infarct (within a few hours of onset) and demyelination plaques.
- Any plane may be selected e.g. sagittal.
- No moving parts, therefore wear is minimal and reliability potentially greater.

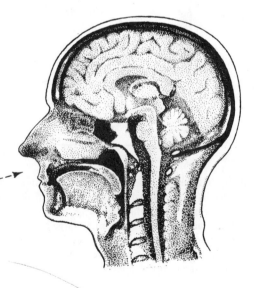

Measurement of Cerebral Blood Flow (CBF)

Cerebral blood flow measurement, although invaluable in increasing knowledge and understanding of many intracranial disease processes, has few direct clinical applications.

Clinical uses:

1. Carotid ligation is occasionally required in the management of intracranial carotid aneurysms. CBF studies before and possibly during operations help minimise the risk of ischaemic complications.

2. The detection of low flow states or impaired autoregulation (page 74) in subarachnoid haemorrhage may guide the timing of operation and indicate the likelihood of ischaemic complications.

3. The identification of haemodynamically significant extracranial stenotic or occlusive carotid artery disease.

Methods:

A solution of radioactive Xenon is injected either intraarterially or intravenously. Alternatively, radioactive Xenon gas is inhaled for a short period. One or more collimators, sited extracranially over each hemisphere, detect the Xenon clearance from the brain over the subsequent ten minutes.

Clearance of Xenon — Inhalation method

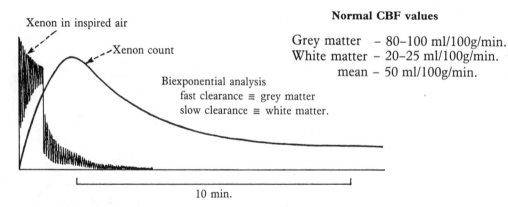

Xenon in inspired air

Xenon count

Biexponential analysis
fast clearance ≡ grey matter
slow clearance ≡ white matter.

10 min.

Normal CBF values

Grey matter   – 80–100 ml/100g/min.
White matter – 20–25 ml/100g/min.
mean – 50 ml/100g/min.

Note: Calculation of CBF assumes a uniform diffusion of Xenon into brain tissue. In the presence of ischaemic/underperfused regions, Xenon will also diffuse from high to low flow areas. This tends to underestimate the flow reduction in these areas.

A collimator detects counts from a large cone-shaped area under its point of application. In normal circumstances fast and slow Xenon clearance reflects grey and white matter respectively. When flow is abnormal, location of the tissues or site involved is less certain.

Collimator

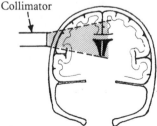

Positron emission tomography accurately measures cerebral blood flow – in particular regional flow – but this technique is not widely available.

Positron Emission Tomography (PET)

This new technique utilises positron emitting isotopes (radionuclides) bound to compounds of biological interest to quantitatively study specific physiological processes. Positron emitting isotopes depend on a cyclotron for production and their half-life is short, thus PET scanners only exist on adjacent sites. This limits availability for routine clinical use but PET scanners provide invaluable research information.

Each decaying positron results in the release of two photons in diametric opposition; these activate two coincidental detectors. Multiple pairs of detectors and computer processing techniques enable quantitative determination of local radioactivity (and density of the labelled compound) for each 'pixel' (a cube of tissue) within the imaged field. Reconstruction using similar imaging techniques to CT scanning produces the positron emission scan.

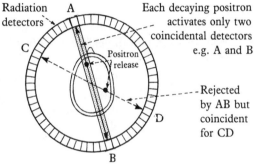

Each detector is linked to several others in a fan shaped distribution

Isotope	Binding Compound		Measurement under study
^{15}Oxygen	Carbon monoxide	– inhalation	– *Cerebral blood volume (CBV)*
^{15}Oxygen	Water	– i.v. bolus	– *Cerebral blood flow (CBF)*
^{18}Fluorine	Fluoro-deoxyglucose	– i.v. bolus	– *Cerebral glucose metabolism (CMRgl)*
^{15}Oxygen	Oxygen	– inhalation	– *Cerebral oxygen utilisation (CMRO$_2$)*
			– *Oxygen extraction factor (OEF)*

Clinical uses:

PET scanning is of particular value in elucidating the relationships between cerebral blood flow, oxygen utilisation and extraction in focal areas of ischaemia or infarction (page 228). Preliminary studies suggest that PET scanning may help identify patients most likely to benefit from extracranial/intracranial anastomosis.

PET scanning has also been used to study patients with dementia and epilepsy and to analyse metabolic activity within brain tumours.

PET scan several days after a left middle cerebral infarct showing a reduction in blood flow.

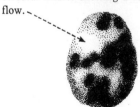

Oxygen utilisation is also reduced with a slight increase in oxygen extraction.

Intracranial Pressure Monitoring

Although CSF pressure may be measured during lumbar puncture, this method is of limited value in intracranial pressure measurement:

— an isolated pressure reading does not indicate the trend in intracranial pressure and pressure waves cannot be monitored.

— lumbar puncture is contraindicated in the presence of an intracranial mass.

— pressure gradients exist between different intracranial and spinal compartments, especially in the presence of brain shift.

Intracranial pressure is measured directly via a catheter inserted into the lateral ventricle. Alternatively, various devices are available to measure pressure on the hemisphere surface, either extradurally or through an opened dura. With these latter techniques, however, damping and pressure gradients may result in inaccuracies.

Technique:

A ventricular catheter is inserted into the frontal horn of the lateral ventricle through a frontal burr hole situated two finger breadths from the midline, behind the hairline and anterior to the coronal suture.

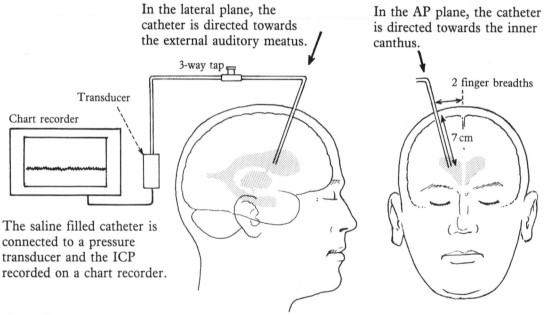

In the lateral plane, the catheter is directed towards the external auditory meatus.

In the AP plane, the catheter is directed towards the inner canthus.

3-way tap

Transducer

Chart recorder

2 finger breadths

7 cm

The saline filled catheter is connected to a pressure transducer and the ICP recorded on a chart recorder.

Complications:

Intracerebral haemorrhage following catheter insertion rarely occurs.

Ventriculitis seldom occurs provided monitoring does not continue for more than 3 days.

Intracranial Pressure Monitoring

NORMAL PRESSURE TRACE   Note waves caused by
pulse pressure and respiration.

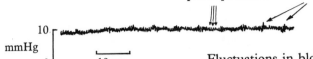

Normal ICP <10 mmHg.

Fluctuations in blood pressure may cause waves of 5–8/min
(Traube-Hering waves).

ABNORMAL PRESSURE TRACE

Look for – *Increase in the mean pressure.*   >20 mmHg – moderate elevation.
>40 mmHg – severe increase in pressure.

N.B.   As ICP increases, the amplitude of the pulse pressure wave increases.

– *β waves*

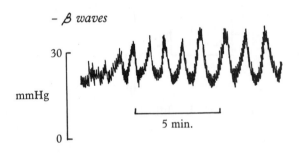

– frequency $\frac{1}{2}$–2/min.
– of variable amplitude.
– often related to respiration.

– *Plateau waves*

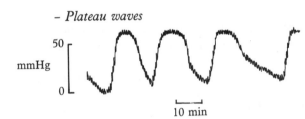

– elevation of ICP over 50 mmHg
lasting 5–20 minutes.
– precede a severe continuous
rise in ICP and precursors of
further clinical deterioration.

CLINICAL USES OF ICP MONITORING

1. Investigation of normal pressure hydrocephalus – the presence of *β* waves for >5% of a
24 hour period suggests impaired CSF absorption and the need for a drainage operation.
2. Post-operative monitoring – a rise in ICP may precede clinical evidence of haematoma
formation or cerebral swelling.
3. Small traumatic haematomas – ICP monitoring may guide management and indicate the
need for operative removal.
4. ICP monitoring is required during treatment aimed at reducing a raised ICP.

Evoked Potentials — Visual, Auditory and Somatosensory

Recording methods

Stimulation of any sensory receptor evokes a minute electrical signal (i.e. microvolts) in the appropriate region of the cerebral cortex. Averaging techniques permit recording and analysis of this signal normally lost within the background electrical activity. When sensitive apparatus is triggered to record cortical activity at a specific time after the stimulus, the background electrical 'noise' averages out i.e. random positive activity subtracts from random negative activity, leaving the signal evoked from the specific stimulus.

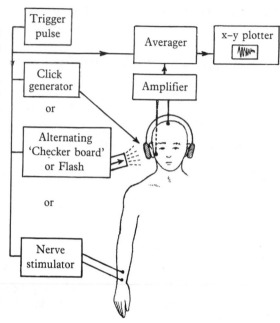

VISUAL EVOKED POTENTIAL (VEP)

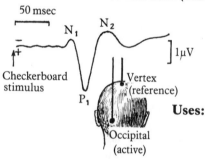

A stroboscopic flash diffusely stimulates the retina; alternatively an alternating checkerboard pattern stimulates the macula and produces more consistent results. The evoked visual signal is recorded over the occipital cortex. The first large positive wave (P_1) provides a useful point for measuring conduction through the visual pathways.

Uses: – *multiple sclerosis detection* – P_1 delayed in 90% of those with established disease.
– *peroperative monitoring* – pituitary surgery.

BRAINSTEM AUDITORY EVOKED POTENTIAL (BAEP)

Electrical activity evoked in the first 10 msec after a 'click' stimulus provides a wave pattern related to conduction through the auditory pathways in the VIII nerve and nucleus (waves I and II) and in the pons and midbrain (waves III–V). Longer latency potentials (up to 500 msec), recorded from the auditory cortex in response to a 'tone' stimulus, are of less clinical value.

Uses: – *hearing assessment* – especially in children.
– *detection of intrinsic and extrinsic brainstem and cerebello-pontine angle lesions* e.g. acoustic tumours.
– *peroperative recording* during acoustic tumour operations.
– *assessment of brainstem function* in coma.

Evoked Potentials — Somatosensory

SOMATOSENSORY EVOKED POTENTIALS (SEP)

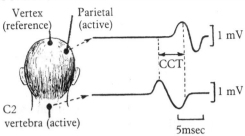

The sensory evoked potential is recorded over the parietal cortex in response to stimulation of a peripheral nerve (e.g. median nerve). Other electrodes sited at different points along the sensory pathway record the ascending activity. Subtraction of the latencies between peaks provides conduction time between these sites.

Central conduction time (CCT)
– conduction time from the dorsal columns (or nuclei) to the parietal cortex.

Uses: – *detection of lesions in the sensory pathways* – brachial plexus injury.
  – spinal cord and brainstem tumours or demyelination.

  – *peroperative recording* – straightening of scoliosis.
  – removal of spinal tumours/AVM } spinal conduction.
  – aneurysm operation with temporary vessel occlusion – CCT.

Myelography

A myelogram outlines the spinal cord and roots and demonstrates the presence or absence of any intraspinal pathology (e.g. disc disease or spondylosis, tumours, abscesses or cysts). A water soluble contrast medium is injected into the subarachnoid space via lumbar puncture (occasionally through a cervical puncture). Under direct screening with an image intensifier, the radiologist controls contrast flow up the spinal canal by varying the degree of patient tilt. X-rays provide a permanent record at the relevant levels.

LUMBO-SACRAL RADICULOGRAM

Lateral/antero-posterior view
Contrast should be screened up to the level of the conus medullaris (L1) to demonstrate any extra- or intradural lesions (see page 381).

Oblique view

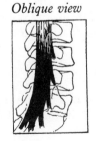

Note contrast filling the nerve roots.

CERVICAL MYELOGRAM

A-P view

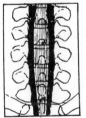

Note the *normal* cervical cord expansion

Lateral view

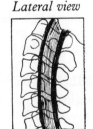

Ensure contrast is screened to the foramen magnum to exclude pathology at this level e.g. Arnold-Chiari malformation.

Problems
– *Arachnoiditis* – previously a major complication with the oil based contrast MYODIL, but rarely occurs with water soluble contrast.
– *Subdural injection* (accidental) – prevents correct interpretation.
– *Haematoma* occurs rarely at the injection site.

Lumbar Puncture

Lumbar puncture permits: – acquisition of cerebrospinal fluid for analysis.
                               – CSF drainage and pressure reduction e.g. in communi-
cating hydrocephalus/CSF fistula.

TECHNIQUE:

1. *Correct positioning of the patient is essential.* Open the vertebral laminae by drawing the knees up to the chest and flexing the neck. Ensure the back is perpendicular to the bed to avoid rotation of the spinal column.

2. Identify the site. The L3/L4 space lies level with the iliac crests and this is most often used, but since the spinal cord ends at L1 any space from L2/L3 to L5/S1 provides a safe approach.

3. Clean the area and insert a few ml of local anaes-thetic.

4. Ensure the stylet of a No18 lumbar puncture needle is fully home (No21 for children) and insert at a slight angle towards the head, so that it parallels the spinous processes. Some resistance is felt as the needle passes through the ligamentum flavum, the dura and arachnoid layers.

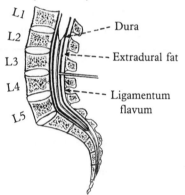

5. Withdraw the stylet and collect the CSF. If bone is encountered, withdraw the needle and reinsert at a different angle. If the position appears correct yet no CSF appears, rotate the needle to free obstructive nerve roots.

A similar technique employing a TUOHY needle allows insertion of intra- or epidural cannula (for CSF drainage or drug instillation) or stimulating electrodes (for pain management).

NOTE: Do not perform lumbar puncture if raised intracranial pressure is suspect. Even a fine needle leaves a hole through which CSF will leak. In the presence of a space-occupying lesion, especially in the posterior fossa, CSF withdrawal creates a pressure gradient which may precipitate tentorial herniation.

CSF COLLECTION

Subarachnoid haemorrhage (SAH) or puncture of a blood vessel by the needle may account for blood stained CSF. To differentiate, collect CSF in three bottles.

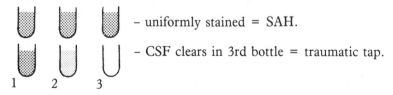

– uniformly stained = SAH.

– CSF clears in 3rd bottle = traumatic tap.

Cerebrospinal Fluid

CSF PRESSURE MEASUREMENT

Check that the patient's head (foramen of Munro) is level with the lumbar puncture needle. Connect a manometer via a 3-way tap to the needle and allow CSF to run up the column. Read off the height.

Normal value: 100–150mm CSF.

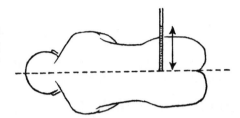

CSF ANALYSIS

Standard Tests

1. Bacteriological   – RBC and differential WBC
   (normal = <5 WBC's per mm^3).
   – gram stain and culture.
   – appearance of supernatant. Xanthochromia (yellow staining) results from subarachnoid haemorrhage with RBC breakdown, high CSF protein or jaundice.

2. Biochemical   – protein   (normal = 0.15–0.45g/l).
   – γ globulin (normal = <12% of total protein).
   – glucose   (normal = 0.45–0.70g/l).

Special Tests

Suspected:

  (i)   Malignant tumour   – cytology.
  (ii) Tubercle   – Ziehl-Neelson stain,
         Lowenstein-Jensen culture.
  (iii) Non-bacterial infection – virology, fungal and parasitic studies.
  (iv) Demyelinating disease   – oligoclonal bands (but not pathognomonic).
  (v)   Neurosyphilis   – Lange's test,
         Wasserman test (WR),
         Venereal Disease Research Lab. (VDRL),
         Treponema Pallidum Immobilisation test (TPI).

Electromyography/Nerve Conduction Studies

Needle electromyography records the electrical activity occurring within a particular muscle.

Nerve conduction studies measure conduction in response to an electrical stimulus.

Both are essential in the investigation of diseases of nerve (neuropathy) and muscle (myopathy).

Repetitive nerve stimulation tests are important in the evaluation of disorders of neuromuscular transmission e.g. myasthenia gravis.

ELECTROMYOGRAPHY

A concentric needle electrode is inserted into muscle. The central – – – – – – wire is the active electrode and the outer casing the reference electrode.

The potential difference between the two electrodes is amplified and displayed on an oscilloscope. An audio monitor enables the investigator to 'hear' the pattern of electrical activity.

Normal muscle at rest is electrically 'silent'; as the muscle gradually contracts, *motor unit potentials* appear...followed by the development of an ...

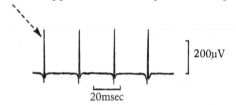

200µV

20msec

... Interference pattern

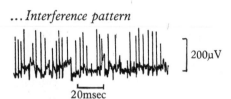

200µV

20msec

The recruitment of more and more motor units prevents identification of individual potentials.

Abnormalities take the form of:
1. Spontaneous activity in muscle when at rest.
2. Abnormalities of the motor unit potential.
3. Abnormalities of the interference pattern.
4. Special phenomena e.g. myotonia.

1. Spontaneous activity at rest

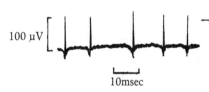

100 µV

10msec

— Fibrillation potentials are due to single muscle fibre contraction and indicate active denervation. They usually occur in neurogenic disorders e.g. neuropathy, motor neurone disease, but can be seen in myopathies.

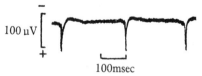

100 µV

100msec

Positive sharp waves

Slow negative waves preceded by sharp positive spikes. Seen in chronically denervated muscle e.g. motor neurone disease, but also in acute myopathy e.g. polymyositis. These waves probably represent injury potentials.

Electromyography/Nerve Conduction Studies

Abnormalities *(continued)*

2. Motor Unit Potential

In myopathies and muscular dystrophies, potentials are polyphasic and of small amplitude and short duration.

In neuropathy, the surviving motor unit potentials are also polyphasic but of large amplitude and long duration.

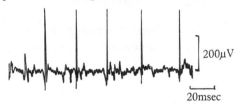

200μV

20msec

The enlarged potentials result from collateral reinnervation.

3. Interference Pattern

In myopathy, recruitment of motor units and the interference pattern remain normal. The interference pattern may even appear to increase due to fragmentation of motor units.

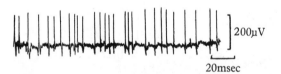

200μV

20msec

In neuropathy, there is a reduction in interference due to a loss of motor units under voluntary control.

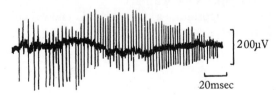

200μV

20msec

4. Myotonia

High frequency repetitive discharge may occur after voluntary movement. The amplitude and frequency of the potentials wax and wane giving rise to the typical 'dive bomber' sound on the audio monitor.

200μV

20msec

Myotonic discharge provoked by moving the needle electrode.

Electromyography/Nerve Conduction Studies

NERVE CONDUCTION STUDIES

Distal latency (latency from stimulus to recording electrodes), *amplitude* of the evoked response and *conduction velocity* all provide information of motor and sensory nerve function.

Conduction Velocity: measurement by stimulating or recording from two different sites along the course of a peripheral nerve.

$$\frac{\text{Distance between two sites}}{\substack{\text{Difference in conduction times}\\ \text{between two sites}}} = \text{Conduction velocity}$$

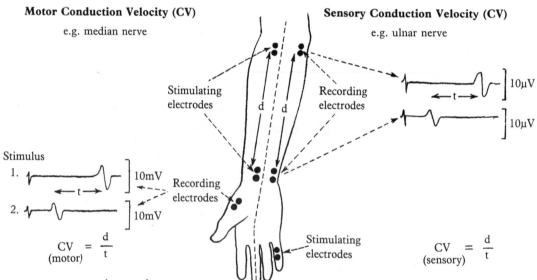

Normal values (Motor)

Ulnar and median nerves	—	50–60 metres per second.
Common peroneal nerve	—	45–55 metres per second.

Motor conduction velocities slow with age.

Body temperature is important; a fall of 1°C slows conduction in motor nerves by approximately 2 metres per second.

Electromyography/Nerve Conduction Studies

REPETITIVE STIMULATION

In the normal subject, repetitive stimulation of a motor nerve at a frequency of <30/second produces a muscle potential of constant form and amplitude. Increasing the stimulus frequency to >30/second results in fatigue manifest by a decline or 'decrement' in the amplitude. In patients with disorders of neuromuscular transmission, repetitive stimulation aids diagnosis:

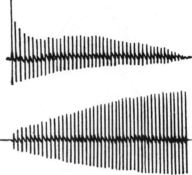

Myasthenia Gravis

A decrementing response occurs with a stimulus rate of 3–5/second.

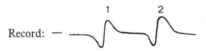

Myasthenic (Eaton Lambert) Syndrome

With a stimulation rate of 20–50/second (i.e. rapid) a small amplitude response increases to normal amplitude – incrementing response.

SINGLE FIBRE ELECTROMYOGRAPHY

A standard concentric needle within muscle will record electrical activity 0.5–1 mm from its tip – sampling from up to 20 motor units. A 'single fibre' electromyography needle with a smaller recording surface detects electrical activity within 300 μm of its tip – sampling 1–3 muscle fibres from a single motor unit.

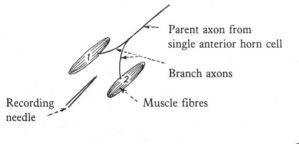

Parent axon from single anterior horn cell

Branch axons

Recording needle

Muscle fibres

Record:

Action potentials recorded from two muscle fibres are not synchronous. The gap between each is variable and can be measured if the first recorded potential is 'locked' on the oscilloscope.

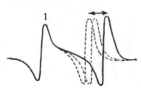

This variability is referred to as JITTER – normally 20–25 μsec (2–5 μsec due to transmission in the branch axon – 15–20 μsec to variation in neuromuscular transmission).

Single fibre electromyography is valuable in the investigation of disorders of neuromuscular transmission as well as studying reinnervation in neuropathies.

Neuro-Otological Tests

AUDITORY SYSTEM

Neuro-otological tests help differentiate conductive, cochlear and retrocochlear causes of impaired hearing. They supplement Weber's and Rinne's test (page 17).

PURE TONE AUDIOMETRY

Thresholds for air and bone conduction are measured in 5dB steps for frequencies up to 8,000 cps.

Pure tone — air conduction

Electromechanical vibrator – bone conduction

Masking noise

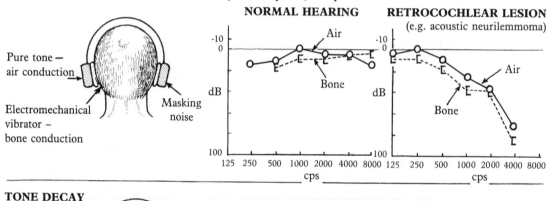

NORMAL HEARING

Air

Bone

dB

125 250 500 1000 2000 4000 8000
cps

RETROCOCHLEAR LESION
(e.g. acoustic neurilemmoma)

Air

Bone

dB

125 250 500 1000 2000 4000 8000
cps

TONE DECAY

Continuous tone applied at 5dB above threshold

Masking noise

When the tone disappears, the intensity is increased by 5dB steps until the sound is heard for a 60 sec period.

Tone decay is the inability to hear *continuous* sound at an intensity above the auditory threshold. It is of most value in detecting retrocochlear lesions.

Conduction deficit — +5dB required
Cochlear deficit — +20dB required

Retrocochlear deficit — >25dB required

SPEECH AUDIOMETRY

Pre-taped words

Masking noise

This tests (i) the sound intensity at which words are perceived.
(ii) the ease with which words are discriminated when presented at a 90dB level above the hearing threshold.

Percentage of words correct

Normal

Conductive

Cochlear

Retrocochlear

Intensity

Eighth nerve lesions markedly reduce speech discrimination, but conductive and cochlear problems have some effect.

LOUDNESS DISCOMFORT

Tones of 100–120dB produce discomfort in normal subjects and in patients with cochlear deafness. This contrasts to patients with conductive or retrocochlear deafness who experience little or no discomfort at high intensity.

Neuro-Otological Tests

LOUDNESS RECRUITMENT

Compares the loudness of pure tones presented alternately to the good and deaf ear at increasing intensities.

Short tones presented alternately to each ear

Tone increased in defective ear until it 'matches' tone in normal ear

Test repeated for several intensity levels

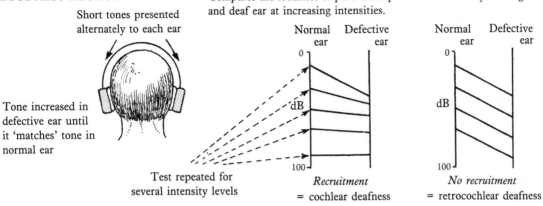

Recruitment
= cochlear deafness

No recruitment
= retrocochlear deafness

With cochlear lesions, at high intensities, the defective ear hears as well as the normal ear indicating loudness recruitment.

N.B. Some retrocochlear lesions (e.g. acoustic nerve tumours) may impair the blood supply or endolymph flow in the cochlea and produce a similar recruitment pattern.

ACOUSTIC IMPEDENCE

An intense acoustic stimulus causes reflex contraction of the stapedius muscle. This in turn causes reduced compliance (increased impedence) of the tympanic membrane.

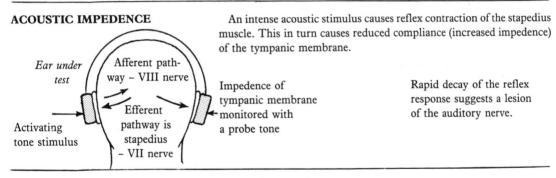

Ear under test

Afferent pathway – VIII nerve

Efferent pathway is stapedius – VII nerve

Activating tone stimulus

Impedence of tympanic membrane monitored with a probe tone

Rapid decay of the reflex response suggests a lesion of the auditory nerve.

AUDITORY BRAIN STEM EVOKED POTENTIAL

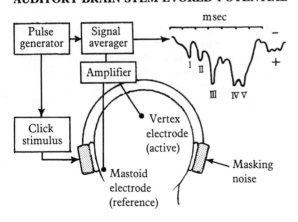

Pulse generator

Signal averager

Amplifier

Click stimulus

Vertex electrode (active)

Mastoid electrode (reference)

Masking noise

msec

Averaging techniques (page 50) permit the recording and analysis of small electrical potentials evoked in response to auditory stimuli. Activity in the first 10msec provides information about the VIII nerve and nucleus (waves I and II) pons and midbrain (waves III–V). Lesions of the VIII nerve diminish the amplitude and/or the latency of wave I or II and all subsequent waves. In comparison, cochlear lesions seldom affect either wave pattern or latency.

59

Neuro-Otological Tests

VESTIBULAR SYSTEM

CALORIC TESTING (VESTIBULO-OCULAR REFLEX)

Compensatory mechanisms may mask clinical evidence of vestibular damage – spontaneous and positional nystagmus. Caloric testing provides useful supplementary information and may reveal undetected vestibular dysfunction.

Method: Water at either 30°C or 44°C is injected into the external auditory meatus. Nystagmus usually develops after a 20sec delay and lasts for more than a minute.

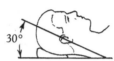

Stimulus is maximal with the head supported 30° from the horizontal (with the lateral semicircular canal in a vertical plane).

Cold water effectively reduces the vestibular output from one side, creating an imbalance and producing eye drift towards the irrigated ear. Rapid corrective movements result in 'nystagmus'. Hot water (44°C) reverses the convection current, increases the vestibular output and changes the direction of the nystagmus.

N.B. Ice water ensures a maximal stimulus when caloric testing for brain death or head injury prognostication.

Time from onset of irrigation to the cessation of nystagmus is plotted for each ear, at each temperature.

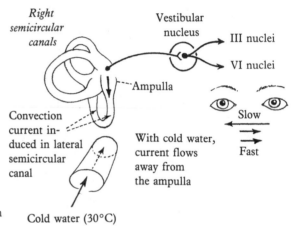

Cold water (30°C)

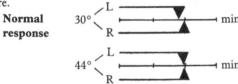

Damage to the labyrinth, vestibular nerve or nucleus results in one of two abnormal patterns, or a combination of both.

Directional preponderance implies a more prolonged duration of nystagmus in one direction than the other and occurs with brain stem, cerebellar and posterior temporal lobe lesions in addition to peripheral lesions.

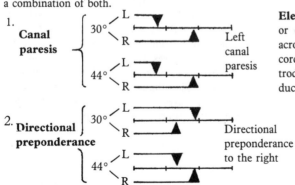

Electronystagmography: optical fixation may reduce or even abolish nystagmus. The potential difference across the eye (the corneo-retinal potential) permits recording of eye movements with laterally placed electrodes and enables detection of spontaneous or reflex induced nystagmus in darkness or with the eyes closed.

SECTION III

Clinical Presentation, Anatomical Concepts and Diagnostic Approach

Headache — General Principles

Headache is a common symptom arising from psychological, otological, ophthalmological, neurological or systemic disease. In clinical practice psychological 'tension' headache is encountered most frequently.

Definition: Pain or discomfort between the orbits and occiput, arising from pain-sensitive structures:

Intracranial
{ Venous sinuses, cortical veins, basal arteries.
Dura of anterior, middle and posterior fossa.
Tentorium.

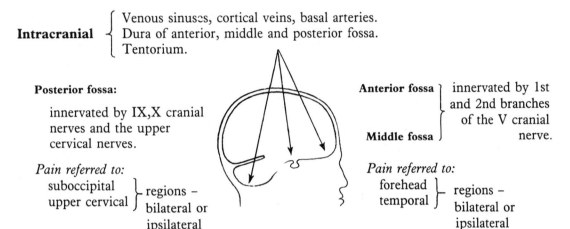

Posterior fossa:

innervated by IX,X cranial nerves and the upper cervical nerves.

Pain referred to:
suboccipital ⎫ regions –
upper cervical ⎭ bilateral or
            ipsilateral

Anterior fossa ⎫ innervated by 1st
          ⎬ and 2nd branches
          ⎪ of the V cranial
Middle fossa ⎭ nerve.

Pain referred to:
forehead ⎫ regions –
temporal ⎭ bilateral or
         ipsilateral

Extracranial pain-sensitive structures are:

Scalp vessels and muscles, orbital contents, mucous membranes of nasal and paranasal spaces, external and middle ear, teeth and gums.

In view of the many causes of head pain an accurate history and examination are essential to direct appropriate investigation and treatment.

Points from the history:
1. *Character* of headache – sharp, dull, stabbing, throbbing.
2. *Site* – unilateral, bilateral, frontal, temporal, occipital.
3. *Mode of onset* – sudden, gradual.
4. *Frequency/duration* – one acute attack, recurrent attacks, chronic.
5. *Timing* – morning, night.
6. *Accompanying symptoms* – vomiting, double vision, watering eye, etc.
7. *Precipitating factors* – posture, exercise, food, hunger, noise, stress, coughing, menstruation, etc.

Examination: Full general examination, including:
                – Ocular – acuity, tenderness, strabismus.
                – Teeth and scalp.
                – Percussion over frontal and maxillary sinuses.
      Full neurological examination.

Headache — Diagnostic Approach

The above clinical features all provide important diagnostic clues. Most information is derived from determining: – whether or not this is the first attack, developing acutely or more gradually (subacute) over several days or weeks.
– whether recurrent attacks have occurred.
– whether attacks have recurred for many years (chronic).
The following table classifies causes in these categories:

ACUTE Cause	Associated features which (if present) aid diagnosis	RECURRENT ATTACKS	Further investigations (if required)
Sinusitis	preceding 'cold' nasal discharge	*	X-ray nasal sinuses
Migraine	visual/neurological aura, nausea, vomiting	*	
Cluster headache	lacrimation, rhinorrhoea	*	
Glaucoma	'misting' of vision 'haloes' around objects	*	Ophthalmological referral
Retrobulbar neuritis	loss of vision (unilateral)		Visual evoked response
Post-traumatic	preceding head injury		Skull X-ray, CT scan
Drugs / toxins	on vasodilator drugs		
Haemorrhage	instantaneous onset vomiting, neck stiffness impaired conscious level		CT scan, lumbar puncture (see page 52)
Infection (meningitis, encephalitis)	as above but more gradual onset with pyrexia	* (if CSF fistula)	
Hydrocephalus	impaired conscious level, leg weakness, impaired upward gaze	*	CT scan
SUBACUTE			
Infection (subacute, chronic meningitis e.g. TB cerebral abscess.)	impaired conscious level, pyrexia, neck stiffness, focal neurological signs		CT scan lumbar puncture
Intracranial tumour Chronic subdural haematoma Hydrocephalus	vomiting, papilloedema, impaired conscious level± focal neurological signs	*	CT scan
Benign intracranial hypertension	vomiting, papilloedema	*	CT scan, ICP monitoring
Temporal arteritis	thickened, tender, scalp arteries		ESR, temporal artery biopsy
CHRONIC			
Tension headache	anxiety, depression	*	
Ocular 'eye strain'	impaired visual acuity	*	Refractive errors
Drugs / toxins	on vasodilator drugs		
Cervical spondylosis	neck, shoulder, arm pain	*	X-ray cervical spine

Headache — Diagnostic Approach

Headache in Children

All causes of adult headache (except retrobulbar neuritis, glaucoma, temporal arteritis and cervical spondylosis) may cause headache in children. In this age group, the commonest type of headache is that accompanying any *febrile illness* or *infection of the nasal passages or sinuses*.

The clinician, however, must not take a complaint of headache lightly; the younger the child, the more likely the presence of an underlying organic disease. Pyrexia may not only represent a mild 'constitutional' upset, but may result from *menigitis, encephalitis* or *cerebral abscess*. The presence of neck stiffness and/or impaired conscious level indicates the need for urgent investigation.

Although *intracranial tumours* are uncommon in childhood, when they occur they tend to lie in the *midline* (e.g. medulloblastoma, pineal region tumours). As a result, obstructive hydrocephalus often develops acutely with headache as a prominent initial symptom.

In a child with 'unexplained' headache, *skull X-ray* and preferrably *CT scan* should be performed:

- if the presentation is acute.
- if the severity progressively increases.
- if school performance declines, or other symptoms e.g. personality change, develop.
- if the head circumference increases.
- if the child is under 5 years.

Headache — Specific Causes

TENSION HEADACHE

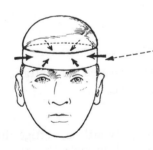

This is a common form of headache experienced by most people at some time of their lives.

Characteristics: Diffuse, dull, aching, 'band-like' headache, worse on touching the scalp and aggravated by noise; associated with 'tension' but not with other physical symptoms.

Duration: Many hours – days.

Frequency: Infrequent or daily; worse towards the end of the day.

May persist over many years.

Mechanism: 'Muscular' due to persistent contraction e.g. clenching teeth, head posture, furrowing of brow.

Treatment: Reassurance.
Benzodiazepines e.g. diazepam.
Antidepressants.

Headache — Specific Causes

MIGRAINE

Migraine is a common familial disorder characterised by *unilateral throbbing headache.*

Onset: – childhood or early adult life.   **Incidence:** – affects 5–10% of the population.
Female:Male ratio: – 2:1.   **Family history:** – obtained in 70% of all sufferers.

Two recognisable forms exist:

CLASSIC MIGRAINE

An *aura* or warning of visual, sensory or motor type followed by headache –

throbbing, unilateral, worsened by bright light, relieved by sleep, associated with nausea and occasionally, vomiting.

COMMON MIGRAINE

The *aura* is absent. The headache has similar features, but it is often poorly localised and its description may merge with that of 'tension' headache.

The aura of classic migraine may take many forms. The visual forms comprise: flashing lights, zig-zags (fortifications), scintillating scotoma (central vision) and may precede visual field defects. Such aura are of retinal or visual (occipital) cortex origin.

The headache is paroxysmal, lasting from 2 to 48 hours and rarely occurring more frequently than twice weekly.

Mechanism:

In the initial aura phase, cerebral arterial *constriction* results in ischaemia of the territory supplied with corresponding clinical manifestations.

Dilatation follows, especially of extracranial scalp vessels, stimulating pain sensitive fibres.

As the attack continues:

Pain-producing substances, NEUROKININS, accumulate in perivascular spaces and perpetuate the headache.

The initial constriction may result from amine release:

SEROTONIN, ADRENALINE, NORADRENALINE —— powerful vasoconstrictors.

Migraine sufferers appear more sensitive to these amines.   An increased concentration of amine metabolites in the urine after an attack supports this hypothesis.

TYPES of 'CLASSIC' MIGRAINE

BASILAR: – Characterised by bilateral visual symptoms, unsteadiness, dysarthria, vertigo, limb parasthesia, even tetraparesis. Loss of consciousness may ensue and precede the onset of headache. This form of migraine frequently affects young women.

HEMIPLEGIC: – Characterised by an aura of unilateral paralysis (hemiplegia) which can persist for some days after the headache has settled. Often misdiagnosed as a 'stroke'. When familial, mendelian dominant inheritance is noted. Recovery is the rule.

OPHTHALMOPLEGIC: – Characterised by extraocular nerve palsies, usually the IIIrd, rarely the VIth. These may result from dilatation of the internal carotid artery with stretching of the III or VI cranial nerve within the cavernous sinus.

Dysphasia, memory disturbance, vertigo or a hemisensory disturbance may also occur.

Headache — Specific Causes

Precipitating factors in Migraine

The migraine sufferer can often identify exogenous factors which induce attacks. Dietary factors include alcohol, chocolate and cheese (high tyramine content). Attacks in women are often more common premenstrually and when on the oral contraceptive. They may disappear in pregnancy. Stress, physical fatigue, exercise, sleep deprivation and minor head trauma may all precipitate attacks.

Diagnosis – from clinical history.   Supported by:
  – a positive family history.
  – the presence of travel sickness or migraine variants (abdominal pains) in childhood.
  – age of onset – childhood, adolescence, early adult life, menopause.

Distinguish from:
– partial (focal) epilepsy (in hemiplegic or hemisensory migraine).
– aneurysmal dilatation (in ophthalmoplegic migraine).
– transient ischaemic attack (in hemiplegic or hemisensory migraine – often difficult in the middle aged).
– arterio-venous malformation – gives well localised headache but not of the 'classic' migraine type.

Management

1. Identification and avoidance of precipitatory factors

2. Prophylaxis

Justification
  frequent and severe attacks.
Commonly used drugs
  Pizotifen (powerful antiserotonin)
  Propranolol (beta adrenergic receptor blocker)
  Methysergide (powerful antiserotonin – use with caution in view of the side effects e.g. retroperitoneal fibrosis).

3. Treatment of an attack

Poor gastro-intestinal absorption of drugs during attack. Metoclopramide will enhance absorption of soluble aspirin etc. Ergotamine tartrate may be used in severe attacks. In a severely prolonged episode (status migrainosus) hydrocortisone i.v. will halt the attack.

CLUSTER HEADACHES (Histamine cephalgia)

Cluster headaches occur less frequently than migraine, and more often in men than women, with onset in early middle age.

Characteristics: Severe unilateral pain around the eye,
  associated with conjunctival injection, lacrimation, rhinorrhoea.
Duration: 10 minutes to 2 hours.
Frequency: Once to many times per day, often wakening from sleep at night. 'Clusters' of attacks separated by weeks or even many months.
  Alcohol may precipitate the attacks.

Mechanism: Serum histamine levels rise during the attacks, hence the alternative name 'histamine cephalgia'
Treatment: Antihistamines give disappointing results. Ergotamine and methysergide are useful prophylactics. Use prednisolone 30mg daily for 10 days in refractory cases.

Headache — Specific Causes

POST-TRAUMATIC HEADACHE

A 'common migraine' or 'tension-like' headache may arise after head injury and accompany other symptoms including light headedness, irritability, difficulty in concentration and in coping with work. Although once thought to have a purely 'psychological' origin, especially with impending litigation, it is now recognised that injuries severe enough to cause loss of consciousness or a period of post-traumatic amnesia, result in some neuronal damage, requiring several weeks to recover.

Treatment: As for tension headache.

GIANT CELL (TEMPORAL) ARTERITIS

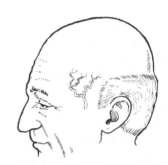

Giant cell arteritis causes headache in the elderly. This is severe and throbbing in nature and overlies the involved vessel – usually the superficial temporal artery, although the condition may affect any extra- or intracranial vessels.
Palpation reveals a thickened, tender, but nonpulsatile artery.

Jaw claudication: pain when chewing or talking due to ischaemia of the masseter muscles is pathognomonic and occurs in a high proportion of patients.
Visual symptoms are common with blindness or diplopia.
Associated systemic symptoms – weight loss, lassitude and generalised muscle aches – polymyalgia rheumatica in one-fifth of cases.
Duration: the headache is intractable, lasting until treatment commences.

Mechanism:

Large and medium sized arteries undergo intense 'giant cell' infiltration, with fragmentation of the lamina and narrowing of the lumen, resulting in distal ischaemia as well as stimulating pain sensitive fibres. Occlusion of important end arteries e.g. the ophthalmic artery, may result in blindness; occlusion of the basilar artery may cause brain stem or bilateral occipital infarction.

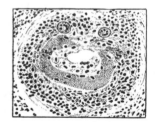

Thickened wall with giant cell infiltrate

Diagnosis: Elevated ESR with a positive temporal artery biopsy.

Treatment: Urgent treatment, prednisolone 60mg daily, prevents visual loss or brain stem stroke as well as relieving the headache. Monitoring the ESR allows gradual reduction in steroid dosage over several weeks to a maintenance level e.g. 5mg daily. Some patients eventually come off steroids; others require life-long treatment.

Headache — Specific Causes

HEADACHE from RAISED INTRACRANIAL PRESSURE

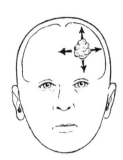

Characteristics:
- generalised.
- aggravated by bending or coughing.
- worse in the morning on awakening; may awaken patient from sleep.
- the severity of the headache gradually progresses.

Associated features:
- vomiting in later stages.
- transient loss of vision (obscuration) with sudden change in posture.
- eventual impairment of conscious level.

Management: further investigations are essential – CT scan.

HEADACHE due to INTRACRANIAL HAEMORRHAGE

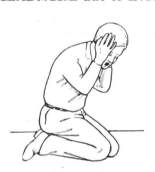

Characteristics:
- instantaneous onset.
- severe pain, spreading over the vertex to the occiput, or described as a "sudden blow to the back of the head".
- patient may drop to his knees or lose consciousness.

Associated features:
- usually accompanied by vomiting.
- focal neurological signs suggest a haematoma.

Management: further investigation – lumbar puncture/CT scan (see Meningism, page 70).

NON-NEUROLOGICAL CAUSES of HEADACHE

Local causes:

SINUSES: Well localised. Worse in morning. Affected by posture e.g. bending. X-ray – sinus opacified. Treatment – decongestants or drainage.

OCULAR: Refraction errors may result in 'muscle contraction' headaches – resolves when corrected with glasses.
Glaucoma does not produce headache without other symptoms e.g. misting of vision, 'haloes'. Cupping seen on fundoscopy.

DENTAL DISEASE: Discomfort localised to teeth. Check for malocclusion.
Check temporomandibular joints.

Systemic causes:
Headache may accompany any febrile illness or may be the presenting feature of accelerated hypertension or metabolic disease e.g. hypoglycaemia, hypercalcaemia.
Many drugs e.g. dipyridamole and toxins e.g. caffeine may also cause headache.

Meningism

Evidence of meningeal irritation caused by infection or subarachnoid haemorrhage results in characteristic clinical features:

SYMPTOMS
1. Headache.
2. Vomiting.
3. Photophobia.

SIGNS

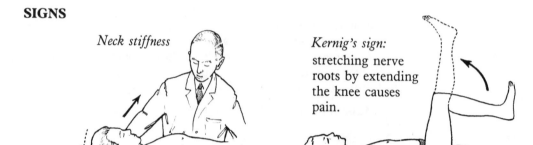

Neck stiffness

Kernig's sign: stretching nerve roots by extending the knee causes pain.

INVESTIGATION

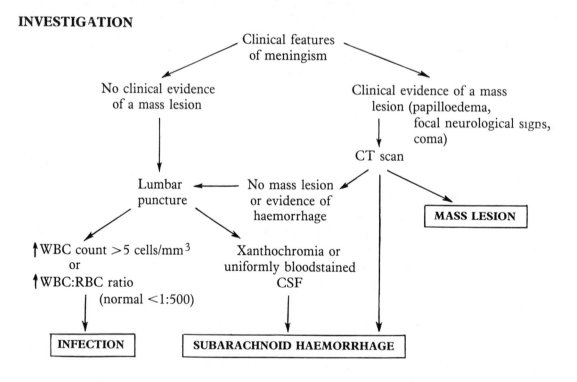

Clinical features of meningism

No clinical evidence of a mass lesion

Clinical evidence of a mass lesion (papilloedema, focal neurological signs, coma)

CT scan

Lumbar puncture ← No mass lesion or evidence of haemorrhage

MASS LESION

↑WBC count >5 cells/mm^3
or
↑WBC:RBC ratio
(normal <1:500)

Xanthochromia or uniformly bloodstained CSF

INFECTION

SUBARACHNOID HAEMORRHAGE

Raised Intracranial Pressure

The skull is basically a rigid structure. Since its contents – brain, blood and cerebrospinal fluid (CSF) – are incompressible, an increase in one constituent or an expanding mass within the skull results in an increase in intracranial pressure (ICP) – the 'Monro Kellie doctrine'.

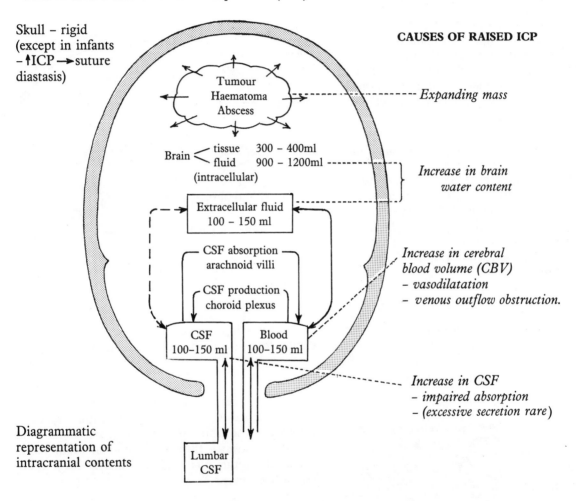

Skull – rigid
(except in infants
– ↑ICP → suture
diastasis)

CAUSES OF RAISED ICP

Tumour
Haematoma
Abscess

------ *Expanding mass*

Brain < tissue   300 – 400ml
        fluid   900 – 1200ml -------
        (intracellular)

} *Increase in brain
water content*

Extracellular fluid
100 – 150 ml

CSF absorption
arachnoid villi

CSF production
choroid plexus

*Increase in cerebral
blood volume (CBV)
– vasodilatation
– venous outflow obstruction.*

CSF   Blood
100–150 ml   100–150 ml

*Increase in CSF
– impaired absorption
– (excessive secretion rare)*

Diagrammatic
representation of
intracranial contents

Lumbar
CSF

Compensatory mechanisms for an expanding
intracranial mass lesion.

Immediate { 1. ↓CSF volume – CSF outflow to the lumbar theca.
            2. ↓Cerebral blood volume.
Delayed —— 3. ↓Extracellular fluid.

71

Raised Intracranial Pressure

CEREBROSPINAL FLUID (CSF)

Secreted at a rate of 500 ml per day from the choroid plexus, CSF flows through the ventricular system and enters the subarachnoid space via the 4th ventricular foramina of Magendie and Luschka.

Under normal conditions, CSF flows freely through the subarachnoid space and is absorbed into the venous system through the arachnoid villi. If flow is obstructed at any point in the pathway, *hydrocephalus* with an associated rise in intracranial pressure develops, as a result of continued CSF production. With an expanding intracranial mass lesion, normal pressure is initially maintained by CSF expulsion to the lumbar theca. Further expansion and subsequent brain shift may obstruct the free flow of CSF not only to the lumbar theca but also to the arachnoid villi, causing an acute rise in intracranial pressure.

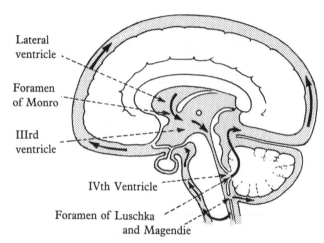

Lateral ventricle

Foramen of Monro

IIIrd ventricle

IVth Ventricle

Foramen of Luschka and Magendie

BRAIN WATER / OEDEMA

Cerebral oedema – an excess of brain water – may develop around an intrinsic lesion within the brain tissue e.g. tumour or abscess or in relation to traumatic or ischaemic brain damage, and contribute to the space-occupying defect.

Different forms of cerebral oedema exist:

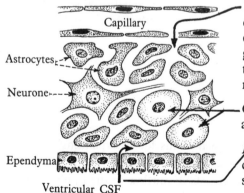

Capillary

Astrocytes

Neurone

Ependyma

Ventricular CSF

Vasogenic: excess fluid (protein rich) passes through defective vessel walls to the extracellular space – especially in the white matter. The extracellular fluid gradually infiltrates throughout normal brain tissue towards the ventricular CSF and this drainage route may aid clearance.

Cytotoxic: fluid accumulates within cells – neurones and glia i.e. intracellular.

Interstitial: when obstructive hydrocephalus develops CSF is forced through to the extracellular space especially in the periventricular white matter.

With *ischaemic* damage, as cell metabolism fails, intracellular Na^+ increases and the cells swell i.e. cytotoxic oedema. Capillary damage follows and vasogenic oedema supervenes.

Raised Intracranial Pressure

CEREBRAL BLOOD FLOW (CBF) / CEREBRAL BLOOD VOLUME (CBV)

Blood flow is dependent on blood pressure and the vascular resistance –

$$\text{Flow} = \frac{\text{Pressure}}{\text{Resistance}}$$

Inside the skull, intracranial pressure must be taken into account –

$$\text{Cerebral Blood Flow (CBF)} = \frac{\text{Cerebral Perfusion Pressure (CPP)}}{\text{Cerebral Vascular Resistance (CVR)}}$$

(i.e. systemic BP – intracranial pressure)

Under normal conditions the cerebral blood flow is coupled to the energy requirements of brain tissue. Various regulatory mechanisms act to maintain a cerebral blood flow sufficient to meet the metabolic demands.

FACTORS AFFECTING THE CEREBRAL VASCULATURE
— Change in extracellular pH or an accumulation of metabolic by-products directly affect the vessel calibre.
— Any change in arteriolar PCO_2 has a direct effect on cerebral vessels, but only a reduction of PO_2 to < 50 mmHg has a significant effect.
— A change in the cerebral perfusion pressure results in a compensatory change in vessel calibre (autoregulation – see below).

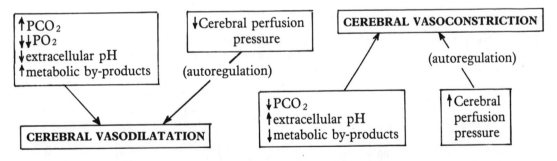

Any change in blood vessel diameter results in considerable variation in cerebral blood volume and this, in turn, directly affects intracranial pressure.

Energy requirements differ in different parts of the brain. In the white matter, flow is 20ml/100g/min, whereas in the grey matter flow is as high as 100ml/100g/min.

73

Raised Intracranial Pressure

Cerebral Blood Flow (continued)

AUTOREGULATION is a compensatory mechanism which permits fluctuation in the cerebral perfusion pressure within certain limits without significantly altering cerebral blood flow.

A drop in cerebral perfusion pressure produces vasodilatation (probably due to a direct 'myogenic' effect on the vascular smooth muscle) thereby maintaining flow; a rise in the cerebral perfusion pressure causes vasoconstriction.

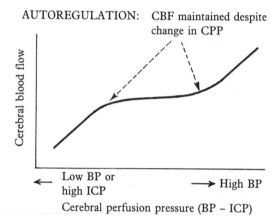

Neurogenic influences appear to have little direct effect on the cerebral vessels but they may alter the range of pressure changes over which autoregulation acts.

Autoregulation fails when the cerebral perfusion pressure falls below 60mmHg or rises above 160mmHg. At these extremes, cerebral blood flow is more directly related to the perfusion pressure.

In damaged brain (e.g. after head injury or subarachnoid haemorrhage), autoregulation is impaired; a drop in cerebral perfusion pressure is more likely to reduce cerebral blood flow and cause ischaemia. Conversely, a high cerebral perfusion may increase the cerebral blood flow, breakdown the blood/brain barrier and produce cerebral oedema as in hypertensive encephalopathy.

INTRACRANIAL PRESSURE (ICP)

Intracranial pressure, measured relative to the foramen of Monro, under normal conditions ranges from 0–135 mm CSF (0–10 mmHg) although very high pressures e.g. 1000 mm CSF may occur transiently during coughing or straining.

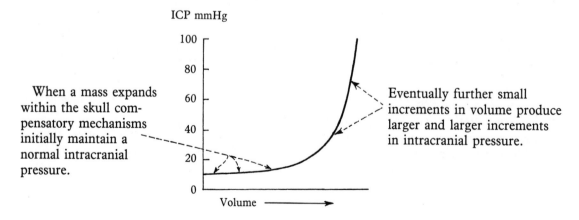

When a mass expands within the skull compensatory mechanisms initially maintain a normal intracranial pressure.

Eventually further small increments in volume produce larger and larger increments in intracranial pressure.

Raised Intracranial Pressure

ICP *(continued)*

When intracranial pressure is monitored with a ventricular catheter, regular waves due to pulse and respiratory effects are recorded (page 49). As an intracranial mass expands and as the compensatory reserves diminish, transient pressure elevations (pressure waves) are superimposed. These become more frequent and more prominent as the mean pressure rises.

Eventually the rise in intracranial pressure and resultant fall in cerebral perfusion pressure reach a critical level and a significant reduction in cerebral blood flow occurs. Electrical activity in the cortex fails at flow rates about 20ml/100g/min. If autoregulation is already impaired these effects develop even earlier. When intracranial pressure reaches the mean arterial blood pressure, cerebral blood flow ceases.

INTERRELATIONSHIPS

Many factors affect intracranial pressure and these should not be considered in isolation. Inter-relationships are complex and feedback pathways may merely serve to compound the brain damage.

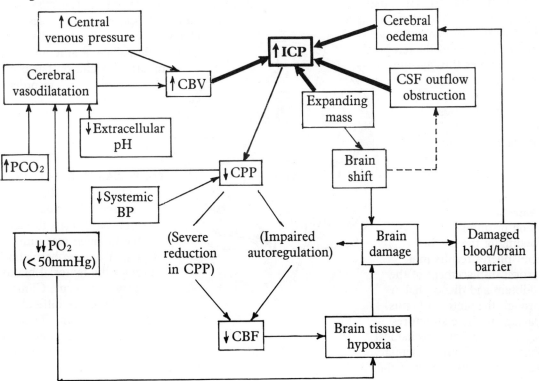

Raised Intracranial Pressure

CLINICAL EFFECTS of RAISED INTRACRANIAL PRESSURE

A raised ICP will produce symptoms and signs but does not cause neuronal damage provided cerebral blood flow is maintained. Damage does however result from brain shift – tentorial or tonsillar herniation.

Clinical features due to ↑ICP:

1. *Headache* — worse in the mornings, aggravated by stooping and bending.
2. *Vomiting* — occurs late in the disease course, often without warning or preliminary nausea i.e. 'projectile'.
3. *Papilloedema* — occurs in a proportion of patients (but not all) with ↑ICP due to obstruction of both axoplasmic and extraaxonal flow. Swelling of the optic disc and retinal and disc haemorrhages result. Vision is only at risk when papilloedema is both severe and prolonged.

BRAIN SHIFT – TYPES

TENTORIAL HERNIATION (lateral): a unilateral expanding mass causes tentorial (uncal) herniation as the medial edge of the temporal lobe herniates through the tentorial hiatus. As the intracranial pressure continues to rise, 'central' herniation follows.

SUBFALCINE 'MIDLINE' SHIFT: occurs early with unilateral space-occupying lesions. Seldom produces any clinical effect, although ipsilateral anterior cerebral artery occlusion has been recorded.

TENTORIAL HERNIATION (central): a midline lesion or diffuse swelling of the cerebral hemispheres results in a vertical displacement of the midbrain and diencephalon through the tentorial hiatus. Damage to these structures occurs either from mechanical distortion or from ischaemia secondary to stretching of the perforating vessels.

TONSILLAR HERNIATION: a subtentorial expanding mass causes herniation of the cerebellar tonsils through the foramen magnum. A degree of *upward* herniation through the tentorial hiatus may also occur. Clinical effects are difficult to distinguish from effects of direct brainstem/midbrain compression.
Unchecked central tentorial herniation will also lead to tonsillar herniation.

Raised Intracranial Pressure

CLINICAL EFFECTS OF BRAIN SHIFT

TENTORIAL HERNIATION – Lateral

The rate of symptom progression is related to the rate of lesion expansion.

The posterior cerebral artery is sometimes occluded but the resultant *homonymous hemianopia* is rarely detected in the acute stage.

Pressure against the reticular formation in the midbrain causes *deterioration of conscious level.*

Pressure from the edge of the tentorium cerebelli on the opposite cerebral peduncle (Kernohan's notch) may produce *limb weakness on the same side* as the lesion i.e. 'false localising sign'.

Basilar artery

Pons

III nerve

Internal carotid artery

Anterior cerebral artery

Compression of the III nerve and oculo-motor nucleus in the midbrain causes – *pupil dilatation and failure to react to light.* *[Ptosis* and *impaired eye movements* are less easy to detect due to the associated depression of conscious level.]*

(Optic nerves and chiasma are not illustrated)

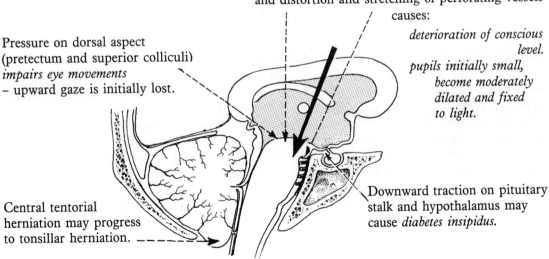

TENTORIAL HERNIATION – Central

Diencephalon and midbrain damage from buckling and distortion and stretching of perforating vessels causes:

deterioration of conscious level.

pupils initially small, become moderately dilated and fixed to light.

Pressure on dorsal aspect (pretectum and superior colliculi) *impairs eye movements* – upward gaze is initially lost.

Downward traction on pituitary stalk and hypothalamus may cause *diabetes insipidus.*

Central tentorial herniation may progress to tonsillar herniation.

Raised Intracranial Pressure

Clinical Effects of Brain Shift *(continued)*

TONSILLAR HERNIATION

A degree of upward cerebellar
herniation is usually present.

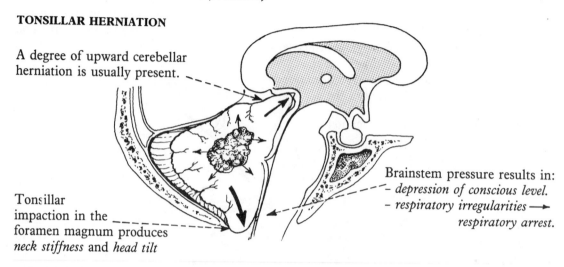

Brainstem pressure results in:
– *depression of conscious level.*
– *respiratory irregularities* →
        respiratory arrest.

Tonsillar
impaction in the
foramen magnum produces
neck stiffness and *head tilt*

An injudicious lumbar puncture in the presence of a subtentorial mass may create a pressure gradient sufficient to induce tonsillar herniation.

NB.   Harvey Cushing described cardiovascular changes – an increase in blood pressure and a fall in pulse rate, associated with an expanding intracranial mass, and probably resulting from direct medullary compression. The clinical value of these observations is often overemphasised. They are often absent; when present they are invariably preceded by a deterioration in conscious level.

INVESTIGATIONS
Patients with suspected raised intracranial pressure require an urgent CT scan.

TREATMENT OF RAISED INTRACRANIAL PRESSURE
When a rising intracranial pressure is caused by an expanding mass or is compounded by respiratory problems, treatment is clear cut; the mass must be removed and blood gases restored to normal levels – by ventilation if necessary.

In some patients, despite the above measures, cerebral swelling may produce a marked increase in intracranial pressure. This may follow removal of a tumour or haematoma or may complicate a diffuse head injury. Artificial methods of lowering intracranial pressure may prevent brain damage and death from brain shift, although their use in some instances is controversial (see page 218).

Intracranial pressure is monitored with a ventricular catheter or surface pressure recording device (see page 48).

Treatment may be instituted when the mean ICP is > 30 mmHg.

Raised Intracranial Pressure

TREATMENT (continued)

Methods of Reducing Intracranial Pressure

MANNITOL INFUSION:

An i.v. bolus of 100 ml of 20% mannitol infused over 15 minutes reduces intracranial pressure by establishing an osmotic gradient between the plasma and brain tissue. *This method 'buys' time prior to craniotomy in a patient deteriorating from a mass lesion.* Mannitol is also used 6 hourly for a 24–48 hour period in an attempt to reduce raised ICP. Repeated infusions however lead to equilibration and a high intracellular osmotic pressure, thus counteracting further treatment. In addition, repeated doses may precipitate lethal rises in arterial blood pressure and acute tubular necrosis. Its use is therefore best restricted for emergency situations.

HYPERVENTILATION:

If the patient is paralysed and hyperventilated – bringing the PCO_2 down to 3.5 kPa, the resultant vasoconstriction and reduction in cerebral blood volume lowers intracranial pressure. (A further drop in PCO_2 risks ischaemic damage due to severe vasoconstriction.) In many patients, however, adaptation to the new PCO_2 level occurs and after several hours the intracranial pressure gradually rises to previous levels.

CSF WITHDRAWAL:

Removal of a few ml. of CSF from the ventricle will immediately reduce the intracranial pressure. Within minutes, however, the pressure will rise and further CSF withdrawal will be required. In practice, this method is of limited value since CSF outflow to the lumbar theca results in a diminished intracranial CSF volume and the lateral ventricles are often collapsed. Continuous CSF drainage may make most advantage of this method.

BARBITURATE THERAPY:

Some workers have advocated barbiturate therapy in the treatment of raised intracranial pressure following brain damage. This reduces neuronal activity and depresses cerebral metabolism; a fall in energy requirements may protect ischaemic areas and subsequent vasoconstriction may reduce cerebral blood volume and intracranial pressure. Although some experimental studies have shown encouraging results, clinical trials have yet to show convincing benefit.

STEROIDS:

There is no doubt that steroids play an important rôle in treating patients with intracranial tumours and surrounding oedema. Cell membranes are stabilised, but it is not certain that their beneficial effect in tumour management is a result of reducing ICP. Steroids appear to be of no value in the treatment of traumatic or ischaemic damage. Experimental evidence suggests that they may help if administered before the damage occurs but clearly this is seldom of practical value.

Coma and Impaired Conscious Level

Many pathological processes may impair conscious level and numerous terms have been employed to describe the various clinical states which result, including obtundation, stupor, semi-coma and deep-coma. These terms result in ambiguity and inconsistency when used by different observers.   Recording conscious level with the *Glasgow coma scale* (page 6) avoids these difficulties and clearly describes the level of consciousness. With this scale:

> COMA = NO SPEECH, NO EYE OPENING, NO MOTOR RESPONSE.

In this section we describe conditions which may present with or lead to coma. Patients experiencing 'transient disturbance of conscious level' require a different approach.

Pathophysiology of coma:

A 'conscious' state depends on intact cerebral hemi-spheres, interacting with the ascending reticular activating system in the brainstem, midbrain, hypothalamus and thal-amus. Lesions diffusely affecting the cerebral hemispheres, or directly affecting the reticular activating system cause impairment of conscious level:

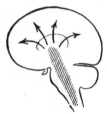

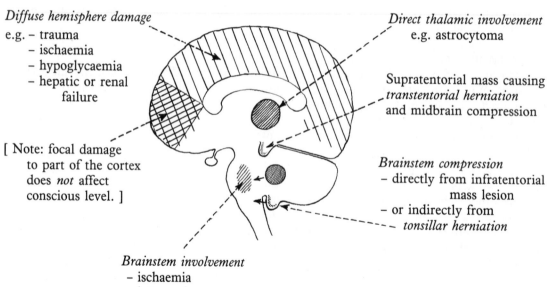

Diffuse hemisphere damage
e.g. – trauma
 – ischaemia
 – hypoglycaemia
 – hepatic or renal
  failure

[Note: focal damage
 to part of the cortex
 does *not* affect
 conscious level.]

Direct thalamic involvement
 e.g. astrocytoma

Supratentorial mass causing
transtentorial herniation
and midbrain compression

Brainstem compression
 – directly from infratentorial
  mass lesion
 – or indirectly from
  tonsillar herniation

Brainstem involvement
 – ischaemia
 – haemorrhage
 – tumour
 – drugs (sedatives, hypnotics)

Coma and Impaired Conscious Level

CAUSES

INTRACRANIAL

TRAUMA

Diffuse white matter injury.
Haematoma – extradural
            – subdural
            – 'burst' lobe

NEOPLASTIC

Tumour with oedema.

OTHER

Epilepsy – post-ictal state.
Hydrocephalus.

VASCULAR

Subarachnoid haemorrhage.
'Spontaneous' intracerebral haematoma.
Cerebral infarct with oedema.
Vertebro-basilar infarct.

INFECTIVE

Meningitis.
Abscess.
Encephalitis.

EXTRACRANIAL

METABOLIC

Hypo/hypernatraemia
Hypo/hyperkalaemia.
Hypo/hypercalcaemia.
Hypo/hyperglycaemia.
Acidosis/alkalosis.
Hypo/hyperthermia.
Uraemia.
Hepatic failure.
Porphyria.

Hypercapnia.
Hypoxia.

ENDOCRINE

Diabetes.
Hypopituitarism.
Adrenal crisis (Addison's disease).
Hypo/hyperparathyroidism.
Hypothyroidism.

RESPIRATORY INSUFFICIENCY

Hypoventilation.
Diffusion deficiency.
Perfusion deficiency.
Anaemia.

DRUGS

Sedatives.
Hypnotics.
Anticonvulsants.
Alcohol.
Anaesthetic agents.

REDUCED CEREBRAL BLOOD FLOW

DECREASED CARDIAC OUTPUT

Vasovagal attack.
Blood loss.
Valvular disease.
Myocardial infarction.
Cardiac arrhythmias.
Hypotensive drugs.

TOXINS

Carbon monoxide.
Heavy metals.

PSYCHIATRIC DISEASE

Hysteria.
Catatonia.

ARTERIAL OCCLUSION

Vertebral artery disease.
Bilateral carotid disease.

Coma and Impaired Conscious Level

Examination of the unconscious patient (see pages 30,31)

DIAGNOSTIC APPROACH

Questioning friends, relatives or the ambulance team, followed by general and neurological examination all provide important diagnostic information.

History	Possible Cause of Coma / Impaired Conscious Level
Head injury leading to admission	→ *Diffuse shearing injury and/or intracranial haematoma.*
Previous head injury (e.g. 6 weeks)	→ *Chronic subdural haematoma.*
Sudden collapse	→ *Intracerebral haemorrhage. Subarachnoid haemorrhage.*
Limb twitching, incontinence	→ *Epilepsy / post-ictal state.*
Gradual development of symptoms	→ *Mass lesion, metabolic or infective cause.*
Previous illness –diabetes	→ *Hypo- or (less likely) hyperglycaemia.*
– epilepsy	→ *Post-ictal state.*
– psychiatric illness	→ *Drug overdose.*
– alcoholism or drug abuse	→ *Drug toxicity.*
– viral infection	→ *Encephalitis.*
– malignancy	→ *Intracranial metastasis.*

General examination

Note the presence of:

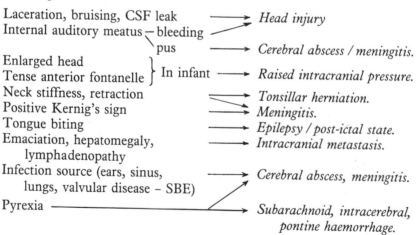

Laceration, bruising, CSF leak → *Head injury*

Internal auditory meatus – bleeding → *Head injury*

⟍ pus → *Cerebral abscess / meningitis.*

Enlarged head / Tense anterior fontanelle } In infant → *Raised intracranial pressure.*

Neck stiffness, retraction → *Tonsillar herniation.*

Positive Kernig's sign → *Meningitis.*

Tongue biting → *Epilepsy / post-ictal state.*

Emaciation, hepatomegaly, lymphadenopathy → *Intracranial metastasis.*

Infection source (ears, sinus, lungs, valvular disease – SBE) → *Cerebral abscess, meningitis.*

Pyrexia → *Subarachnoid, intracerebral, pontine haemorrhage.*

Coma and Impaired Conscious Level

DIAGNOSTIC APPROACH (*continued*)

General examination (*continued*)

Possible Cause of Coma / Impaired Conscious Level

Hypotension / Blood loss
Cardiac arrhythmias ⟶ Reduced cardiac output ⟶ *Cerebral ischaemia.*
Valvular disease ⟶ Emboli
Respiratory insufficiency

Smell of alcohol ⟶ *Alcohol abuse.*
Needle marks on limbs ⟶ *Drug abuse.*
'Snout' rash ⟶ *Solvent abuse.*

Neurological examination:

Signs of raised intracranial pressure (ICP)
  – papilloedema ⟶ *Intracranial mass lesion.*
  – tense anterior fontanelle *Hydrocephalus.*
        (in infants)

Neurological signs
  – unilateral, dilated, fixed pupil ⟶ *Diffuse cerebral swelling e.g. anoxia.*
  – bilateral dilated, fixed pupils ⟶ *Drugs – glutethimide* ⎫ *overdose.*
                              sympathomimetics ⎭

  – pinpoint pupils ⟶ *Drugs – opiates*
                             parasympathomimetics.
                             Pontine haemorrhage.

  – eye movements absent   pupils fixed ⟶ *Severe - trauma*
    (spontaneous or reflex)   *- ischaemia*
                        pupils   *- haemorrhage.*
                        usually   *Drugs (transient effect).*
                        reacting ⟶ *Hypoxic/hepatic encephalopathy.*

  – asymmetric limb response ⟶ *Focal brain damage e.g.*
    (i.e. hemi/monoparesis)
                                               - tumour.
                                               - trauma.
                                                   - haematoma.
                                                   - encephalitis.

⎡ NB - *hepatic encephalopathy* ⎤ ⎫ *occasionally produce*
⎢   - *hypoglycaemia* ⎥ ⎬ *asymmetrical responses*
⎣   - *uraemia.* ⎦ ⎭

Symmetrical limb responses ⎫
Reacting pupils   ⎬ ⟶ Suggests a *metabolic encephalopathy*
Full eye movements   ⎭   *or drug toxicity.*
Subhyaloid haemorrhage (on fundoscopy) ⟶ *Subarachnoid haemorrhage.*

Coma and Impaired Conscious Level

Investigations:

The sequence of investigations depends on the clinical findings:

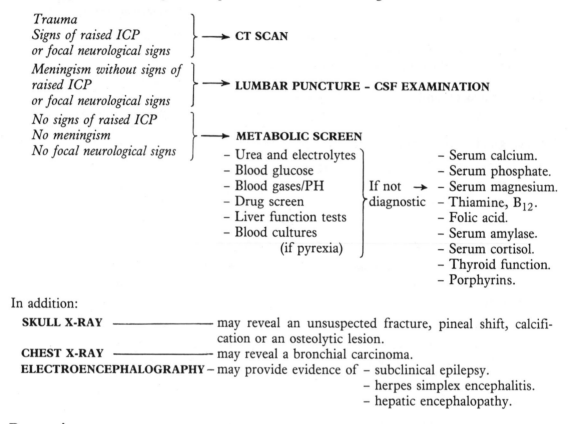

Trauma
Signs of raised ICP
or focal neurological signs } ⟶ **CT SCAN**

Meningism without signs of
raised ICP
or focal neurological signs } ⟶ **LUMBAR PUNCTURE – CSF EXAMINATION**

No signs of raised ICP
No meningism
No focal neurological signs } ⟶ **METABOLIC SCREEN**

– Urea and electrolytes
– Blood glucose
– Blood gases/PH
– Drug screen
– Liver function tests
– Blood cultures
     (if pyrexia)

If not ⟶
diagnostic

– Serum calcium.
– Serum phosphate.
– Serum magnesium.
– Thiamine, B_{12}.
– Folic acid.
– Serum amylase.
– Serum cortisol.
– Thyroid function.
– Porphyrins.

In addition:

SKULL X-RAY ——————— may reveal an unsuspected fracture, pineal shift, calcification or an osteolytic lesion.

CHEST X-RAY ——————— may reveal a bronchial carcinoma.

ELECTROENCEPHALOGRAPHY – may provide evidence of – subclinical epilepsy.
                                             – herpes simplex encephalitis.
                                             – hepatic encephalopathy.

Prognosis:

Although *conscious level examination* does not aid diagnosis, it plays an essential rôle in patient management and along with the *duration of coma, pupil response* and *eye movements* provides valuable prognostic information.

84

Transient Loss of Consciousness

Many conditions causing coma may also transiently affect a patient's conscious level. This results from:

Reduction in cerebral arterial oxygen supply
— *Cardiac arrhythmias* \} *reduced*
— *Vasovagal attack* \} *cardiac output*
— *Vertebro-basilar attack*
— *Basilar migraine*

Reduction in cerebral glucose supply — *Hypoglycaemia*
Abnormal electrical activity — *Epilepsy*

Clinical details – see page 94.

Drug abuse – *solvents* or *barbiturates* may cause transient, intermittent confusion.

DIAGNOSTIC APPROACH

HISTORY:

The patient's own description of the attack or that of an eye witness may virtually establish the diagnosis. Prodromal features of pallor, nausea and sweating accompany *vasovagal attacks*. Clonic/tonic movements occur shortly after the onset of an *epileptic 'grand mal' attack* (but may also occur at the end of a vasovagal attack or cardiac arrhythmia).

Palpitations, sweating, behavioural disturbances and seizures may precede loss of consciousness from *hypoglycaemia*. Vertigo and scintillating teichopsia often precede *basilar migraine;* a throbbing headache follows the period of loss of consciousness.

ELECTROENCEPHALOGRAPHY (EEG) – may reveal a focal disturbance – *epilepsy.*

ELECTROCARDIOGRAPHY (ECG) – may reveal a *cardiac arrythmia.*

BLOOD GLUCOSE – may indicate *hypoglycaemia.*

If an eye witness' account and the above tests provide no evidence of the cause, proceed to:

1. **TELEMETRIC EEG and ECG MONITORING** over a 24 hour period.
2. **72 HOUR FAST** – if symptoms appear, check **blood glucose** and **insulin** levels.

Confusional States and Delirium

Of all acute medical admissions, 5–10% present with a **confused verbal response** i.e. disorientation in time and/or place. Most are easily distracted, have slowed thought processes and a limited concentration span. Some may lose interest in the examination to the point of drifting off to sleep.

Perceptual disorders (illusions and hallucinations) may accompany the confused state – **delirium**. This is often associated with withdrawal and lack of awareness or with restlessness and hyperactivity.

Primary neurological disorders contribute to only 10% of those patients presenting with an acute confusional state. In the elderly, post-operative disorientation is particularly common and multiple factors probably apply; in these patients the prognosis is good.

DIAGNOSTIC APPROACH

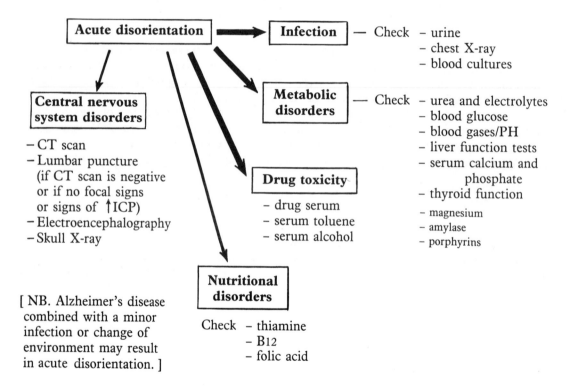

Acute disorientation ⟶ **Infection** — Check – urine
– chest X-ray
– blood cultures

Central nervous system disorders

– CT scan
– Lumbar puncture
(if CT scan is negative
or if no focal signs
or signs of ↑ICP)
– Electroencephalography
– Skull X-ray

Metabolic disorders — Check – urea and electrolytes
– blood glucose
– blood gases/PH
– liver function tests
– serum calcium and
phosphate
– thyroid function
– magnesium
– amylase
– porphyrins

Drug toxicity

– drug serum
– serum toluene
– serum alcohol

Nutritional disorders

Check – thiamine
– B12
– folic acid

[NB. Alzheimer's disease combined with a minor infection or change of environment may result in acute disorientation.]

Epilepsy

Definitions:

A seizure or epileptic attack is the consequence of a paroxysmal uncontrolled discharge of neurones within the central nervous system. The clinical manifestations range from a major motor convulsion to a brief period of lack of awareness.

The *prodrome* refers to mood or behavioural changes which may precede the attack by some hours.

The *aura* refers to the symptom immediately before loss of consciousness and will localise the attack to its point of origin within the nervous system.

The *ictus* refers to the attack or seizure itself.

The *postictal period* refers to the time immediately after the ictus during which the patient may be confused, disorientated and demonstrate automatic behaviour.

The characteristics of the attack which suggest epilepsy are the stereotyped and uncontrollable nature.

History:

Epilepsy has been described since ancient times. The 19th century neurologist Hughlings-Jackson suggested 'a sudden excessive disorderly discharge of cerebral neurones' as the causation of the attack. Berger (1929) recorded the first electroencephalogram (EEG) and not long after, it was appreciated that certain seizures were characterised by particular EEG abnormalities.

Incidence and Course:

5 per cent of the population will suffer a single seizure at some time. In 0.5 per cent of the population this will be recurrent, and in these 10 per cent will experience episodes which are partially resistant to treatment. Most epileptics have few seizures and permanent or prolonged remission, the average duration of epilepsy being 10 years.

30 per cent of epileptics develop attacks before the age of 4 years and 90 per cent before 25 years.

EPILEPSY IS A SYMPTOM OF NUMEROUS DISORDERS, BUT IN 50 PER CENT OF SUFFERERS THE CAUSE REMAINS UNCLEAR DESPITE CAREFUL HISTORY TAKING, EXAMINATION AND INVESTIGATION.

Epilepsy — Classification

The modern classification of the epilepsies is based upon the *nature* of the attack rather than the presence or absence of an underlying cause. The use of the electroencephalogram (EEG) has greatly increased our understanding of the source or 'point of origin' of any particular type of epileptic attack.

Attacks which begin **focally** from a single location within one hemisphere are thus distinguished from those of **generalised** nature which probably commence in deeper midline structures and project to both hemispheres simultaneously.

CORTICAL ORIGIN

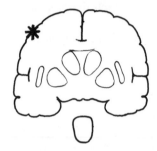

Partial (focal) seizures
  Simple partial seizure:
    Motor
    Sensory

  Complex partial seizure,
    Syn. Psychomotor temporal
            lobe epilepsy.

Focal EEG abnormality

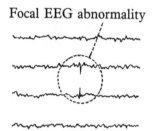

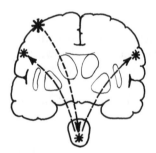

Partial seizures progressing to generalised tonic/clonic (grand mal) epilepsy.

  Simple
    or   ⟶   progressing
  Complex partial

Focal ⟶ generalised
EEG abnormality

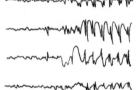

SUBCORTICAL ORIGIN

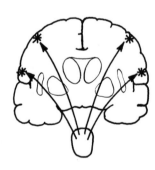

Generalised seizures
  Absences (petit mal)
  Tonic seizures
  Tonic/clonic seizures (grand mal)
  Akinetic seizures
  Infantile spasms

Generalised
EEG abnormality

The Partial Seizures

SIMPLE MOTOR SEIZURES

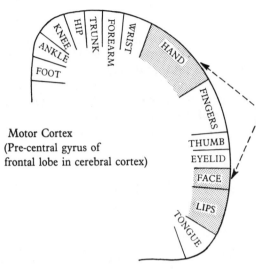

Motor Cortex
(Pre-central gyrus of
frontal lobe in cerebral cortex)

These arise in the frontal motor cortex with movements occurring in contralateral face, trunk or limbs.

The **Jacksonian** motor seizure consists of a 'march' of involuntary movement from one muscle group to the next.

Movement is clonic (shaking) and usually begins in hand or face — these having the largest representative cortical area.

Motor seizures with the above 'march' are quite rare, usually they are less localised, involving many muscle groups simultaneously and are tonic (rigid) or clonic.

After a motor seizure the affected limb(s) may remain weak for some hours before return of function occurs — **Todd's Paralysis.**

Adversive Seizures

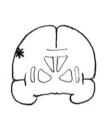

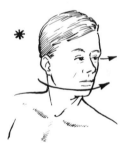

The patient is aware of movement of the head. Attacks often progress to loss of consciousness and tonic/clonic epilepsy.

The patient's eyes and head turn away from the site of the focal origin. The site of origin is usually in the supplementary motor cortex of the frontal lobe with involvement of frontal 'gaze centre'.

Some authorities, however, doubt the localising value of such an attack.

SIMPLE SENSORY SEIZURES   These arise in the sensory cortex, the patient describing numbness or tingling in an extremity or on the face. A 'march' similar to the Jacksonian motor seizure may occur. Motor symptoms occur concurrently — the limb appears weak without involuntary movement.

The representation of limbs, trunk etc. in the post-Rolandic sensory cortex is similar to that of the motor cortex.

Visual and auditory simple partial seizures also occur but are rare.

Motor and sensory seizures indicate structural brain disease, the focal onset localising the lesion i.e. focal onset in the leg may indicate a parasagittal lesion such as a meningioma. **Full investigation is mandatory.**

The Partial Seizures

COMPLEX PARTIAL SEIZURES

These attacks originate within the temporal lobe and are characterised by a complex aura (initial symptom) and occasionally a confused manner during the episode.

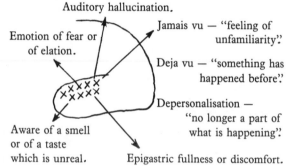

INFERIOR HORN OF
LATERAL VENTRICLE

HIPPOCAMPUS

TEMPORAL
LOBE

PONS

Coronal section through the pons showing medial aspect of the temporal lobe and hippocampus.

Complex partial seizures are synonymous with **psychomotor epilepsy** and **temporal lobe epilepsy.**

The epileptic 'focus' lies in the medial part of the temporal lobe, hippocampus or lateral surface of the lobe.

The nature of the attack: The 'psychic' manifestations of complex partial seizures are many and represent derangement of normal temporal lobe function (see Higher cortical dysfunction).

Formed visual hallucination.
Auditory hallucination.

Emotion of fear or of elation.

Jamais vu — "feeling of unfamiliarity".

Deja vu — "something has happened before".

Depersonalisation — "no longer a part of what is happening".

Aware of a smell or of a taste which is unreal.

Epigastric fullness or discomfort.

One or many of these disturbances occur in complex partial seizures and often are recognised as such only by their repetitive, uncontrollable and inappropriate nature, the sufferer not realising immediately that something is wrong.

The patient appears 'glazed' or 'distant' and may fail to respond to questions or commands. 'Eye staring' and a motor component of a primitive nature can occur with:

    Champing of teeth, swallowing,

    Smacking with lips or

    Semipurposeful movements of the limbs.

A period of automatic behaviour may then ensue — AUTOMATISM — during which the patient behaves inappropriately and may even become violent when restrained. He may wander away from the scene of the attack.

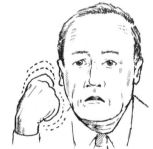

Confusion is common on recovery. Headache after an attack is frequent. The whole episode may last for seconds but occasionally may be prolonged and a rapid succession of attacks may occur. Attacks show an increased incidence in adolescence and early adult life. A history of birth trauma or febrile convulsions in infancy may be obtained. Lesions in the hippocampus occur as a result of anoxia or the convulsion itself and act as a source of further epilepsy. When surgery is carried out hippocampal sclerosis is often found. Occasionally other pathologies are identified such as hamartomas, vascular malformations and low grade malignant astrocytomas.

Partial Progressing to Generalised Seizures

As will be seen later, the seizure discharge has the capacity to spread from its point of origin and excite other structures. When spread occurs to the subcortical structures (thalamus and upper reticular formation) their excitation releases a discharge which spreads back to the whole cerebral cortex of both hemispheres, resulting in tonic/clonic epilepsy.

This chain of events is reflected in the electroencephalogram (EEG).

The symptoms (aura) before the tonic/clonic convulsion give a clue to the site of the initial discharge (simple partial or complex partial).

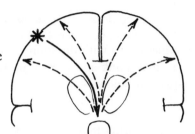

An eye witness account is important as the aura may be forgotten by the patient because of retrograde amnesia.

The TONIC/CLONIC ATTACKS

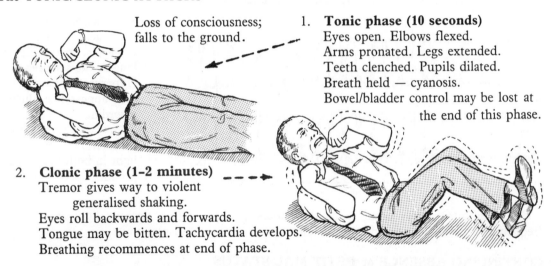

Loss of consciousness; falls to the ground.

1. **Tonic phase (10 seconds)**
   Eyes open. Elbows flexed.
   Arms pronated. Legs extended.
   Teeth clenched. Pupils dilated.
   Breath held — cyanosis.
   Bowel/bladder control may be lost at the end of this phase.

2. **Clonic phase (1–2 minutes)**
   Tremor gives way to violent generalised shaking.
   Eyes roll backwards and forwards.
   Tongue may be bitten. Tachycardia develops.
   Breathing recommences at end of phase.

The patient then sleeps with stertorous respiration and cannot be roused. On regaining consciousness the patient is confused and headache is present. He may feel exhausted for hours or even several days afterwards. Muscles may ache as a result of violent movement and muscle damage occurs with elevation of the muscle enzyme creatinine phosphokinase (CPK). Trauma occurs frequently, either as a result of the fall or as a result of the movements e.g. posterior dislocation of the shoulder.

The differentiation of these attacks from hysteria will be discussed later.

Generalised Seizures

Generalised seizure attacks arise from subcortical structures and take the following forms:

ABSENCES (Syn: Petit mal)

Onset in childhood (between 4 and 12 years of age).

Family history in 40% of patients.

When absences are associated with **myoclonus** and **drop** or **akinetic attacks**, this suggests primary childhood myoclonic epilepsy which has a poorer prognosis.

The absence may occur many times a day with duration of 5-15 seconds.

The patient stares vacantly, eyes may blink and myoclonic jerks occur.

Attacks may be induced by hyperventilation.

Frequent episodes lead to falling off in scholastic performance.

Attacks rarely present beyond adolescence.

In 30% of children, adolescence may bring tonic/clonic seizures (**Grand mal**).

Distinction of Absences from Complex Partial Seizures is easy; the latter are longer — 30 seconds or more — and followed by headache, lethargy, confusion and automatism.

The ELECTROENCEPHALOGRAM (EEG) is diagnostic.

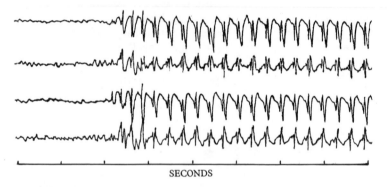

SECONDS

3 per second spike and wave activity occurs in all leads, persisting as long as the seizure.
Hyperventilation evokes this appearance during recording.
Similarly photic stimulation — flashing a light in both eyes — may produce spike and wave discharge.

Clinically, attacks may occur when the patient is exposed to a flashing light at a critical frequency, e.g. disco lights, adjusting a television set or visual display units.

CONTINUING ABSENCE or PETIT MAL STATUS

Long periods of clouding of consciousness with continuing "spike and wave" activity on the EEG.

TONIC SEIZURES

Sudden sustained muscular contraction associated with immediate loss of consciousness.

Tonic episodes occur as frequently as tonic/clonic episodes in children and should alert the physician to a possible anoxic aetiology.

In adults, tonic attacks are rare.

92

Generalised Seizures

TONIC/CLONIC SEIZURES (Syn: Grand mal)

It is the absence of a focal onset which may distinguish this *primary* generalised seizure from that *secondary* to a focal onset.

The *epileptic cry* must not be confused with an aura of focal onset. This results from tonic contraction of respiratory muscles with partial closure of vocal cords. The tonic phase is associated with rapid neuronal discharge. The clonic phase begins as neuronal discharge slows.

The ELECTROENCEPHALOGRAM during an attack is, not surprisingly, marred by movement artefact. 10–14 c.p.s. spike activity may be seen.

When the seizure ends, the record may be 'silent' and then gradually pick up. Slow rhythm may persist for some hours — postictal changes.

The record between attacks may be normal or slow with occasional clinically silent bursts of seizure activity.

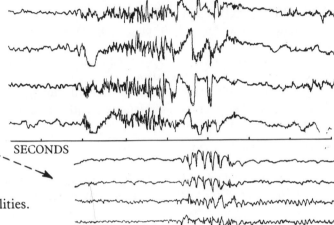

SECONDS

SECS

Again, hyperventilation or photic stimulation may bring out abnormalities.

AKINETIC SEIZURES

A sudden fall to the ground without warning. Akinetic seizure may occur in patients with absence (petit mal) but also in middle aged women. In the latter case, consciousness is retained and it seems unlikely that these attacks are 'true epilepsy'.

INFANTILE SPASMS

These occur in the first few months of life.

Repetitive shock-like flexion of neck and trunk with flexion of knees (Salaam attacks) characterise this disorder.

Infants will show a progressive mental deterioration unless attacks are controlled.

The EEG shows continuous irregular spike and wave activity called HYPSARRHYTHMIA.

Steroids, if given early, may reduce the frequency and duration of infantile spasms.

Two types of infantile spasm are recognised:

1. Of unknown etiology with normal development leading up to the onset.
2. With a definable cause — perinatal cerebral injury, congenital abnormality.

40% make a good recovery (attend normal school).

The **REFLEX EPILEPSIES** are a rare group of seizure disorders in which tonic/clonic or complex partial seizures are evoked by sensory stimuli. A primary generalised seizure induced by photic stimulation may be regarded as a reflex epilepsy, but the term is usually reserved for:

1. **Musicogenic epilepsy** in which certain musical themes or tones 'trigger' seizures.
2. **Reading epilepsy** in which reading a passage will evoke involuntary jaw movements followed by a seizure.
3. **Arithmetical epilepsy** in which performing calculations will 'trigger' seizures.

Epilepsy — Differential Diagnosis

The diagnosis of epilepsy is a clinical one depending on the patient's account of attacks and reports from witnesses.

Impairment of consciousness occurs in: **Vasovagal syncope, Cardiac arrhythmias, Migraine** (Basilar migraine), **Hypoglycaemia, Episodic confusion, Pseudoseizures.**

Hysterical and malingering **pseudo-seizures** cause diagnostic difficulties especially when occurring in a patient who has also known genuine epilepsy.

SYNCOPE (VASOVAGAL) ATTACKS

These attacks occur usually when the patient is standing and result from reduced cerebral blood flow.

Prodromal pallor, nausea and sweating occur; if the patient sits down, the attack may pass off or proceed to brief loss of consciousness.

Rigidity and clonic movements may occur if impaired cerebral blood flow is maintained.

Mechanism: Peripheral vasodilatation with drop in blood pressure followed by vagal overactivity with fall in heart rate.

Syncopal attacks occur in hot, crowded rooms (e.g. classroom) or in response to pain or emotional disturbance.

The presence of rigidity and clonic movements leads to confusion with epilepsy. The performing of an EEG in this situation may cloud the issue.

CARDIAC ARRHYTHMIAS

Seen in situations such as Complete Heart Block (Adams–Stokes attacks).

Prolonged arrest of cardiac rate or critical reduction will lead progressively to loss of consciousness — tonic jerks — cyanosis/stertorous respiration — fixed pupils and extensor plantar responses.

On recovery of normal cardiac rhythm, the degree of persisting neurological damage depends upon the duration of the episode and the presence of pre-existing cerebrovascular disease. In suspected patients, electrocardiography is mandatory. Continuous (24 hours) ECG monitoring may be necessary.

MIGRAINE

Basilar migraine ia a rare disorder in young women with a prodrome of severe vertigo or scintillating teichopsia followed by unconsciousness. Tonic clonic movements do not occur and a severe throbbing headache is present on awakening.

HYPOGLYCAEMIA

Amongst other neuroglycopenic manifestations, seizures or intermittent behavioural disturbances may occur. A rapid fall of blood sugar is associated with symptoms of catecholamine release e.g. palpitations, sweating etc. In 'atypical' seizures such a metabolic cause should be excluded preferably by blood sugar estimation when symptomatic.

EPISODIC CONFUSION

Intermittent confusional episodes in persons on drugs such as barbiturates or toxins such as solvent abuse.

Epilepsy – Differential Diagnosis

PSEUDOSEIZURES

A difficult distinction is between genuine epilepsy and attention seeking, hysterical or malingering episodes in which violent shaking and feigned loss of consciousness occurs (pseudoseizures). Often known epileptics will also manifest such attacks.

The following aids distinction:

Pseudoseizures	Genuine seizures
Pupils remain unchanged.	Pupils dilate.
Blood pressure/heart rate do not alter.	Blood pressure/heart rate increase.
Plantar responses down going.	Extensor plantar responses.
May show facial cyanosis but not nail beds.	Face and nail beds cyanosed.

Biochemical Tests

Pseudoseizures	Genuine seizures
pO_2 and pH unaltered.	pO_2 and pH lowered.
Creatine phosphokinase normal.	Creatine phosphokinase elevated.
Serum prolactin levels normal.	Marked elevation of serum prolactin.

Electroencephalogram

Pseudoseizures	Genuine seizures
Muscle artefact.	Muscle artefact and seizure activity.

CAUTION: The postictal confusional state may result in behaviour so bizarre that a pseudo-seizure is wrongly suspected.

Epilepsy – Causation

Epilepsy is a symptom of disease rather than a disease itself. The investigation of epilepsy depends on knowledge of potential causes.

Partial seizures with or without **secondary generalisation.**

NEWBORN	INFANCY	CHILDHOOD	ADOLESCENCE and ADULTHOOD
Hypocalcaemia. Hypoglycaemia. Asphyxia. Hyperbilirubinaemia. Water intoxication. Inborn errors of metabolism. Trauma. Intracranial haemorrhage (Vit K deficiency, thrombocytopaenia, etc.).	Febrile convulsions. Inborn errors of metabolism. Congenital defects. CNS infection.	Trauma. Congenital defects. Arterio-venous malformation. CNS infection.	Trauma. Neoplasm. Withdrawal from drugs/ alcohol. Arterio-venous malformation. CNS infection.
		LATE ADULT	Trauma. Neoplasm. Drug/alcohol withdrawal. Vascular disease. Degenerative disease. CNS infection.

The cause is not usually evident and scarring in the temporal lobe is assumed.

Once epilepsy has been 'triggered' by a specific cause at a given period it may persist throughout life e.g. febrile convulsion in infancy or neonatal asphyxia may be the cause of complex partial seizures which reappear some years later.

Other general medical conditions may be associated with seizures e.g. metabolic diseases, collagen vascular disorders.

Epilepsy

Generalised Epilepsies
There appears to be no clearly definable cause. Genetic factors play a role; concordance in monozygote twins being 75% for petit mal. An autosomal dominant gene would appear responsible for spike and wave abnormalities seen in the EEG's of parents and siblings of patients with generalised epilepsy. The defect is assumed to be metabolic though its nature is unknown.

Epilepsy – Investigation

With an incidence of 0.5% of the population, selectivity in investigation is necessary. CT scanning could not realistically be carried out in all patients.

The concern of the clinician is that epilepsy may be symptomatic of a cerebral lesion.

Investigations serve to: 1. Define cause.   2. Aid clinical diagnosis in difficult cases.

ROUTINE INVESTIGATION

Haematology.
Biochemistry. (esp. Calcium)
Skull X-ray.
Chest X-ray.
Electroencephalography.

When onset is late   (outwith early adolescence) and/or focal signs on examination and/or very focal disturbance on EEG and/or simple partial seizures i.e.
       Jacksonian motor seizures
–investigation should proceed to exclude
       structural intracranial lesion.

Computed Tomographic brain scan should be performed.
Occasionally angiography may also be necessary if a vascular malformation is suspect.

Late onset epilepsy with no history of birth complications, febrile convulsion or trauma especially when episodes are simple partial and, to a lesser extent, complex partial, **requires full investigation.**

If unselected cases of epilepsy have CT scanning the incidence of abnormal scans is small.

In focal attacks, such as simple motor seizures, the number of abnormal scans approaches 50% on initial examination and will increase with follow up.

When a patient presents with status epilepticus as the first manifestation of epilepsy, a frontal structural pathology must be suspected and CT scanning again carried out.

Finally, it must be remembered that subarachnoid haemorrhage, cerebral haemorrhage and infarction may present wit a seizure.

INVESTIGATIONS TO AID DIAGNOSIS

In doubtful cases, if the EEG is normal, it is often best to wait and see whether further attacks occur and, if so, obtain an eye witness account.

When episodes are frequent and troublesome, special EEG techniques may be applied:
    Sleep recordings.
    Recordings after activation with procyclidine.
    Recordings with special electrodes to look at the medial surface of the temporal lobe
      (sphenoidal and nasopharyngeal electrodes).
    Prolonged ambulatory recording may be invaluable in difficult cases.

The value of the EEG in epilepsy should be tempered by the knowledge that even in clear cut cases it may be normal.

Epilepsy — Treatment

The majority of patients respond to drug therapy (anticonvulsants). In intractable cases surgery may be necessary.

Drug treatment should be simple, preferably using one anticonvulsant (monotherapy). Polytherapy is to be avoided especially as drug interactions occur between major anticonvulsants.

Treatment is aimed at rendering the patient 'fit free', though not always achieved. If the patient goes three years without an attack, withdrawal of therapy should be considered; an EEG should preferably be performed and should show no 'discharge'. Withdrawal should be carried out only if the patient is satisfied that a further fit would not ruin employment etc. (e.g. car driver). The risk of teratogenicity is well known (6%) especially with phenytoin, but not prescribing drug therapy in pregnancy is perhaps more risky to the fetus than continuation. All anticonvulsants probably have some risk of producing fetal abnormalities, though these are usually mild.

A common problem in epilepsy clinics is non-compliance with drug therapy. The introduction of assay of blood anticonvulsant levels has led to:

1. Identification of non-compliers.
2. Tailoring of drug dose to patient's requirements.
3. The realisation of failure with therapeutic levels of one anticonvulsant and thus the logical change to another.

The commonest anticonvulsants in present clinical use are:

Carbamazepine   Sodium valproate   Clonazepam   Ethosuximide
Phenobarbitone   Primidone   Phenytoin

Sodium valproate is the first-line drug in the treatment of the generalised epilepsies with ethosuximide in childhood.

Carbamazepine is the first-line drug in the treatment of partial seizures and partial seizures with secondary generalisation.

	Sodium Valproate	Phenobarbitone	Phenytoin	Carbamazepine
Mode of Action	Unclear	Depressant effect on neuronal membranes	Prevents propagation of discharge. Effect on G.A.B.A.	Unclear.
Metabolised	Liver. Protein bound. Short variable half life.	Liver or excreted in urine unchanged. Long half life (60 hours).	Liver. Can saturate enzyme systems Long half life.	Liver. Enzyme inducer. Short half life (10 hours).
Dose (ADULT)	2–3 x daily. 600mg to 3g total daily dose.	Can be given as single dose e.g. 90mg at night.	Can be given as single dose e.g. 150-400mg at night.	2–3 x daily. 600mg to 1.2g total daily dose.
Side effects	Gastro-intestinal upset. Thrombocytopenia. Drug induced hepatitis. Hair loss. Tremor/chorea.	Sedation. Depression. Behavioural disturbance in children. Skin rashes. Withdrawal seizures.	Gum hypertrophy. Acne. Coarsening of facial characteristics. At toxic levels — Nystagmus. Ataxia. Diplopia. Neuropathy.	Gastro-intestinal upset. Ataxia. Skin rash. Agranulocytosis. Antidiuretic effect.

Epilepsy — Surgical Treatment

In some patients, despite adequate drug administration (checked by serum levels), recurrent seizures prevent a normal life style; of these a proportion may benefit from operation provided seizures arise from a single focus. Theoretically, removal of the focus abolishes the partial seizure and prevents progression to a generalised seizure.

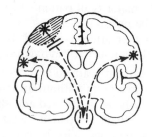

Extensive EEG investigation, both before and often during operation, helps to localise the site of the primary focus.

CT scanning may reveal an underlying structural abnormality (e.g. tumour, AVM or hamartoma) increasing the likelihood of improvement after operative removal. The discovery of a structural abnormality may in itself indicate the need for operation. In many patients with a temporal focus, temporal lobectomy reveals scarring of the most medial aspect – 'medial temporal sclerosis'. It is not known whether this is the cause of the epilepsy or the result of anoxia during repeated attacks.

Operation is contraindicated in patients with severe mental retardation or with an underlying psychiatric problem.

Operative techniques:

RESECTION

Temporal or other cortical resection incorporating the eliptogenic focus.

This is the most commonly employed technique. Over half obtain good results, become seizure free or acquire easier control.

Subtotal or total hemispherectomy in children with major irreversible damage to the whole hemisphere.

Good seizure control results, but morbidity and mortality are high.

Stereotactic lesions — Numerous different target sites have been tried in an attempt to prevent generalised spread.

Results are generally inconclusive, but the limbic targets (amygdala, fornix and anterior commissure) may produce some benefit.

Corpus callosum – section Prevents spread to opposite hemisphere.

Good results, but risk of neuropsychological upset.

Status Epilepticus

A succession of tonic/clonic convulsions, one after the other with a gap between each, is referred to as **serial epilepsy.**

When consciousness does not return between attacks the condition is then termed **status epilepticus.** This state may be life threatening with the development of pyrexia, deepening coma and circulatory collapse.

Status epilepticus may occur with any pathology though frontal lesions are more common; following head injury; when drug therapy is changed (especially when phenobarbitone is withdrawn); or, in some cases, for no discernable reason.

TREATMENT

There is no completely satisfactory approach.

> NOTE: ALL DOSE REGIMES APPLY TO ADULTS AND NOT TO CHILDREN.

General:

    Establish an air way.

    O_2 inhalation 8 litres/minute.

    I.v. infusion: 500ml 5% dextrose/0.9N saline.

    Vital signs recorded regularly — especially temperature.

        Prevent hyperthermia (sponging, etc.).

Specific:

    DIAZEPAM 5mg i.v. followed, after 2 minutes' gap, by further 5mg i.v.

    Effective for 10–20 minutes then seizures may return.

    Beware respiratory depression with repeated injections.

    Diazepam precipitates in i.v. infusion and should be

        given directly into the blood stream.

    If not controlled then proceed to longer acting drug.

    PHENYTOIN does not depress respiration.

    Loading dose: 15mg/kg given slowly i.v. at rate of 50mg/min.

    There is a risk of cardiac arrhythmia — use an ECG monitor.

    Contraindicated where known cardiac conduction defect or history of recent myocardial infarction.

    Maintenance, 500mg i.v. or orally, daily.

    If condition persists 30 minutes after loading dose, Phenobarbitone may be added, 200-300mg i.v. given at rate of 50mg/min.

    Respiration should be monitored.

At this point seizures should be controlled.

    120mg phenobarbitone i.m. 4 hourly and 500mg phenytoin i.v. daily should be given until oral therapy can be initiated.

In resistant cases, thiopentone or althesin may be used with assisted ventilation.

Throughout treatment the patient should receive the previously established anticonvulsant treatment, especially when using drugs (e.g. diazepam) which have only a temporary effect.

Status Epilepticus

Electrolytes as well as calcium and blood glucose should be checked initially and throughout. Blood gases should be estimated if clinically indicated.

Other drugs may be used in the management of status epilepticus e.g.:

Heminevrin,   Lorazepam,
Clonazepam,   Lignocaine,
                     Paraldehyde.

The foregoing regime, however, should control most cases of status epilepticus.

Absence status responds well to diazepam.

Complex partial seizure status may respond to 'loading' with phenytoin or simply increasing the existing therapy. Neither of these situations is as life threatening as status epilepticus.

Withdrawal of drug treatment

Epilepsy is not necessarily a life-long disorder and once a patient has been 2–3 years without an attack following recurrent seizures, an attempt should be made to withdraw drug treatment. The patient must be fully agreeable and accept the consequences which a further attack might have on employment and driving. 50% of persons within 2 years of withdrawing treatment will have sustained a further attack.

Epilepsy and Pregnancy

The frequency of seizures may decrease or decline in pregnancy. The patient may present with the first seizure during pregnancy (when investigation is limited) or during the puerperium. Tumours or arteriovenous malformations can enlarge in pregnancy and produce such seizures; however, these causes are rare and most attacks idiopathic. Cortical venous thrombosis and systemic lupus erythematosus should be considered as alternative explanations.

The Febrile Convulsion

Febrile convulsions occur in the immature brain as a response to high fever, probably as a result of water and electrolyte disturbance.
No particular infection can be incriminated.
Usually occurs between 6 months and 3 years of age.
Rare after 5 years of age.
Recurrent in 50% of patients.

Long term follow up suggests a liability to develop seizures in later life (unassociated with fever) especially in males.
The duration of seizure, number of seizures and positive family history all increase risk.

Treatment is aimed at preventing a prolonged seizure by sponging the patient and using rectal diazepam.
The role of prophylaxis after one seizure is debatable.

Disorders of Sleep

PHYSIOLOGY

Sleep results from activity in certain sleep producing areas of the brain rather than from reduced sensory input to the cerebral cortex.

Stimulation of these areas produces sleep; damage results in states of persistent wakefulness.

Pontine
reticular formation
raphe nuclei
Medullary

Two forms of sleep are recognised:

	1. **Rapid eye movement (REM) sleep**	2. **Non-rapid eye movement (NonREM) sleep**
Characterised by:	– Rapid conjugate eye movement. – Fluctuation of temperature, BP, heart rate and respiration. – Muscle twitching. – Presence of dreams.	– Absence of eye movement. – Stability of temperature, BP, heart rate and respiration. – Absence of muscle twitching. – Absence of dreams.
Originates in:	– Pontine reticular formation.......	– Mid-line pontine and medullary nuclei (raphé nuclei).
Mediated by:	– Noradrenaline.................	– Serotonin.

The **Electroencephalogram** shows characteristic patterns which correspond to the type and depth of sleep.

REM sleep — A low voltage record dominated by fast activity.

NonREM sleep
  Drowsy — A low voltage record with slower rhythms.

  Intermediate — Sharp waves evident on vertex leads (V waves) and waxing and waning sleep spindles.

  Deep — A high voltage record dominated by slow activity.

The Sleep pattern

In adults nonREM and REM sleep alternate throughout the night.

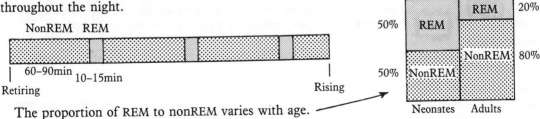

NonREM REM

60–90min 10–15min

Retiring   Rising

50% REM REM 20%

     NonREM 80%

50% NonREM

Neonates Adults

The proportion of REM to nonREM varies with age.

In view of the important rôle of serotonin and noradrenaline in sleep, it is understandable that drugs may affect the duration and/or content of sleep.

Disorders of Sleep

NARCOLEPSY and CATAPLEXY

Narcolepsy:

An irresistible desire to sleep in inappropriate circumstances and places. Attacks occur suddenly, when seated; of brief duration unless patient remains undisturbed.

Cataplexy:

Sudden loss of postural tone. The patient crumples to the ground. Consciousness is preserved. Emotion – laughter or crying – will precipitate an attack.

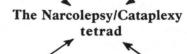

The Narcolepsy/Cataplexy tetrad

Only 10% of patients manifest the complete tetrad.

Sleep paralysis:

On awakening, the patient is unable to move. This may last for 2–3 minutes.

Hypnagogic Hallucinations

Vivid dreams or hallucinations occur as the patient falls asleep or occasionally when apparently awake.

Males are affected more than females.

Onset is in adolescence/early adult life. The disorder is life long but becomes less troublesome with age. It may have a familial incidence or may occur after head injury, with multiple sclerosis or with hypothalamic tumours. The cause remains unknown, though the presence of certain histocompatibility antigens (DR2) in sufferers does suggest an immunological basis.

Diagnosis:

The diagnosis is dependent upon the clinical history. The electroencephalogram may help, showing a REM pattern with daytime sleep and at the onset of nocturnal sleep.

Treatment:

Drugs which inhibit REM sleep may benefit: – amphetamines.
– clomipramine.
– pemoline.

NIGHT TERRORS (Pavor nocturnus)

These occur in children, shortly after falling asleep and during deep to intermediate nonREM sleep. The child awakes in a state of fright with a marked tachycardia, yet in the morning cannot recollect the attack. Such attacks are not associated with psychological disturbance, are self limiting and if necessary will respond to diazepam.

NIGHTMARES

These occur during REM sleep. Drug or alcohol withdrawal promotes REM sleep and is often associated with vivid dreams.

SOMNAMBULISM (Sleep walking)

Sleep walking varies from just sitting up in bed to walking around the house with the eyes open, performing complex major tasks. Episodes occur during intermediate or deep nonREM sleep. In childhood, somnambulism is associated with night terrors and bed wetting, but not with psychological disturbance. In adults, there is an increased incidence of psychoneurosis.

Disorders of Sleep

SLEEP STARTS

On entering sleep, sudden jerks of the arms or legs commonly occur and are especially frequent when a conscious effort is made to remain awake e.g. during a lecture. This is a physiological form of myoclonus.

HYPERSOMNIA

Lesions which affect the structures in the floor of the third ventricle may produce excessive sleepiness e.g. tumours or encephalitis, and are often associated with diabetes insipidus.

Systemic disease such as myxoedema may result in hypersomnia, as may conditions which produce hypercapnia – chronic bronchitis, or primary muscle disease e.g. dystrophia myotonica.

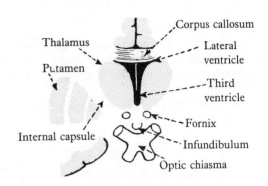

SLEEP APNOEA SYNDROMES

Respiratory rate fluctuates during REM sleep with occasional short episodes of apnoea. These are normal physiological events.

Sleep apnoea may also result from central reduction of respiratory drive or a mechanical obstruction of the airway.

Central causes:

Brain stem medullary infarction or following cervical/foramen magnum surgery.

Mechanical causes:

Obesity.   Tonsillar enlargement.
Myxoedema.   Acromegaly.

When breathing ceases, the resultant hypercapnia and hypoxia eventually stimulate respiration.

Patients may present with daytime sleepiness, nocturnal insomnia and early morning headache. Snoring and restless movements are characteristic. In severe cases of sleep apnoea, hypertension may develop with right heart failure secondary to pulmonary arterial hypertension. Polycythaemia and left heart failure may ensue.

Treatment depends on aetiology. Mechanical airway obstruction should be relieved; drugs such as theophylline are occasionally helpful

The *Pickwickian syndrome:*   sleep apnoea associated with obesity, named after the Dickens' fat boy who repeatedly fell asleep.

Higher Cortical Dysfunction

Specific parts of the cerebral hemispheres are responsible for a certain aspect of function. In normal circumstances these functions are integrated and the patient operates as a whole. Damage to part of the cortex will result in a characteristic disturbance of function. Interruption by disease of 'connections' between one part of the cortex and another will 'disconnect' function.

General Anatomy

Brodmann, on the basis of histological differences, divided the cortex into 47 areas. Knowledge of these areas is not practical, though they are referred to often in some texts.

6 layers can be recognised in the cerebral cortex superficial to the junction with the underlying white matter.

The relative preponderance of each layer varies in different regions of the cortex and appears to be related to function.

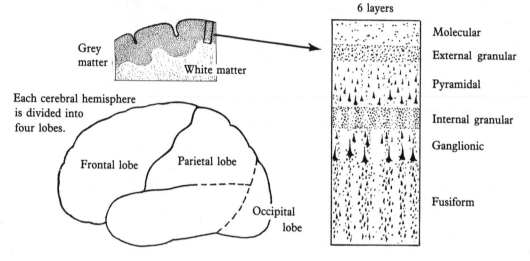

The frontal motor cortex – dominated by pyramidal rather than granular layers – AGRANULAR CORTEX.

The parietal sensory cortex – dominated by granular layers – GRANULAR CORTEX.

The largest cells of the agranular cortex are the giant cells of Betz. These give rise to some of the motor fibres of the corticospinal tract.

Right and Left Hemisphere Function

Unilateral brain damage reveals a difference in function between hemispheres. The left hemisphere is 'dominant' in right-handed people. In left-handed subjects the left hemisphere is also dominant in the majority (up to 75%), the right hemisphere being dominant in the remainder.

Hand preference may be hereditary but, in some cases, disease of the left hemisphere in early life determines left-handedness.

Higher Cortical Dysfunction

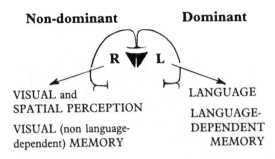

Non-dominant   **Dominant**

R L

VISUAL and
SPATIAL PERCEPTION

VISUAL (non language-
dependent) MEMORY

LANGUAGE

LANGUAGE-
DEPENDENT
MEMORY

Hemisphere dominance may be demonstrated by the injection of sodium amytal into the internal carotid artery. On the dominant side this will produce an arrest of speech for up to 30 seconds – the WADA TEST. Such a test may be important before temporal lobectomy for epilepsy when handedness/hemisphere dominance is in doubt.

Frontal Lobes

<u>Lateral surface</u>

Superior
frontal gyrus
and sulcus

Middle
frontal
gyrus

Inferior
frontal gyrus

Pre-central
gyrus

Central sulcus
separates frontal
from parietal lobe
posteriorly

Lateral sulcus
separates frontal
from temporal lobe inferiorly

<u>Orbital surface</u>

Olfactory
bulb

Olfactory
nerve

Orbital
sulci

Stem of
lateral sulcus

<u>Medial surface</u>

Cingulate
sulcus

Central sulcus

Paracentral lobule

Corpus callosum

Frontal lobe function

1. Pre-central gyrus – motor cortex
   contralateral movement – face, arm,
   leg, trunk.
2. Broca's area – dominant hemisphere –
   expressive centre for speech.
3. Supplementary motor area –
   contralateral head and eye turning.
4. Pre-frontal areas –
   'personality', initiative.
5. Paracentral lobule –
   cortical inhibition of bladder and
   bowel voiding.

105

Frontal Lobes

Impairment of frontal lobe function

1. Pre-central gyrus — Monoplegia or hemiplegia depending on extent of damage.
Anteriorly placed lesion – more spastic.

2. Broca's area
(Inferior part of dominant frontal lobe)
Results in Broca's dysphasia (see page 119) (motor or expressive).

3. Supplementary motor area — Paralysis of head and eye movement to opposite side.
Head turns 'towards' diseased hemisphere and eyes look in the same direction.

Representation of the opposite half of the body is similar to that of the motor cortex.

(After PENFIELD)

4. Pre-frontal areas
(The vast part of the frontal lobes anterior to the motor cortex as well as undersurface (orbital) of frontal lobes.)
— Damage is often bilateral e.g. infarction, following haemorrhage from anterior communicating artery aneurysm, neoplasm, trauma or anterior dementia.
— Results in a change of personality with antisocial behaviour/loss of inhibitions.
Inappropriate jocularity (WITZELSUCHT).
The patient loses initiative and becomes disinterested and unconcerned.

An extreme of this state is AKINETIC MUTISM where, as a result of bilateral damage to the orbital surface of the frontal lobes, the patient appears awake but does not vocalise, is incontinent and makes minimal motor response to painful stimulation.

Pre-frontal lesions are also associated with:

1. Primitive reflexes – grasp, pout, etc. (see page 341).
2. Disturbance of gait – 'frontal ataxia'.
3. Resistance to passive movements of the limbs – PARATONIA.

Unilateral lesions may show minor degrees of such change.

5. Paracentral lobule

Damage to the posterior part of the superior frontal gyrus results in incontinence of urine and faeces – 'loss of cortical inhibition'. This is particularly likely with ventricular dilatation and is an important symptom of Normal Pressure Hydrocephalus.

Parietal Lobes

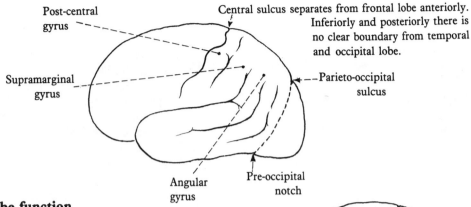

Post-central gyrus

Central sulcus separates from frontal lobe anteriorly. Inferiorly and posteriorly there is no clear boundary from temporal and occipital lobe.

Supramarginal gyrus

Parieto-occipital sulcus

Angular gyrus

Pre-occipital notch

Parietal lobe function

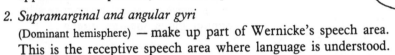

1. *Post-central gyrus* (Granular cortex)
   The sensory cortex receives afferent pathways for appreciation of posture, touch and passive movement.

2. *Supramarginal and angular gyri*
   (Dominant hemisphere) — make up part of Wernicke's speech area. This is the receptive speech area where language is understood.

3. The *non-dominant* parietal lobe is important in the concept of body image and the awareness of the external environment. The ability to construct shapes etc. results from such visual/proprioceptive skills.

4. The *dominant* parietal lobe is implicated in the skills of handling numbers/calculation.

5. The *visual pathways* – the fibres of the optic radiation (lower visual field) – pass deep through the parietal lobe.

Impairment of parietal lobe function

1. Disease of *either dominant or non-dominant* sensory cortex (post-central gyrus) will result in contralateral disturbance of cortical sensation:

   Postural sensation disturbed.

   Sensation of passive movement disturbed.

   Accurate localisation of light touch may be disturbed.

   Discrimination between one and two points (normally 4 mm on finger tips) is lost.

   Appreciation of size, shape, texture and weight may be affected, with difficulty in distinguishing coins placed in hand, etc (astereognosis).

   Perceptual rivalry (sensory inattention) is characteristic of parietal lobe disease. Presented with two stimuli, one applied to each side (e.g. light touch to the palm of the hand) simultaneously, the patient is only aware of that one contralateral to the normal parietal lobe. As the gap between application of stimuli is increased (approaching 2–4 seconds) the patient becomes aware of both.

2. *Supramarginal and angular gyri* - receptive dysphasia (see page 119).

Parietal Lobes

3. *Non-dominant*   4. *Dominant*

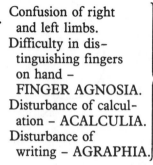

No longer aware of opposite (left sided) limbs – even when densely hemiparetic; denies weakness – ANOSOGNOSIA.

Difficulty in dressing e.g. getting arm into pyjamas – DRESSING APRAXIA.

Disturbance of geographical memory – GEOGRAPHICAL AGNOSIA (e.g. patient cannot find his bed in ward).

Cannot copy geometrical pattern – CONSTRUCTIONAL APRAXIA.

Confusion of right and left limbs. Difficulty in distinguishing fingers on hand – FINGER AGNOSIA. Disturbance of calculation – ACALCULIA. Disturbance of writing – AGRAPHIA.

These comprise GERSTMANN's SYNDROME

5. Damage to the *optic radiation* deep in the parietal lobe will produce a lower homonymous quadrantanopia.

Temporal Lobes

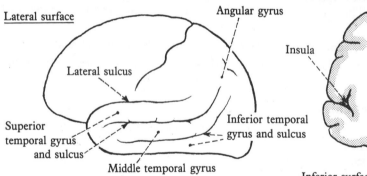

Lateral surface

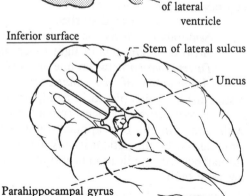

Coronal section

Inferior surface

Anteriorly, the temporal lobe is separated from the frontal lobe by the lateral sulcus. Posteriorly and superiorly, separation from occipital and parietal lobes is less clearly defined.

The lateral sulcus is deep and contains 'buried' temporal lobe. The buried island of cortex is referred to as the INSULA.

The temporal lobe also has a considerable inferior and medial surface in contact with the middle fossa.

Temporal Lobes

Temporal lobe function

1. *The auditory cortex* lies within the insula (Heschl's gyrus).
   The *dominant* hemisphere is important in the hearing of language.
   The *non-dominant* hemisphere is important in the hearing of sounds, rhythm and music.
   Close to the auditory cortex labyrinthine function is represented.

2. *The middle and inferior temporal gyri* are concerned with learning and memory (see later).

3. *The limbic lobe:* the inferior and medial portions of the temporal lobe, including the hippocampus and parahippocampal gyrus.
   The sensation of olfaction is mediated through this structure as well as emotional/affective behaviour.
   Olfactory fibres terminate in the uncus.
   The limbic lobe or system also incorporates inferior frontal and medial parietal structures and will be discussed later.

4. *The visual pathways* pass deep in the temporal lobe around the posterior horn of the lateral ventricle.

Impairment of temporal lobe function

1. *Auditory cortex*
   Cortical deafness: Bilateral lesions are rare but may result in complete deafness of which the patient may be unaware.
   Lesions which involve surrounding association areas may result in difficulty in hearing spoken words (dominant) or difficulty in appreciating rhythm/music (non-dominant) – *AMUSIA*.
   Auditory hallucinations may occur in temporal lobe disease e.g. complex partial seizures.

2. *Middle and inferior temporal gyri*
   Disturbance of memory/learning will be discussed later.
   Disordered memory may occur in complex partial seizures

   either after the event – postictal amnesia

   or in the event – deja vu, jamais vu.

3. *Limbic lobe* damage may result in:
   - Olfactory hallucination with complex partial seizures.
   - Aggressive or antisocial behaviour.
   - Inability to establish new memories (see later).

4. Damage to *optic radiation* will produce an upper homonymous quadrantanopia.

Dominant hemisphere lesions are associated with Wernicke's dysphasia.

Occipital Lobe

The occipital lobe merges anteriorly with the parietal and temporal lobes.

On the medial surface the calcarine sulcus extends forwards and the parieto-occipital sulcus separates occipital and parietal lobes.

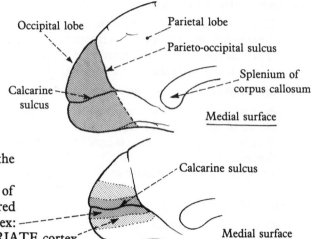

Occipital lobe function

The occipital lobe is concerned with the perception of vision (the visual cortex).

The visual cortex lies along the banks of the calcarine sulcus — this area is referred to as the STRIATE cortex: above and below this lies the PARASTRIATE cortex.

The *striate* cortex is the primary visual cortex and when stimulated by visual input relays information to the *parastriate* – association visual cortex. This, in turn, connects with the parietal, temporal and frontal lobes both on the same side and on the opposite side (through the posterior part of the corpus callosum) so that the meaning of a visual image may be interpreted, remembered, etc.

The visual field is represented upon the cortex in a specific manner (page 127).

Impairment of occipital lobe function

A cortical lesion will result in a homonymous hemianopia with or without involvement of the macula, depending on the posterior extent of the lesion.

When only the occipital pole is affected, a central hemianopia field defect involving the macula occurs with a normal peripheral field of vision.

Cortical Blindness

Extensive bilateral cortical lesions of the striate cortex will result in cortical BLINDNESS. In this, the pupillary light reflex is normal despite the absence of conscious perception of the presence of illumination (light reflex fibres terminate in the midbrain).

ANTON's Syndrome

Involvement of both the striate and the parastriate cortices affects the interpretation of vision. The patient is unaware of his visual loss and denies its presence. This denial in the presence of obvious blindness characterises Anton's syndrome.

Cortical blindness occurs mainly in vascular disease (posterior cerebral artery) but also following hypoxia and hypertensive encephalopathy or after surviving tentorial herniation.

Occipital Lobe

Visual Hallucinations are common in migraine when the occipital lobe is involved; also in epilepsy when the seizure source lies here.

Hallucinations of occipital origin are elementary – unformed – appearing as patterns (zig-zags, flashes) and fill the hemianopic field, whereas hallucinations of temporal lobe origin are formed, complex and fill the whole of the visual field.

Visual Illusions also may occur as a consequence of occipital lobe disease. Objects appear smaller (MICROPSIA) or larger (MACROPSIA) than reality. Distortion of a shape may occur or disappearance of colour from vision.

These illusions are more common with non-dominant occipital lobe disease.

Prosopagnosia: The patient, though able to see a familiar face e.g. a member of the family, cannot name it. This is usually associated with other disturbances of 'interpretation' and naming with intact vision such as colour agnosia (recognition of colours and matching of pairs of colours). Bilateral lesions at occipito-temporal junction are responsible.

Higher Cortical Dysfunction   The DISCONNECTION SYNDROMES

Cortical function is described, on the previous pages, 'lobe by lobe'. These functions integrate by means of connections between hemispheres and lobes. Lesions of these connecting pathways disorganise normal function, resulting in recognisable syndromes – the Disconnection syndromes.   APRAXIA is a feature of some of these disorders.   IDEOMOTOR APRAXIA – language in the form of a command cannot alone initiate and direct the performance of a learned motor task e.g. "Shake your fist", "Wave good-bye with your hand" – though these tasks can be performed spontaneously. Apraxia is not associated with motor weakness or incoordination.

The connecting pathways may be divided into:

*Intra*hemispheric: lying in the subcortical white matter and linking parts of the same hemisphere.

*Inter*hemispheric: traversing the corpus callosum and linking related parts of the two hemispheres.

The Intrahemispheric Disconnection Syndromes

1. Conduction Aphasia

Lesion of the arcuate fasciculus linking Wernicke's and Broca's speech areas.
Characterised by:
Fluent dysphasic speech. Good comprehension of written/spoken material. Poor repetition.

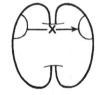

2. Pure word deafness

Lesion of the connection between the primary auditory cortex (Herschl's gyrus) and auditory association cortex.
Characterised by:
Impaired comprehension of spoken word. Self initiated language is normal. The patient seems deaf but audiometry is normal.

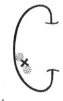

3. Buccal lingual and 'sympathetic' apraxia.

Involves the links between left and right association motor cortices in the subcortical region.
Characterised by:
Right brachiofacial weakness and apraxia of tongue, lip and left limb movements.

Pre-motor
motor cortex
Broca's area

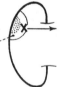

The Interhemispheric Disconnection Syndromes

1. Left side apraxia

Lesion of the anterior corpus callosum with interruption of the connections between the left and right association motor cortices.
Characterised by:
Apraxia of left sided limb movements.

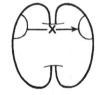

2. Pure word blindness or alexia without agraphia

Lesion of the posterior corpus callosum and dominant occipital lobe with interruption of connections between the visual cortex and the angular gyrus/Wernicke's area.
Characterised by:
Inability to read, to name colours, to copy writing, but with normal spontaneous writing and the ability to identify colours.

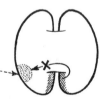

3. Agenesis of the corpus callosum

This is a developmental disorder with no connection between the two hemispheres.
Characterised by:
A failure to name an object presented visually or by touch to the non-dominant hemisphere. (The right and left visual fields cannot match presented objects.)

Higher Cortical Dysfunction — Memory

Memory is the ability to retain and recall information and experiences.

It involves *Registration* — a confused patient cannot register new information.
Retention — affected in disorders such as KORSAKOFF's psychosis.
Recall — rarely organically disordered.
Reproduction — language dependent.

The **Limbic system** contains structures important in memory.

The *hippocampus,* a deep structure in the temporal lobe, ridges the floor of the lateral ventricle. Fimbriae of the hippocampus connect this structure to the *fornix.*

There appears to be a loop from hippocampus ⟶ fornix ⟶ mamillary body ⟶ thalamus ⟶ cingulate gyrus ⟶ back to hippocampus.

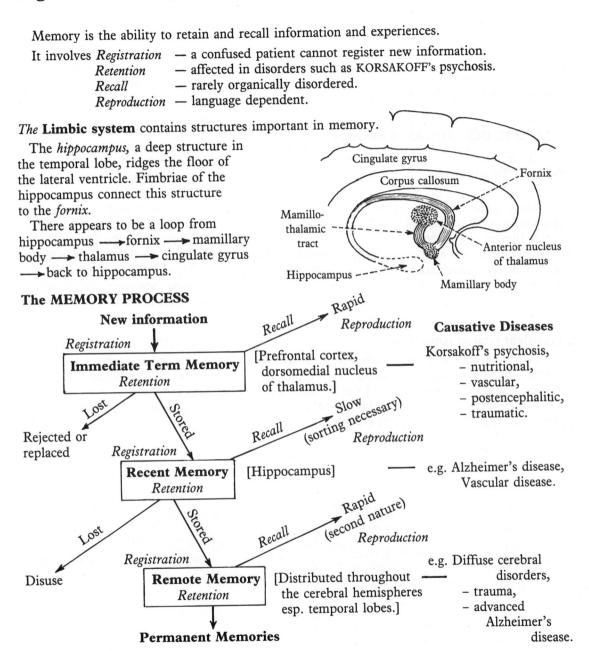

The MEMORY PROCESS

New information

Registration

Immediate Term Memory
Retention

Recall → **Rapid** *Reproduction*

[Prefrontal cortex, dorsomedial nucleus of thalamus.]

Causative Diseases

Korsakoff's psychosis,
– nutritional,
– vascular,
– postencephalitic,
– traumatic.

Lost → Rejected or replaced

Stored

Registration

Recent Memory
Retention

[Hippocampus]

Recall → **Slow** (sorting necessary) *Reproduction*

e.g. Alzheimer's disease, Vascular disease.

Lost → Disuse

Stored

Registration

Remote Memory
Retention

[Distributed throughout the cerebral hemispheres esp. temporal lobes.]

Recall → **Rapid** (second nature) *Reproduction*

e.g. Diffuse cerebral disorders,
– trauma,
– advanced Alzheimer's disease.

Permanent Memories

There is great individual variability between the extent of the lesion and the degree of memory disturbance. Also, reproduction of lesions in experimental animals does not always appear to affect memory.

Higher Cortical Dysfunction — Memory

TESTS of Memory (See Examination, page 9) aim to distinguish loss of immediate, recent or remote memory.

Disorders may be further classified into those which affect memories established before the injury or damage – RETROGRADE AMNESIA, and those established following the injury or damage – ANTEGRADE AMNESIA.

SPECIFIC DISORDERS of Memory

Korsakoff's psychosis

An inability to acquire new memories, with some impairment of memory prior to onset of illness (Retrograde amnesia).

Confabulation – a false description of present events and circumstances – is usually present

Lesion

Hippocampus and limbic structures, especially the dorsomedial nucleus of the thalamus.

Etiology

Bilateral posterior cerebral occlusion.

Herpes simplex encephalitis.

Tuberculous meningitis.

Wernicke-Korsakoff syndrome.

Third ventricular tumours.

Dementias (posterior type) in which temporal lobes are involved early.

Transient Global Amnesia.

This is a condition of middle-late age in which total amnesia for recent events occurs with normal function during this period i.e. the patient may go to work and behave normally. Recurrent attacks are uncommon. Episodes may last for some hours.

Pathogenesis is unknown but presumed vascular (bilateral hippocampal ischaemia seems probable). The condition appears benign.

Disorders of Speech and Language

Introduction

Disturbed speech and language are important symptoms of neurological disease. The two are not synonymous. Language is a function of the dominant cerebral hemisphere and may be divided into (a) *emotional* – the instinctive expression of feelings representing the earliest forms of language acquired in infancy and (b) *symbolic* or *propositional* – conveying thoughts, opinions and concepts. This language is acquired over a twenty year period and is dependent upon culture, education and normal cerebral development.

An understanding of disorders of speech and language is essential, not just to the clinical diagnosis but also to improve communication between patient and doctor. All too often patients with language disorders are labelled 'confused' as a consequence of superficial evaluation.

DYSARTHRIA

Dysarthria is a *disturbance of articulation* in which the content of speech – language – is unaffected.

Mechanism of articulation

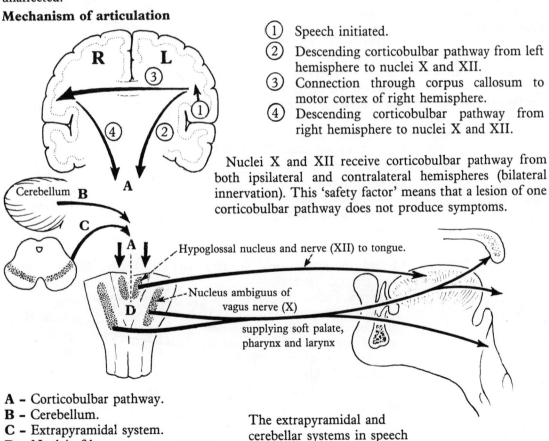

① Speech initiated.

② Descending corticobulbar pathway from left hemisphere to nuclei X and XII.

③ Connection through corpus callosum to motor cortex of right hemisphere.

④ Descending corticobulbar pathway from right hemisphere to nuclei X and XII.

Nuclei X and XII receive corticobulbar pathway from both ipsilateral and contralateral hemispheres (bilateral innervation). This 'safety factor' means that a lesion of one corticobulbar pathway does not produce symptoms.

Hypoglossal nucleus and nerve (XII) to tongue.

Nucleus ambiguus of vagus nerve (X) supplying soft palate, pharynx and larynx

A – Corticobulbar pathway.
B – Cerebellum.
C – Extrapyramidal system.
D – Nuclei of lower motor neurones of X, XII cranial nerves.

The extrapyramidal and cerebellar systems in speech modulate articulatory muscle action.

Disorders of Speech — Dysarthria

DIAGNOSTIC APPROACH

Listen to spontaneous speech and ask the patient to read aloud. Observe:
lingual consonants – *'ta ta ta'* (made with the tongue), labial consonants – *'mm mm mm'* (made with the lips), guttural consonants – *'ga ga ga'* (laryngeal and pharyngeal/palatal).

Difficulty with articulation

= DYSARTHRIA

N.B.   Beware misinterpretation, dialect or poorly fitting teeth.

Speech hoarse and strained; labial consonants especially affected.

Associated contralateral hemiparesis or dysphasia → SPASTIC DYSARTHRIA (Cortical origin)
e.g. Middle cerebral artery occlusion. Neoplasm.

Other signs of pseudobulbar palsy (impaired chewing, swallowing). → SPASTIC DYSARTHRIA (Corticobulbar origin)
e.g. Bilateral small vessel occlusion. Motor neurone disease.

Speech slow and monotonous with abnormal separation of syllables – *'scanning speech';* at times may sound explosive – **Associated signs of cerebellar disease.** → ATAXIC DYSARTHRIA
(Lesion in cerebellar vermis and paravermis)
e.g. Multiple sclerosis. Hereditary ataxias.

Soft and monotonous with poor volume and little inflection – **Associated signs of extrapyramidal disease.** → HYPOKINETIC (slow) HYPERKINETIC (fast) DYSARTHRIA (Lesion of the extrapyramidal system)
e.g. Parkinson's disease. Huntington's chorea.

Labial consonants first affected, later gutterals. *Nasal speech* and progression to total loss of articulation *(anarthria).* **Associated signs of l.m.n. weakness of X and XII.** → FLACCID DYSARTHRIA (Involvement of X and XII nuclei or emergent nerves to muscles of articulation,)
e.g. Motor neurone disease. Bulbar poliomyelitis. Cranial polyneuritis.

Many diseases affect multiple sites and a 'mixed' dysarthria occurs.

For example, multiple sclerosis with corticobulbar and cerebellar involvement will result in a mixed spastic/ataxic dysarthria.

Disorders of Speech — Dysphonia

Sound is produced by the passage of air over the vocal cords.
Respiratory disease or vocal cord paralysis results in a disturbance of this facility – *Dysphonia*.
A complete inability to produce sound is referred to as *Aphonia*.

DIAGNOSTIC APPROACH

If, despite attempts, there is deficient sound production then examine the vocal cords by *indirect laryngoscopy*.

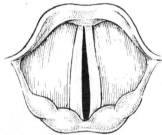

Causative Diseases
e.g.

Medullary damage.
– infarction
– syringobulbia

Paralysis of both vocal cords
Patient speaks in whispers
and inspiratory stridor is present.

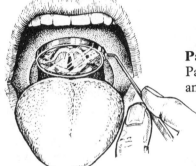

Normal abduction of vocal cords – *'Ahh'*

Mirror held in posterior pharynx

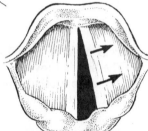

e.g.

Recurrent laryngeal
nerve palsy
– following thyroid
surgery
– bronchial neoplasm
– aortic aneurysm.

Paralysis of right vocal cord
which does not move with *'Ahh'*
while left abducts. When patient
says *'E'* normal cord will move
towards paralysed cord.
Voice is hoarse and nasal.

Spastic Dysphonia
Sounds as though speaking
while being strangled!
Similar to writer's cramp.
No known pathological cause.

OTHER DISORDERS OF SPEECH

MUTISM — An absence of any attempt at oral communication. It may be associated with bilateral frontal lobe or third ventricular pathology (see Akinetic mutism).

ECHOLALIA — Constant repetition of words or sentences heard in severe dementing illness.

PALILALIA — Repetition of last word or words of patient's speech. Heard in extrapyramidal disease.

LOGORRHOEA – Prolonged speech monologues; associated with deep cortical lesion.

Disorders of Language — Dysphasia

Dysphasia is a loss of production or comprehension of spoken and/or written language.

Hand preference is associated with 'hemisphere dominance'. In right handed people the left hemisphere is dominant; in left handed people the left hemisphere is dominant in most, though 25% have a dominant right hemisphere.

The cortical centres for language reside in the dominant hemisphere.

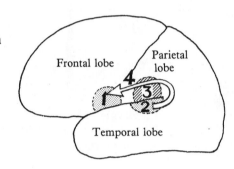

1 BROCA's AREA

Executive or motor area for the production of language – lies in the inferior part of the frontal lobe on the lateral surface of the cerebral hemisphere abutting the mouth of the Sylvian fissure.

2 and **3** RECEPTIVE AREAS

Here the spoken word is understood and the appropriate reply or action initiated. These areas lie at the posterior end of the Sylvian fissure on the lateral surface of the hemisphere.

The temporal lobe receptive area (**2**) lies close to the auditory cortex of the transverse gyrus of the temporal lobe. The parietal lobe receptive area (**3**) lies within the angular gyrus.

Receptive and expressive areas must be linked in order to integrate function. The link is provided by (**4**), the ARCUATE FASCICULUS, a fibre tract which runs forwards in the subcortical white matter.

Dysphasia may develop as a result of vascular, neoplastic, traumatic infective or degenerative disease of the cerebrum when language areas are involved.

Disorders of Language – Dysphasia

DIAGNOSTIC APPROACH

Listen to content and fluency of speech. Test comprehension i.e. simple then complex commands

Non-fluent, hesitant speech; may be confined to a few repeated utterances or, in less severe cases, is of a 'telegraphic' nature with articles and conjunctions omitted.
Good comprehension.
Handwriting poor.
Look for coexisting right arm and face weakness.

→ BROCA's DYSPHASIA
(Motor or expressive dysphasia)

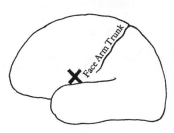

Causative Diseases

Vascular disease.
Neoplasm.
Trauma.
Infective disease.
Degenerative
    disease.

Comprehension impaired.
Speech non-sensical but fluent.
  neologisms –non-existent words.
  paraphrasia –half right words.
Patient unaware of language
        problem.
Handwriting poor

Differentiate from confused patient – construction of words and sentences is normal.

→ WERNICKE's DYSPHASIA
(Sensory or receptive dysphasia)

Parietal

Temporal

Vascular disease.
Neoplasm.
Trauma.
Infective disease.
Degenerative
    disease.

Speech non-sensical but fluent (neologisms and paraphrasia) yet comprehension is normal.
Repetition is poor.

→ CONDUCTION DYSPHASIA

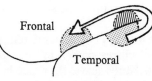

Frontal

Temporal

Vascular disease.
Neoplasm.
Trauma.
Infective disease.
Degenerative
    disease.

Non-fluent speech and impaired comprehension.
Often associated with hemiplegia/hemianaesthesia and visual field deficit.

→ GLOBAL DYSPHASIA
Damage involving a large area of the dominant hemisphere.

Vascular disease.
Neoplasm.
Trauma.
Infective disease.
Degenerative
    disease.

Impairment of Vision

ANATOMY and PHYSIOLOGY

Anatomically the visual system is contained in the supratentorial compartment. It is composed of peripheral receptors in the retina, central pathways and cortical centres. The control of ocular movement and pupillary responses are closely integrated. The eye is the peripheral receptor organ concerned with the presentation of light stimuli to the retina.

The Retina   3 distinct layers of the retina are identified:

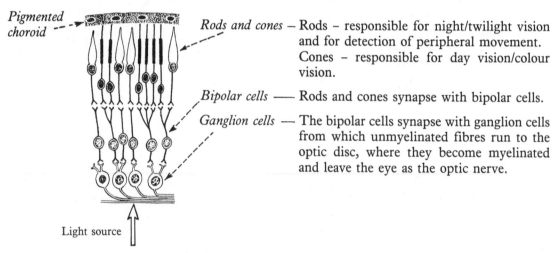

Pigmented choroid

Rods and cones – Rods – responsible for night/twilight vision and for detection of peripheral movement. Cones – responsible for day vision/colour vision.

Bipolar cells —— Rods and cones synapse with bipolar cells.

Ganglion cells —— The bipolar cells synapse with ganglion cells from which unmyelinated fibres run to the optic disc, where they become myelinated and leave the eye as the optic nerve.

Light source

The *macular region* of the retina is its most important area for visual acuity. Here, cones lie in the greatest concentration whereas rods are more numerous in the surrounding retina.

The optic nerve leaves the orbit through the *optic foramen* and passes posteriorly to unite with the opposite optic nerve at the *optic chiasma*. Here, partial decussation occurs (axons from ganglion cells on the nasal side of the retina cross over to the opposite side).

The *optic tract* consisting of ipsilateral temporal and contralateral nasal fibres passes to the *lateral geniculate body*. A few fibres leave the tract before the lateral geniculate body and pass to the *superior colliculus* (fibres concerned with pupillary light reflex).

Axons of cell bodies in the lateral geniculate body make up the *optic radiation*. This enters the hemisphere in the most posterior part of the internal capsule, courses deep in parietal and temporal lobes and terminates in the *calcarine cortex* of the occipital lobe.

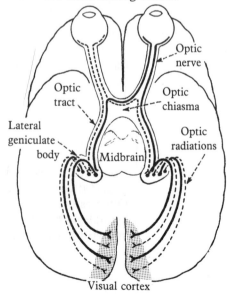

Optic nerve

Optic tract

Optic chiasma

Lateral geniculate body

Optic radiations

Midbrain

Visual cortex

120

Impairment of Vision

CLINICAL APPROACH and DIFFERENTIAL DIAGNOSIS

Patients presenting with visual impairment require a systematic examination, not only of *vision*, but also of the *pupillary response, eye movements,* and, unless the cause clearly lies within the globe, a *full neurological examination.*

The findings aid localisation of the lesion, e.g.

Impairment of vision + impaired pupil response indicates a lesion anterior to the lateral geniculate body.

A homonymous hemianopia + receptive dysphasia indicates a parieto-temporal lesion.

Refractive errors are excluded by testing visual acuity through a pinhole or by correcting a lens deformity (page 10).

Four types of refractive error exist:

PRESBYOPIA – failure of accommodation with age.
HYPERMETROPIA (long sightedness) – short eyeball.
MYOPIA (short sightedness) – long eyeball.
ASTIGMATISM – variation in corneal curvature.

If this examination is normal, then the lesion lies in the retina, visual pathways or visual cortex.

Examine the globe and anterior chamber.

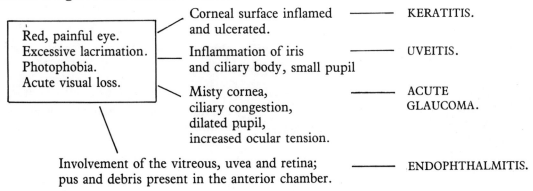

Red, painful eye.
Excessive lacrimation.
Photophobia.
Acute visual loss.

Corneal surface inflamed and ulcerated. ——— KERATITIS.

Inflammation of iris and ciliary body, small pupil ——— UVEITIS.

Misty cornea, ciliary congestion, dilated pupil, increased ocular tension. ——— ACUTE GLAUCOMA.

Involvement of the vitreous, uvea and retina; pus and debris present in the anterior chamber. ——— ENDOPHTHALMITIS.

Examine the lens with an ophthalmoscope.

Opacification indicates CATARACT

121

Impairment of Vision

Clinical Approach and Differential Diagnosis *(continued)*

Examine the posterior segment of the eye with an ophthalmoscope.

Pupil dilatation may be required.

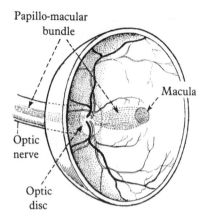

Papillo-macular bundle

Macula

Optic nerve

Optic disc

In the normal fundus, the *disc* is pale with a central cup and reddish-brown surrounding retina. Arteries and veins emerge from the optic disc. The *macula* is darker than the rest of the fundus and lies on the temporal side of the disc. One-third of all retinal fibres arise from the small macular region and pass to the optic nerve head (disc) as the *papillo–macular bundle*. The macula is the region of sharpest vision (cone vision), whereas peripheral vision (rod vision) serves the purpose of perception of movement and directing central/macular vision. The optic nerve head contains no rods or cones and accounts for the physiological *blind spot* in normal vision. The macular fibres being so functionally active, are the most susceptible to damage and produce a specific defect in the visual field – a SCOTOMA.

Retinal abnormality with acute impairment of vision

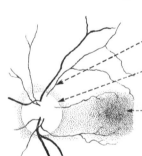

Arteries: narrow – branch occlusion, one vessel absent, embolus may be visualised.

→ ARTERIAL OCCLUSION
Confirm with visual field examination.

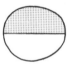

Altitudinal field defect

Look for embolic source e.g. carotid stenosis.

Disc: white.
Retina: pale and oedematous.
After a few days the macular area becomes cherry red in appearance. (Retina thinned here and the choroid shows through.)

Loss of retinal colour (becomes milky white) and macular blush.

→ CENTRAL RETINAL ARTERY OCCLUSION

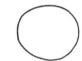

Disc margin blurred.

Loss of physiological 'central cup'.

Veins enlarged.

Radial streaks and corrugated appearance of the retina.

Haemorrhages may appear.

PAPILLITIS: *visual acuity severely affected* due to associated inflammation of the optic nerve (Retrobulbar neuritis).

PAPILLOEDEMA: *visual acuity normal* (unless in late stage when the macular area is affected by haemorrhage. Physiological blind spot is enlarged).

Impairment of Vision

Clinical approach and Differential diagnosis *(continued)*

N.B. Distinguish:

> HYPERMETROPIC patients who have a pale indistinct disc often difficult to differentiate from early papilloedema.
> HYPERTENSIVE RETINOPATHY – superficial haemorrhages and 'cotton wool' exudates.
> PSEUDOPAPILLOEDEMA – 'DRUSEN' – colloid bodies near the optic disc which raise the disc and blur the margin. This is a variant of normal.

Separation of the superficial retina from the pigment layer ⟶ RETINAL DETACHMENT (traumatic or spontaneous).

Retinal abnormalities with gradual impairment of vision.

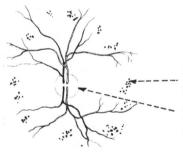

Disc white like a 'tennis ball' with 'punched out' margins: blood supply is less prominent and the number of arteries reduced.

⟶ OPTIC ATROPHY

primary (optic nerve disease): *compression, toxins, ischaemia, optic neuritis.*

secondary (following papilloedema):

↓

visual field charting (see later) may help differentiate cause.

N.B. Any disease of the optic nerve or anterior visual pathway causing loss of vision will eventually result in optic atrophy.

Pigmentary deposits in the periphery of the retina. ⟶ RETINITIS PIGMENTOSA

Progressive pallor of the optic disc.

Areas of white sclera exposed along with areas of proliferation of retinal pigmentory epithelium – follows atrophy of the choroid. ⟶ CHOROIDITIS

Occurs in *toxoplasmosis* and in *high (progressive) myopia* near the disc or macula with loss of central vision.

Field examination reveals a patchy loss.

LEFT   RIGHT

Fixation point

Blind spot

Impairment of Vision

Clinical approach and Differential diagnosis *(continued)*

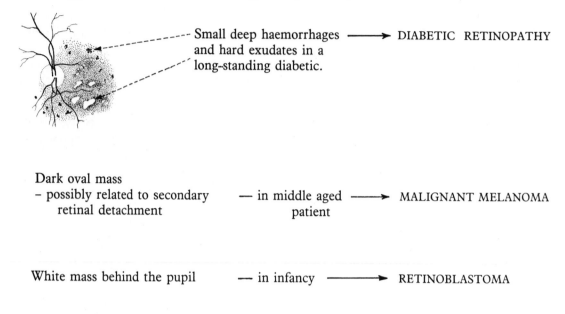

Small deep haemorrhages and hard exudates in a long-standing diabetic. ⟶ DIABETIC RETINOPATHY

Dark oval mass
– possibly related to secondary retinal detachment   — in middle aged patient ⟶ MALIGNANT MELANOMA

White mass behind the pupil   — in infancy ⟶ RETINOBLASTOMA

Examine the visual fields

If ophthalmoscopic examination is normal or if optic atrophy is evident, then visual field examination is essential. Visual confrontation is useful for detecting large defects, but smaller defects require visual field charting with a Bjerrum screen and/or perimeter (page 11).

In interpreting the physical findings of examination it is important to remember that the ocular system *reverses* the image. The nasal side of the fundus picks up the temporal image and vice versa. Damage, therefore, to the nasal side of the retina will produce a temporal visual field defect.

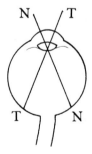

Impairment of Vision

Clinical approach and Differential diagnosis *(continued)*

Central scotoma Characteristic of most optic nerve lesions.

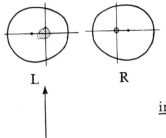

L   R

RETROBULBAR NEURITIS – associated papillitis may be evident on fundoscopy; may be first sign of *multiple sclerosis.*

OPTIC NERVE COMPRESSION

X-ray optic foramen ——————— orbital lesion (usually with
CT scan (orbital/intracranial)   – *tumour*   (proptosis)
                                        – *granuloma*

intracranial lesions
– *tumour* e.g. meningioma
    (chordoma, dermoid)
– *granuloma* e.g. tuberculoma
    (rare)   sarcoid
– *aneurysm* e.g. anterior communicating,
                            ophthalmic

lesion within optic canal
– *tumour* e.g. meningioma
– *granuloma*
– *hyperostosis* e.g. Paget's
    disease, fibrous dysplasia

→ angiography confirms

Pupil response
may be impaired
(Marcus-Gunn
pupil)

OPTIC NERVE GLIOMA → CT scan → exploration
LEBER's OPTIC ATROPHY – large bilateral scotoma

Centro-caecal scotoma

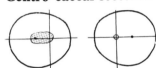

The scotoma extends to involve the blind spot.
Characteristic of toxic amblyopia
– alcohol, tobacco.

Arcuate scotoma

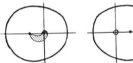

The scotoma extends from the blind spot following the course of nerve fibres.
Characteristic of glaucoma, seen also in small lesions close to the optic disc such as choroiditis.

Mononuclear blindness

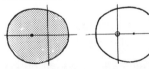

The end result of an inflammatory, vascular or compressive optic nerve lesion.

Direct pupillary response absent; consensual present.

Junctional scotoma

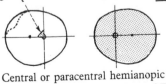

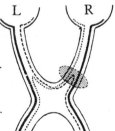

L   R

— indicates the presence of an *optic nerve lesion immediately anterior to the chiasma.*
Nasal fibres not only decussate in the chiasma, but also loop forward into the opposite optic nerve.
This lesion emphasises the importance of examining the 'normal' eye in monocular impairment of vision.

Central or paracentral hemianopic scotoma –'Junctional scotoma of Traquair'.

Often associated with peripheral temporal field defect.

Impairment of Vision

Clinical approach and Differential diagnosis *(continued)*
Bitemporal hemianopia/quadrantanopia

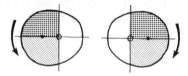 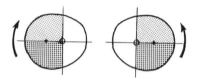

Involvement of the upper quadrants first indicates compression of the optic chiasma from below and suggests:

- PITUITARY ADENOMA

- NASOPHARYNGEAL CARCINOMA

- SPHENOID SINUS MUCOCELE

Involvement of the lower quadrants first indicates compression of the optic chiasma from above and suggests:

- CRANIOPHARYNGIOMA

- THIRD VENTRICULAR TUMOUR

The optic chiasma is closely associated with the pituitary fossa.

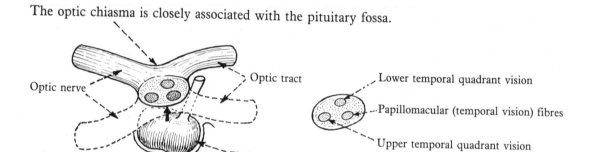

Homonymous Hemianopia

An incongruous homonymous hemianopia (i.e. one eye more affected than the other) suggests a lesion of the OPTIC TRACT near the chiasma.

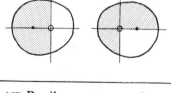

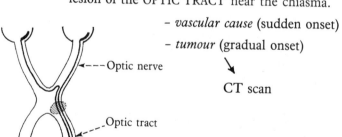

- *vascular cause* (sudden onset)

- *tumour* (gradual onset)

CT scan

The 'incongruous' defect occurs as a result of rotation of nasal and temporal fibres.

NB Pupil response may be impaired when light is shone from affected field.

Impairment of Vision

Congruous homonymous hemianopia (Fields can be exactly superimposed)

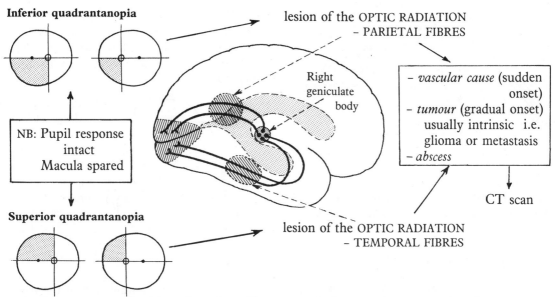

Inferior quadrantanopia

lesion of the OPTIC RADIATION
– PARIETAL FIBRES

Right
geniculate
body

- *vascular cause* (sudden
onset)
- *tumour* (gradual onset)
usually intrinsic i.e.
glioma or metastasis
- *abscess*

CT scan

NB: Pupil response
intact
Macula spared

Superior quadrantanopia

lesion of the OPTIC RADIATION
– TEMPORAL FIBRES

At the temporo-parietal junction where fibres meet, lesions produce a complete 'homonymous hemianopia'.

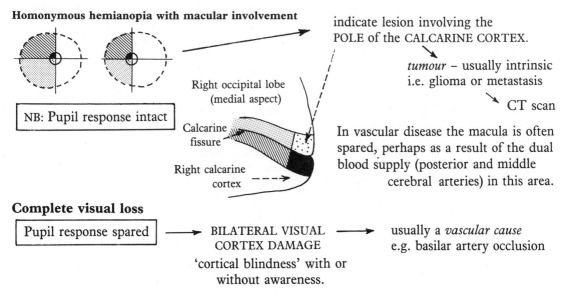

Homonymous hemianopia with macular involvement

indicate lesion involving the
POLE of the CALCARINE CORTEX.

tumour – usually intrinsic
i.e. glioma or metastasis

CT scan

NB: Pupil response intact

Right occipital lobe
(medial aspect)

Calcarine
fissure

Right calcarine
cortex

In vascular disease the macula is often
spared, perhaps as a result of the dual
blood supply (posterior and middle
cerebral arteries) in this area.

Complete visual loss

Pupil response spared $\longrightarrow$ BILATERAL VISUAL $\longrightarrow$ usually a *vascular cause*
CORTEX DAMAGE   e.g. basilar artery occlusion

'cortical blindness' with or
without awareness.

The interpretation of the visual image and its integration with other cortical functions is discussed under 'Higher Cortical Function'.

Disorders of Smell

The OLFACTORY (I) cranial nerve conveys the sensation of smell.

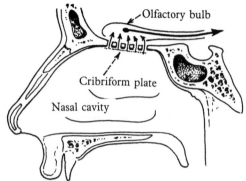

A number of fine nerves arising from receptor cells in the nasal mucosa pierce the *cribriform plate* of the ethmoid bone. These pass to the *olfactory bulb* where they synapse with neurones of the olfactory tract.

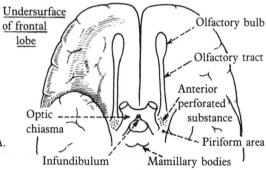

The neurones pass back in the olfactory tract to the *piriform area* of the temporal lobe and the *amygdaloid nucleus*.

A loss of the sense of smell is called ANOSMIA.

Differential diagnosis

IMPAIRMENT or LOSS OF SMELL – unilateral or bilateral

- TEMPORARY — *Upper respiratory tract infection:* inflammation of the nasal mucosa is the commonest cause of impairment or loss of smell.

- TEMPORARY/PERMANENT
  - *Head injury:* anosmia may occur with or without evidence of cribriform plate fracture. Recovery is usual.
  - *Viral infections:* any viral illness may cause anosmia which can be permanent.
  - *Drugs:* penicillamine treatment.
  - *Endocrine disease:* Addison's disease and thyrotoxicosis.
  - *Tumours:* Olfactory groove meningioma.
    - Frontal bone osteoma.
    - Pituitary tumours.
    - Frontal lobe glioma.
    - Frontal lobe abscess.
  - *Aneurysm of the circle of Willis:* Anterior communicating, Ophthalmic.
  - *Raised intracranial pressure:* without local damage to olfactory structures, may rarely cause anosmia.

OLFACTORY HALLUCINATIONS — Complex partial seizures often associated with dream-like states. — *Temporal lobe disease* (hippocampus pirifirm area): Anosmia does not occur since cortical representation is bilateral.

Pupillary Disorders

ANATOMY / PHYSIOLOGY

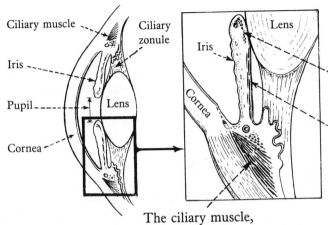

The iris controls the size of the pupil. It contains two groups of smooth muscle fibre:

1. *Sphincter pupillae;* a circular constrictor, innervated by the *parasympathetic* nervous system.
2. *Dilator pupillae;* a radial dilator, innervated by the *sympathetic* nervous system.

The ciliary muscle, through the ciliary zonule, controls the degree of convexity of the lens.

Pathway of pupillary constriction and the light reflex (parasympathetic).

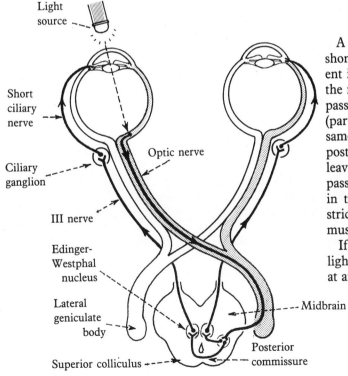

A stimulus, such as a bright light shone in the left eye, will send an afferent impulse along the OPTIC NERVE to the midbrain; here a second order fibre passes to the *Edinger Westphal nucleus* (part of the III nerve nucleus) on the same and opposite side (through the posterior commissure). Efferent fibres leave in the OCULOMOTOR NERVE, pass to the ciliary ganglion and thence, in the short ciliary nerve, to the constrictor fibres of the sphincter pupillae muscle.

If all pathways are intact, shining a light in one eye will constrict *both pupils* at an equal rate and to a similar degree.

Pupillary Disorders

Pathway of pupillary dilatation (sympathetic)

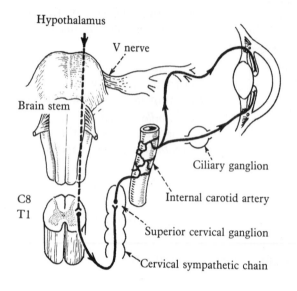

Sympathetic fibres descend from the hypothalamus through the lateral aspect of the brain stem into the spinal cord. The pupillary fibres pass out in the anterior roots of C8, T1, enter the sympathetic chain and, in the superior cervical ganglion, give rise to postganglionic fibres which ascend on the wall of the internal carotid artery to enter the cranium. The fibres eventually leave the intracranial portion of the internal carotid artery and pass directly through the ciliary ganglion to the iris or join the cranial nerves III, IV, V, and VI, running to the eye and iris. Sudomotor fibres (concerned with sweating) run up the external carotid artery to the dermis of the face.

Interruption of sympathetic supply affects:
1. Pupillary dilatation.
2. Levator palpebrae muscle (30% supplied by sympathetic).
3. Orbital involuntary muscle.
4. Vasoconstrictor fibres to orbit, eyelid and face.

Mechanism of Accommodation

When gaze is focused on a near object the medial rectus muscles contract and the pupil constricts (accommodation for near vision).

The pathway is poorly understood but must involve the visual cortex, Edinger-Westphal nuclei and both medial rectus components of the III nerve nucleus in the midbrain.

Inability of the pupil to accommodate need not always be associated with impairment of convergence, though usually this is the case.

Pupillary Disorders

PUPIL DILATATION – Causes

III nerve lesion ——

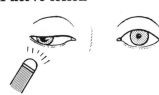

Examination of the light reflex (page 12) distinguishes lesions of the optic (II) and oculomotor (III) nerves.

Failure of the pupil to constrict when light is shone into either the affected or the contralateral eye indicates a III nerve lesion.

Look for – PTOSIS – 70% of levator palpebrae muscle is supplied by the oculomotor nerve.

– IMPAIRED EYE MOVEMENTS.

Causes of a III nerve lesion are described on page 140.

In comatose patients, pupil dilatation and failure to react to light is the simplest way of detecting a III nerve lesion; after head injury or in patients with raised intracranial pressure this is an important sign of transtentorial herniation.

The Tonic Pupil – Adie's Pupil

This is a benign condition usually affecting young women. Onset is usually acute and unilateral in 80%.

The pupil dilates and the patient complains of mistiness in the affected eye.

Pupil constriction to both direct and consensual light is often absent but very slow pupillary constriction occurs with accommodation.

When accommodation is relaxed –
slow dilatation occurs ----

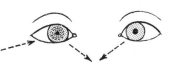

Occasionally the pupil appears completely unreactive to both light and accommodation. When the pupil is associated with reduced or absent limb reflexes this is termed the HOLMES-ADIE syndrome.

Diagnosis: confirmed by pupillary response to pilocarpine (0.1 or 0.05%) – the tonic pupil will constrict (denervation hypersensitivity); the normal eye is not affected.

The cause is unknown; the lesion may lie in the midbrain or ciliary ganglion.

Drugs:

Mydriatic drops
Glutethamide ⎬ overdose produces large unreactive pupils.
Amphetamine

N.B. Pupils are often large in childhood and may fluctuate in size in response to fatigue and excitement.

Pupillary Disorders

PUPIL CONSTRICTION – Causes

Horner's syndrome

Lesion

MYOSIS – the affected pupil is smaller than the opposite pupil. It does not dilate when the eye is shaded.

PTOSIS – the affected eyelid droops and may be slightly raised voluntarily. Ptosis is less marked than with a III nerve palsy.

ENOPHTHALMOS – backward displacement of the eyeball into the orbit.

DISTURBANCE OF SWEATING – depends on the site of the lesion. Absence of sweating occurs when the lesion is proximal to fibre separation along the internal and external carotid artéries.

Horner's syndrome may result from sympathetic damage at the following sites:

Pre-ganglionic
- *Brain stem* – Intrinsic tumour e.g. glioma.
  - Vascular lesion.
  - Syringobulbia.
- *Cervical cord* – Intrinsic tumour e.g. glioma.
  - Syringomyelia.
- *Anterior roots C8, T1* – Tumour e.g. neurofibroma.
  - Lower brachial plexus palsy.
- *Cervical sympathetic chain* – Carcinoma of the apex of the lung – PANCOAST SYNDROME.

Post-ganglionic – Internal carotid occlusion.
- Middle fossa lesions – tumour, granuloma.

Distinguish peripheral and central lesions by instilling drugs e.g. 1% cocaine in eyes.

Pre-ganglionic lesions	*Post-ganglionic lesion*
Right sided Horner's	Right sided Horner's
Cocaine acts at the adrenergic nerve endings and, by preventing adrenaline reuptake, causes pupil dilatation when the lesion is preganglionic.	When the lesion is postganglionic, cocaine has no effect because there are no nerve endings on which the drug may act.

Investigative approach: depends on associated signs. Chest X-ray is mandatory.

Raeder's syndrome: a painful 'Horner's syndrome' with associated involvement of one or several cranial nerves (II – VI) as well as the orbital sympathetic supply (page 152).

Pupillary Disorders

Pupil constriction – causes *(continued)*

The Argyll-Robertson Pupil

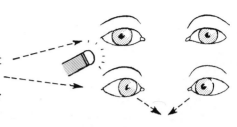

A *small pupil, irregular* in shape, which does not react to light but does react to accommodation.

It responds inadequately to pupillary dilator drugs.

Argyll-Robertson pupils are usually synonymous with *syphilitic infection* but they may also result from *any midbrain lesion – neoplastic, vascular, encephalitic or demyelinative*.

The Argyll-Robertson pupil has also been described in *diabetes* and in *alcoholic neuropathy* as well as following infectious mononucleosis. The lesion could lie in the midbrain, involving fibres passing to the Edinger-Westphal nucleus, in the posterior commissure or, alternatively, in the ciliary ganglion. A central lesion seems most likely.

Investigative approach: – look for associated signs of neurosyphilis.
                              – blood serology – VDRL, TPHA.

Drugs: *Opiate* overdosage produces small unreactive pupils.

N.B. In the elderly the pupils become small.

Other Pupillary Disorders

Failure of Accommodation and Convergence

Impaired accommodation and convergence are of limited diagnostic value since other clinical features are usually more prominent.

Causes: – extrapyramidal disease e.g. Parkinson's.
               – tumours of the pineal region.

The Marcus Gunn Pupil   (Pupillary escape)

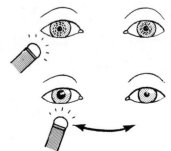

Illumination of one eye normally produces pupillary constriction with a degree of waxing and waning (hippus).

When afferent transmission in the optic nerve is impaired, this 'escape' becomes more evident.

If the light source is 'swung' from eye to eye, dwelling 4 seconds on each, the affected pupil may eventually, paradoxically, dilate – a 'Marcus Gunn' pupil.

The swinging light test is a sensitive test of optic nerve damage.

Diplopia — Impaired Ocular Movement

Diplopia or double vision results from impaired ocular movement.

RELATED ANATOMY and PHYSIOLOGY

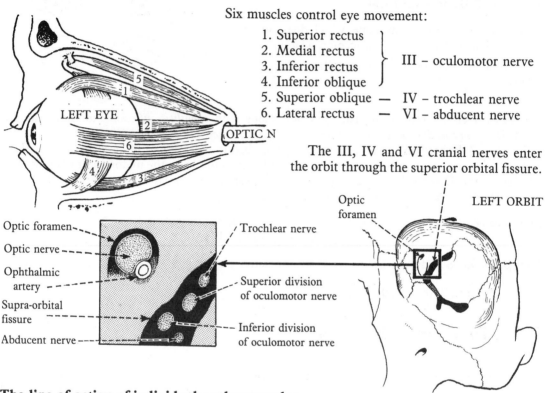

Six muscles control eye movement:

1. Superior rectus ⎫
2. Medial rectus ⎪
3. Inferior rectus ⎬ III – oculomotor nerve
4. Inferior oblique ⎭
5. Superior oblique — IV – trochlear nerve
6. Lateral rectus — VI – abducent nerve

The III, IV and VI cranial nerves enter the orbit through the superior orbital fissure.

The line of action of individual ocular muscles

Eye movements result from a continuous interplay of all the ocular muscles, but each muscle has a direction of maximal efficiency.

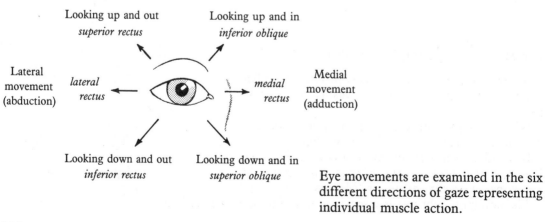

Eye movements are examined in the six different directions of gaze representing individual muscle action.

Diplopia — Impaired Ocular Movement

The line of action of individual ocular muscles *(continued)*

As a result of the angle of insertion into the globe, the inferior and superior recti and the oblique muscles also have a rotatory or torsion effect.

When the eye is turned out, the oblique muscles rotate the globe; when turned in the inferior or superior recti rotate the globe.

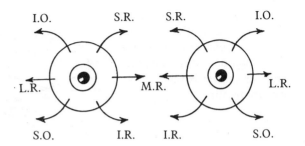

The OCULOMOTOR (III) nerve

The oculomotor nucleus lies in the *ventral periaqueductal grey matter* at the level of the *superior colliculus*. Nerve fibres pass through the *red nucleus* and *substantia nigra* and emerge medial to the *cerebral peduncle*.

The nucleus has a complex structure:

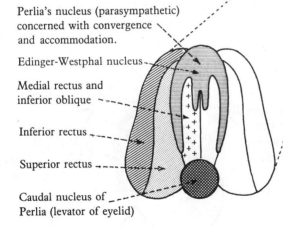

Perlia's nucleus (parasympathetic) concerned with convergence and accommodation.

Edinger-Westphal nucleus

Medial rectus and inferior oblique

Inferior rectus

Superior rectus

Caudal nucleus of Perlia (levator of eyelid)

The nucleus is a paired structure which lies close to the midline, the portion representing the medial rectus abutting its neighbour.

Diplopia — Impaired Ocular Movement

III nerve *(continued)*

On leaving the brain stem
the nerve passes through the
interpeduncular cistern close to
the posterior communicating artery
and runs towards the
cavernous sinus.

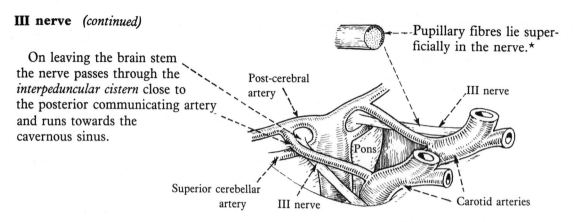

*This explains early pupillary involvement with III nerve compression and pupillary sparing with nerve infarction in hypertension and diabetes.

The nerve runs within the lateral wall of the
cavernous sinus
and then finally through the *superior
orbital fissure* into the *orbit*.

Here it divides into:

1. Superior branch to the levator of the
   eyelid and the superior rectus.
2. Inferior branch to the inferior oblique,
   medial and inferior recti.

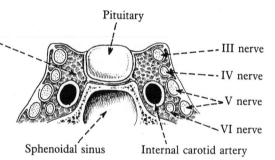

The TROCHLEAR (IV) nerve

This nerve supplies the *superior oblique muscle* of the eye.

The nucleus lies in the midbrain at the level of the
inferior colliculus, near the ventral *peri-aqueductal
grey matter*. The nerve passes laterally and dorsally
around the central grey matter and decussates
in the dorsal aspect of the brain stem in close
proximity to the *anterior medullary velum* of
the cerebellum.

Emerging from the brain stem the nerve
passes laterally around the *cerebral
peduncle* and pierces the dura to lie in
the lateral wall of the *cavernous sinus*.
Finally, it passes through the *superior
orbital fissure* into the orbit.

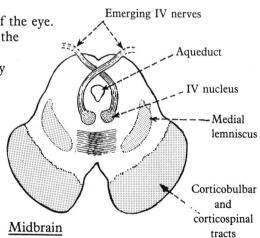

Midbrain

Diplopia — Impaired Ocular Movement

The ABDUCENS (VI) nerve

This nerve supplies the *lateral rectus muscle* of the eye.

The nucleus lies in the floor of the IV ventricle within the lower portion of the *pons*. The axons pass ventrally through the pons without decussating.

Note the close association of the VI and VII nuclei.

Emerging from the brain stem the nerve runs up anterior to the pons for approximately 15 mm before piercing the dura overlying the *basilar portion* of the *occipital bone*.

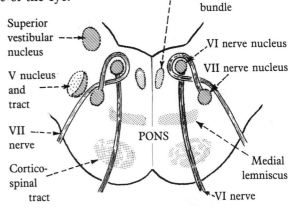

Under the dura the nerve runs up the *petrous portion* of the *temporal bone* and from its apex passes on to the lateral wall of the *cavernous sinus* and finally through the *superior orbital fissure*.

Note the long intracranial course and the proximity of the VI to the V cranial and greater superficial petrosal nerves at the apex of the petrous temporal bone.

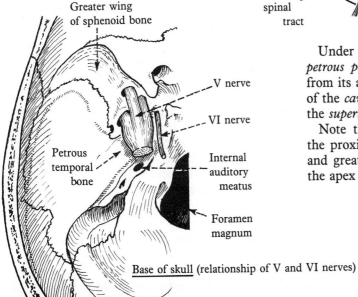

Base of skull (relationship of V and VI nerves)

DIPLOPIA

When the eyes fix on an image, impairment of movement of one eye results in projection of the image upon the macular area in the normal eye and to one side of the macula in the paretic eye; two images of the single object are thus perceived.

Paralysis of right lateral rectus

The image seen by the paretic eye is the *false image;* that seen by the normal eye is the *true image.* The false image is always *outermost;* this may lie in the vertical or the horizontal plane.

Diplopia — Impaired Ocular Movement

Clinical assessment   **Investigations**

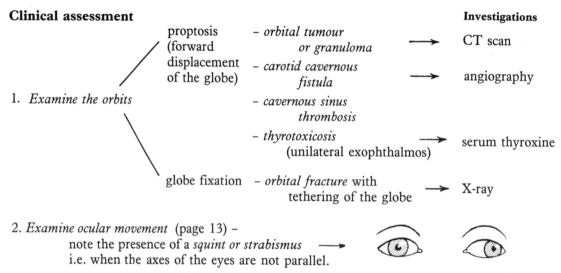

1. *Examine the orbits*

proptosis (forward displacement of the globe)
- *orbital tumour or granuloma* ⟶ CT scan
- *carotid cavernous fistula* ⟶ angiography
- *cavernous sinus thrombosis*
- *thyrotoxicosis* (unilateral exophthalmos) ⟶ serum thyroxine

globe fixation — *orbital fracture* with tethering of the globe ⟶ X-ray

2. *Examine ocular movement* (page 13) –
note the presence of a *squint or strabismus* ⟶
i.e. when the axes of the eyes are not parallel.

Differentiate

CONCOMITANT squint – an ocular disorder. The eyes adopt an abnormal position in relation to each other and the deviation is constant in all directions of gaze. Such squints are usually 'convergent' and develop in the first few years of life before binocular vision is established. Suppression of vision from one eye *(amblyopia ex anopsia)* results in *absence of diplopia.* Occasionally patients subconsciously alternate vision from one eye to the other, retaining equal visual function in both – *strabismus alternans.* Correction of an underlying hypermetropia with convex lenses may offset the tendency for the eyes to converge.

PARALYTIC squint –
(a) affected eye shows limited movement.
(b) angle of eye deviation and diplopia greatest when looking in the direction controlled by the weak muscle.
(c) diplopia is always present.
(d) the patient may assume a head tilt posture to minimise the diplopia.
  Paralytic squint results from disturbance of function of nerves or muscles.

III NERVE LESION

In the primary position, the affected eye deviates laterally (due to unopposed action of the lateral rectus) and PTOSIS and
PUPIL DILATATION are evident.

(Ptosis may be complete, unlike the partial ptosis of a Horner's syndrome.)

Diplopia — Impaired Ocular Movement

IV NERVE LESION

The eyes appear conjugate in the primary position.

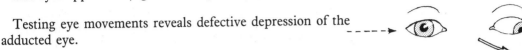

Testing eye movements reveals defective depression of the adducted eye.

Symptomatically the patient complains of double vision when looking downwards e.g. when descending stairs or reading, and the head may tilt to the opposite side to minimise the diplopia.

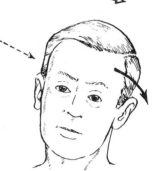

A IV nerve palsy is difficult to detect when associated with a III nerve palsy. If inward rotation (intorsion) is absent on looking downwards when eye is abducted, then a IV nerve palsy coexists with the III nerve palsy.

VI NERVE LESION

The eyes appear conjugate in the primary position.

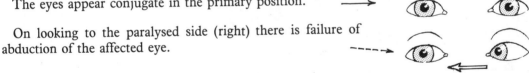

On looking to the paralysed side (right) there is failure of abduction of the affected eye.

Diplopia is horizontal (true and fake image side by side) and is present only when looking to the paralysed side and is maximal at the extreme of binocular lateral vision.

NOTE: In partial oculomotor palsies, the patient may be aware of diplopia, although eye movements appear normal. When this occurs:
- check diplopia is 'true' by noting its disappearance on covering one eye.
- determine the direction of maximal image displacement and the eye responsible for the outermost image (see page 14).

This information is sufficient to differentiate a III, IV and VI nerve lesion.

OCULAR MUSCLES

If the limitation of eye movement is not restricted to one muscle, or group of muscles with a common innervation, and affects both eyes, look for:
- involvement of extraocular muscles
   (levator palpebrae superioris,
      orbicularis oculi)

   myasthenia gravis
   ocular myopathy
- signs of fatigue on repeated testing

Diplopia — Impaired Ocular Movement

CAUSES OF III NERVE LESION

MIDBRAIN

When BILATERAL → oculomotor nucleus

When III nerve lesion is associated with

TREMOR → red nucleus
or
CONTRALATERAL HEMIPARESIS → cerebral peduncles
(WEBER's SYNDROME)

infarction, demyelination, intrinsic tumour e.g. glioma, basilar aneurysm compression.

ORBITAL FISSURE/ORBIT

Look for PROPTOSIS and associated involvement of the IV,VI and FIRST DIVISION of the V NERVES

- *orbital tumour,*
  granuloma,
- *periostitis.*

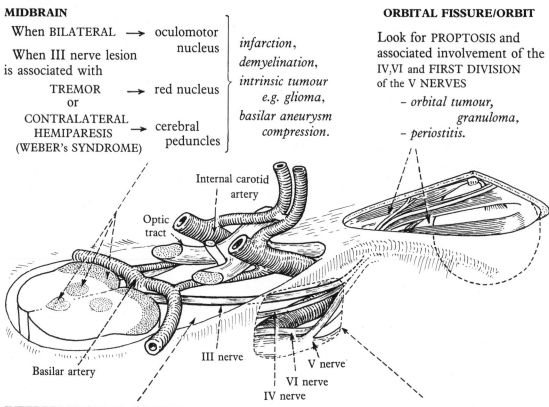

Internal carotid artery

Optic tract

Basilar artery

III nerve

V nerve

VI nerve

IV nerve

INTERPEDUNCULAR CISTERN

When III nerve lesion is associated with:

DETERIORATION OF CONSCIOUS LEVEL → *transtentorial herniation.*

RETRO-ORBITAL PAIN ± SUB-ARACHNOID HAEMORRHAGE → *aneurysm compression (posterior communicating or basilar aneurysm).*

MENINGISM + OTHER CRANIAL NERVE PALSIES → *basal meningitis*
- TB, syphilitic, bacterial.
- carcinomatous.

PUPIL REACTION SPARED SUDDEN ONSET → *nerve trunk infarction especially if hypertension, diabetes, polyarteritis nodosa, SLE.*

CAVERNOUS SINUS

Look for associated involvement of IV, VI and 1st DIVISION OF V NERVE,

- *tumour*
  - *pituitary adenoma,*
  - *meningioma,*
  - *metastasis,*
  - *nasopharyngeal carcinoma,*
- *intracavernous aneurysm.*
- *cavernous sinus thrombosis.*

140

Diplopia — Impaired Ocular Movement

CAUSES OF IV NERVE LESION

MIDBRAIN

When IV nerve lesion is associated with:

CONTRALATERAL
  HEMIPARESIS,
CONTRALATERAL
  HEMISENSORY LOSS } nuclear or intramedullary lesion } *infarction, demyelination, intrinsic tumour e.g. glioma*

ORBITAL FISSURE
ORBIT
CAVERNOUS SINUS } *Causes as for III nerve lesion*

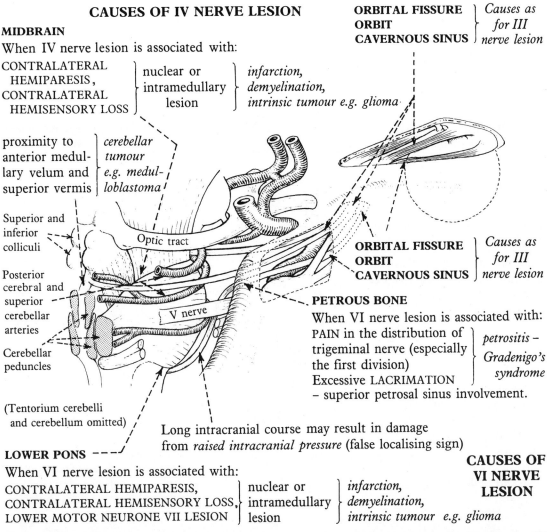

proximity to anterior medullary velum and superior vermis } *cerebellar tumour e.g. medulloblastoma*

Superior and inferior colliculi

Optic tract

Posterior cerebral and superior cerebellar arteries

Cerebellar peduncles

V nerve

**ORBITAL FISSURE
ORBIT
CAVERNOUS SINUS** } *Causes as for III nerve lesion*

PETROUS BONE

When VI nerve lesion is associated with:
PAIN in the distribution of trigeminal nerve (especially the first division) } *petrositis – Gradenigo's syndrome*
Excessive LACRIMATION
– superior petrosal sinus involvement.

(Tentorium cerebelli and cerebellum omitted)

Long intracranial course may result in damage from *raised intracranial pressure* (false localising sign)

LOWER PONS

When VI nerve lesion is associated with:

CONTRALATERAL HEMIPARESIS,
CONTRALATERAL HEMISENSORY LOSS,
LOWER MOTOR NEURONE VII LESION } nuclear or intramedullary lesion } *infarction, demyelination, intrinsic tumour e.g. glioma*

**CAUSES OF
VI NERVE
LESION**

NOTE: Infective or carcinomatous meningitis and nerve trunk infarction may also involve the IV and VI nerves, although less often than the III nerve.

Investigative approach

Impaired ocular movement from III, IV or VI nerve lesions requires full investigation with *straight X-rays, CT scan* and where appropriate *CSF cytology*. Unexplained III nerve lesions require *angiography;* only in elderly hypertensive or diabetic patients with pupillary sparing may angiography be omitted.

When myopathy or myasthenia gravis is suspected then appropriate investigations – receptor antibodies, EMG studies and occasionally muscle biopsy – may be necessary.

Disorders of Gaze

ANATOMY and PHYSIOLOGY
Two cortical centres of ocular control are recognised:
    1. Middle gyrus of frontal lobe (frontal eye field).
    2. Occipital cortex.

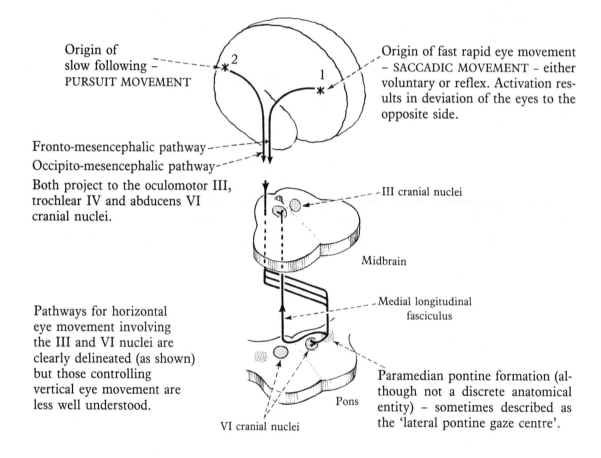

Origin of slow following – PURSUIT MOVEMENT

Origin of fast rapid eye movement – SACCADIC MOVEMENT - either voluntary or reflex. Activation results in deviation of the eyes to the opposite side.

Fronto-mesencephalic pathway
Occipito-mesencephalic pathway
Both project to the oculomotor III, trochlear IV and abducens VI cranial nuclei.

III cranial nuclei

Midbrain

Pathways for horizontal eye movement involving the III and VI nuclei are clearly delineated (as shown) but those controlling vertical eye movement are less well understood.

Medial longitudinal fasciculus

Paramedian pontine formation (although not a discrete anatomical entity) – sometimes described as the 'lateral pontine gaze centre'.

Pons

VI cranial nuclei

Note that the cortical descending pathways from one side activate the ipsilateral III nucleus and the contralateral VI nucleus thus swinging the direction of gaze to the opposite side.

It is important to distinguish between *saccadic* and *pursuit* movement. When following an object a slow pursuit movement maintains the image on the macular area of the retina. To fixate on a new object, rapid saccadic movement aligns the new target on the macular area. When locked in to the new target, pursuit movement maintains fixation.

Eye movement occurs voluntarily in a conjugate (parallel) manner in any direction. Eye movements also occur reflexly to auditory or labyrinthine stimulation.

142

Disorders of Gaze

Gaze disorders usually follow vascular episodes (infarct or haemorrrhage) but may also occur in traumatic, inflammatory or neoplastic disease.

CONJUGATE DEVIATION of the EYES
Occurring during a seizure

Eyes deviated towards the affected limbs.

  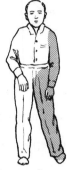

Indicates an epileptic focus in the frontal lobe contralateral to the direction of eye deviation.

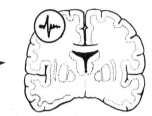

Accompanying a hemiparesis.

Eyes deviated *away* from the hemiparetic limb.

  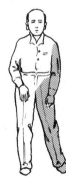

Indicates a lesion in the frontal lobe *ipsilateral* to the direction of eye deviation.

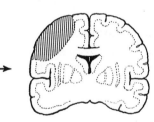

Eyes deviated *towards* the hemiparetic limb.

  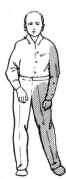

Indicates a lesion in the pons *contralateral* to the direction of eye deviation.

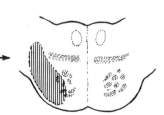

Disorders of Gaze

PARINAUD's SYNDROME

A syndrome characterised by impaired ocular mobility and pupillary responses.

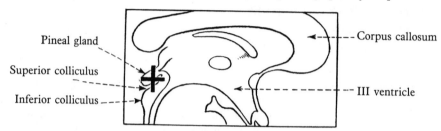

The lesion affects the midbrain tectum (✚)
- Upward gaze and convergence are lost.
- The pupils are dilated and the response to light and accommodation is impaired.

Causes: Third ventricular or pineal tumours. Wernicke's encephalopathy. Encephalitis rarely.

ATAXIC NYSTAGMUS (Internuclear ophthalmoplegia)

This disorder, due to damage to the medial longitudinal bundle, is dealt with on page 173. It is an *inter*nuclear disorder of eye movement.

OCULAR APRAXIA

Bilateral prefrontal motor cortex damage will produce this unusual finding in which the patient does not move the eyes voluntarily to command, yet has a full range of random eye movement.

Facial Pain and Sensory Loss

The fifth cranial nerve subserves facial sensation and innervates the muscles of mastication.

Anatomy:

The anatomical arrangement of the trigeminal central connections are complex.

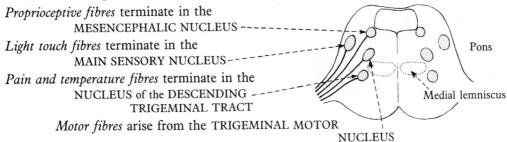

Proprioceptive fibres terminate in the
MESENCEPHALIC NUCLEUS

Light touch fibres terminate in the
MAIN SENSORY NUCLEUS

Pain and temperature fibres terminate in the
NUCLEUS of the DESCENDING
TRIGEMINAL TRACT

Motor fibres arise from the TRIGEMINAL MOTOR
NUCLEUS

Pons

Medial lemniscus

Longitudinal arrangement of the Trigeminal Nuclei (Sensory paths)

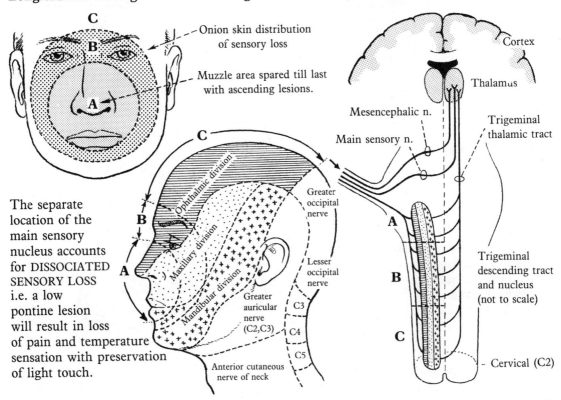

C

B

A

Onion skin distribution
of sensory loss

Muscle area spared till last
with ascending lesions.

The separate
location of the
main sensory
nucleus accounts
for DISSOCIATED
SENSORY LOSS
i.e. a low
pontine lesion
will result in loss
of pain and temperature
sensation with preservation
of light touch.

C

Ophthalmic division

B

Maxillary division

A

Mandibular division

Greater
occipital
nerve

Lesser
occipital
nerve

Greater
auricular
nerve
(C2,C3)

C3

C4

C5

Anterior cutaneous
nerve of neck

Cortex

Thalamus

Mesencephalic n.

Main sensory n.

Trigeminal
thalamic tract

A

B

C

Trigeminal
descending tract
and nucleus
(not to scale)

Cervical (C2)

Note the topographical arrangement of the descending nucleus. A cervical lesion extending up in the brain stem e.g. syringomyelia ⟶ syringobulbia produces a characteristic 'onion skin' distribution of pinprick and temperature loss, and spares the muzzle area until last.

Facial Pain and Sensory Loss

The peripheral course of the V nerve

The nerve roots emerge from the lateral aspect of the brain stem at the midpontine level and run to the Gasserian ganglion. This contains the bipolar sensory nuclei and lies on the apex of the petrous bone in the middle fossa. It gives off the three divisions of the trigeminal nerve. Each division exits through its own foramen and supplies a specific area of the face.

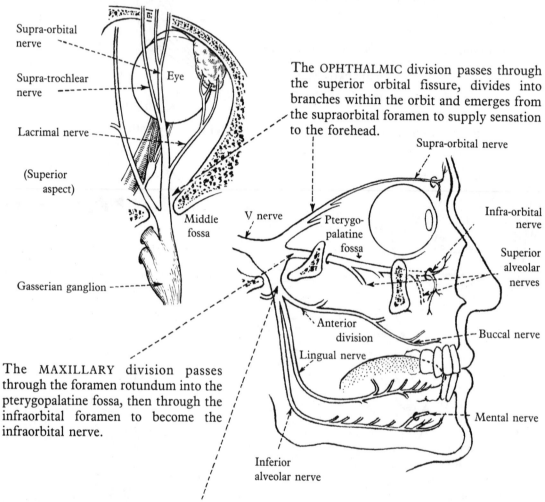

Supra-orbital nerve

Supra-trochlear nerve

Lacrimal nerve

Eye

(Superior aspect)

Middle fossa

Gasserian ganglion

V nerve

The OPHTHALMIC division passes through the superior orbital fissure, divides into branches within the orbit and emerges from the supraorbital foramen to supply sensation to the forehead.

Supra-orbital nerve

Pterygo-palatine fossa

Infra-orbital nerve

Superior alveolar nerves

Anterior division

Lingual nerve

Buccal nerve

Mental nerve

Inferior alveolar nerve

The MAXILLARY division passes through the foramen rotundum into the pterygopalatine fossa, then through the infraorbital foramen to become the infraorbital nerve.

The MANDIBULAR division exits from the foramen ovale. The anterior trunk incorporates the motor division of the V nerve, innervating the muscles of mastication – masseter, pterygoids and temporalis – as well as supplying sensation to the cheek and gums (buccal nerve).

The lingual branch of the posterior trunk supplies sensation to the anterior two-thirds of the tongue (and is joined by the chordi tympani from the facial nerve carrying salivary secretomotor fibres and taste to the anterior two-thirds of the tongue).

146

Facial Pain and Sensory Loss

Examination of facial sensation:

This should include examination of the *corneal reflex* and *masticatory muscle function* (page 15).

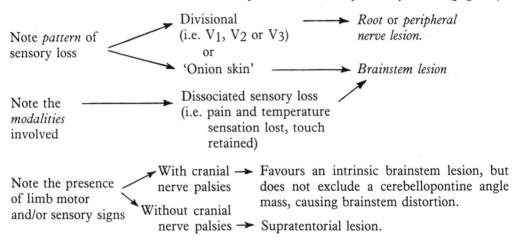

Note *pattern* of sensory loss → Divisional (i.e. V₁, V₂ or V₃) → *Root* or *peripheral nerve lesion.*

or

'Onion skin' → *Brainstem lesion*

Note the *modalities* involved → Dissociated sensory loss (i.e. pain and temperature sensation lost, touch retained)

Note the presence of limb motor and/or sensory signs → With cranial nerve palsies → Favours an intrinsic brainstem lesion, but does not exclude a cerebellopontine angle mass, causing brainstem distortion.

Without cranial nerve palsies → Supratentorial lesion.

Causes of V nerve lesions:

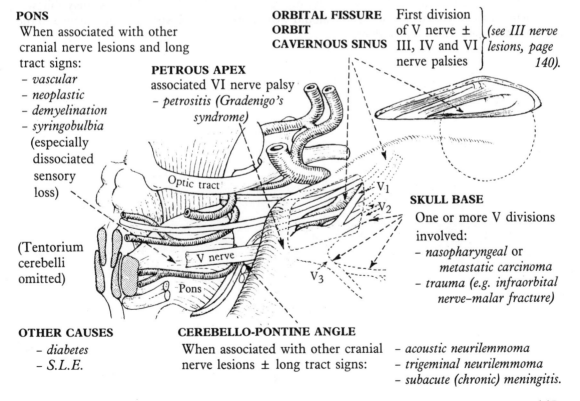

PONS
When associated with other cranial nerve lesions and long tract signs:
- *vascular*
- *neoplastic*
- *demyelination*
- *syringobulbia*
  (especially dissociated sensory loss)

(Tentorium cerebelli omitted)

PETROUS APEX
associated VI nerve palsy
- *petrositis (Gradenigo's syndrome)*

Optic tract

V nerve

Pons

ORBITAL FISSURE First division
ORBIT of V nerve ±
CAVERNOUS SINUS III, IV and VI nerve palsies } (*see III nerve lesions, page 140).*

V₁

V₂

V₃

SKULL BASE
One or more V divisions involved:
- *nasopharyngeal* or *metastatic carcinoma*
- *trauma (e.g. infraorbital nerve–malar fracture)*

OTHER CAUSES
- *diabetes*
- *S.L.E.*

CEREBELLO-PONTINE ANGLE
When associated with other cranial nerve lesions ± long tract signs:

- *acoustic neurilemmoma*
- *trigeminal neurilemmoma*
- *subacute (chronic) meningitis.*

Facial Pain and Sensory Loss

HERPES ZOSTER INFECTION

Herpes zoster may affect the Gasserian ganglion, causing inflammation and nerve cell necrosis. Herpetic skin eruptions result and cover either the whole trigeminal area or one individual division – usually the ophthalmic division. Rarely trigeminal motor paralysis occurs. 'Scarring' in the ganglion after recovery probably explains the frequent post-herpetic neuralgia.

TRIGEMINAL NEUROPATHY:

This painful condition causes a progressive sensory loss in one or more trigeminal divisions with trophic ulceration of the nasal ala. Such sensory disturbance may occur in systemic lupus erythematosus but usually the cause is unexplained. The condition runs a slow protracted course.

GRADENIGO's SYNDROME:

Infection involving the inferior petrosal sinus (usually extending from the middle ear) may produce V and VI nerve damage causing diplopia, facial pain and sensory loss.

NEUROPATHIC KERATITIS

Corneal anaesthesia from a central or peripheral V nerve lesion may lead to a neuropathic keratitis. The corneal surface becomes hazy, ulcerated and infected and blindness may follow.

Patients with absent corneal sensation should wear a protective perspex shield, attached to the side of spectacles, when out of doors.

Facial Pain — Diagnostic Approach

Pain in the face may result from many different disorders and often presents as a diagnostic problem to the neurologist or neurosurgeon.

Consider:

1. Site of Pain

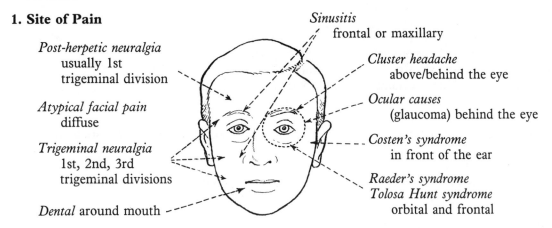

Post-herpetic neuralgia
    usually 1st
    trigeminal division

Atypical facial pain
    diffuse

Trigeminal neuralgia
    1st, 2nd, 3rd
    trigeminal divisions

Dental around mouth

Sinusitis
    frontal or maxillary

Cluster headache
    above/behind the eye

Ocular causes
    (glaucoma) behind the eye

Costen's syndrome
    in front of the ear

Raeder's syndrome
Tolosa Hunt syndrome
    orbital and frontal

2. Quality of Pain

Trigeminal neuralgia	– sharp, stabbing, shooting, paroxysmal.
Atypical facial pain	– dull, persisting.
Post-herpetic neuralgia	– dull, burning, persisting, occasional paroxysm.
Dental	– dull.
Sinusitis	– sharp, boring, worse in the morning.
Ocular	– dull, throbbing.
Costen's syndrome	– severe aching, aggravated by chewing.
Cluster headache	– sharp, intermittent.

3. Associated symptoms/signs

Trigeminal neuralgia	– often no neurological deficit, but occasional blunting of pin-prick over involved region.
Atypical facial pain	– accompanying features of depressive illness.
Post-herpetic neuralgia	– occasional evidence of scarring.
Dental	– swelling of lips/face.
Sinusitis	– puffy appearance around eyes, tenderness to percussion over involved sinus.
Ocular	– glaucoma: associated visual symptoms – blurring/haloes/loss.
Costen's syndrome	– tenderness over temperomandibular joints
Cluster headache	– associated lacrimation/rhinorrhoea.

Attention to site, quality and associated symptoms and signs should result in the diagnosis.

Facial Pain — Trigeminal Neuralgia

TRIGEMINAL NEURALGIA (Tic Douloureux)

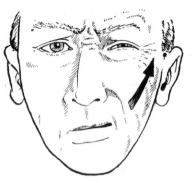

Trigeminal neuralgia is characterised by paroxysmal attacks of severe, short, sharp, stabbing pain affecting one or more divisions of the trigeminal nerve. The pain involves the second or third divisions more often than the first; it rarely occurs bilaterally, and never simultaneously on each side. Paroxysmal attacks last for several days or weeks; they are often superimposed on a more constant ache. When the attacks settle, the patient may remain pain free for many months.

Chewing, speaking, washing the face, tooth brushing, cold winds or touching a specific 'trigger spot' e.g. upper lip or gum may all precipitate an attack of pain.

Trigeminal neuralgia more commonly affects females and patients over 50 years of age.

Aetiology:

In many patients the cause of trigeminal neuralgia remains unexplained as do the long periods of remission. Several predisposing factors are recognised:

Root compression – *tumours* of the cerebello-pontine angle lying against the V nerve roots e.g. meningioma, epidermoid cyst, frequently present with trigeminal neuralgia.

– *arterial vessels* often abut and sometimes clearly indent the trigeminal nerve roots, but this mechanism cannot apply to all patients.

Demyelination – the incidence of trigeminal neuralgia is increased in patients with demyelinating disease.

MANAGEMENT

Drug therapy

CARBAMAZEPINE proves effective in most patients (and helps confirm the diagnosis). Provided toxicity does not become troublesome i.e. drowsiness, ataxia, the dosage is increased until pain relief occurs (600–1600 mg/day).

If pain control is limited, other drugs – CLONAZEPAM, PHENYTOIN – may occasionally benefit.

Persistence of pain on full drug dosage or an intolerance of the drugs, indicates the need for further measures.

Facial Pain — Trigeminal Neuralgia

MANAGEMENT (continued)
Operative therapy:

Peripheral nerve techniques:
Nerve block with alcohol or phenol provides temporary relief (up to one year). *Avulsion* of the supra- or infraorbital nerves gives more prolonged pain relief.

Trigeminal ganglion/root injection:
Alcohol or phenol injection into the trigeminal ganglion effectively produces pain relief, but area control is limited and the risk of corneal anaesthesia, ulceration and scarring is high.

Glycerol injection into Meckel's cave has recently been found to produce pain relief without causing any permanent sensory deficit.

Trigeminal root section:
Through either a subtemporal (extra- or intradural) or posterior fossa approach, the appropriate trigeminal root is identified and divided.

Microvascular decompression:
Exploration of the cerebellopontine angle reveals blood vessels in contact with the trigeminal nerve roots in 85–90%. Separation of these structures and insertion of a non absorbable sponge produces pain relief in most patients, without the associated problems of nerve destruction.

Radiofrequency thermocoagulation:
The site of facial 'tingling' produced by electrical stimulation of a needle inserted into the trigeminal ganglion, accurately identifies the location of the needle tip. When the site of tingling corresponds to the trigger spot or site of pain origin, radiofrequency thermocoagulation under general anaesthetic, produces a permanent lesion – usually resulting in analgesia of the appropriate area with retention of light touch.

Results and Complications:

Pain relief: accurate comparison of the wide variety of techniques used for trigeminal neuralgia is difficult; all but peripheral nerve avulsion appear to produce similar results. Approximately 80–85% of patients remain pain free for a 5 year period. Results of peripheral nerve avulsion are less satisfactory with pain recurring in 50% within 2 years.

Dysaesthesia/Anaesthesia dolorosa: this troublesome sensory disturbance follows any destructive technique to nerve or root in 5–30% of patients. Microvascular decompression avoids this problem and as yet the incidence appears very low with glycerol injection.

Corneal anaesthesia: this occurs most frequently following phenol or alcohol injection into the trigeminal ganglion, but is also a problem when root section or thermocoagulation involves the first division.

Mortality: microvascular decompression and open root section carry a low mortality rate (1–3%), but this must not be ignored when comparing results with safer methods.

Treatment selection: This largely depends on the surgeon's personal preference and experience.

V_2 and V_3 pain – thermocoagulation provides good results with minimal risk.

V_1 pain – microvascular decompression does not endanger corneal sensation.

The recent introduction of glycerol injection may prove optimal for pain in all distributions – especially in the frail and elderly who tolerate alternative procedures less well.

151

Facial Pain — Other Causes

Temporomandibular joint dysfunction (Costen's syndrome)

 Aching pain occurring in front of the ear, aggravated by chewing; due to malalignment of one temporomandibular joint as a consequence of dental loss with altered 'bite' or involvement of the joint in rheumatoid arthritis.
This condition requires dental treatment with realignment.

Raeder's syndrome (The paratrigeminal syndrome)

Pain in 1st and 2nd trigeminal divisions, maximal around the eye and associated with a sympathetic paresis (ptosis and small pupil). Sweating in the lower face is preserved. Associated with lesions of the middle fossa e.g. nasopharyngeal carcinoma, granulomas.

Tolosa Hunt syndrome

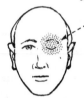 Severe orbital pain with the development of ocular palsies as well as loss of 1st division trigeminal sensation.
Caused by lesions involving the superior orbital fissure – granulomas or osteitis.

Atypical facial pain

The patient, often a young or middle aged woman, experiences a dull, persistent pain, spreading diffusely over one or both sides of the face. These symptoms often result from an underlying depression and may respond well to antidepressant therapy.

'Cluster' headaches – see page 67.

Facial Weakness

Related Anatomy

The facial (VII) nerve contains mainly motor fibres supplying the muscles of facial expression, but also visceral efferent (parasympathetic) and visceral afferent (taste) fibres.

The motor nucleus lies in the lower pons medial to the descending nucleus and tract of the Vth cranial nerve. Axons from the motor nucleus wind around the nucleus of the VIth cranial nerve. The facial nerve and its sensory root (*nervus intermedius*) exit from the lateral aspect of the brain stem and cross the cerebellopontine angle immediately adjacent to the VIII cranial nerve. They enter the internal auditory meatus and, passing through the facial canal of the temporal bone, lie in close proximity to the inner ear and tympanic membrane. The facial nerve gives off several branches before exiting from the skull through the stylomastoid foramen.

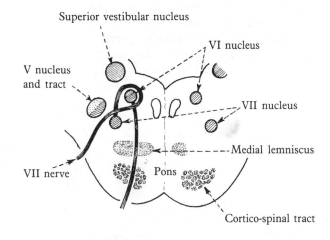

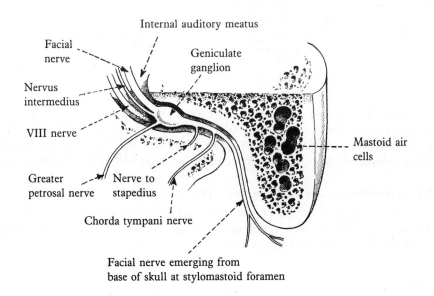

Facial Weakness

Visceral efferent and visceral afferent fibres arise and terminate in the superior salivary nucleus and nucleus/tractus solitarius respectively.

They run together as nervus intermedius and accompany the facial nerve to the internal auditory meatus. The parasympathetic fibres (visceral efferent) pass in the greater petrosal nerve to the sphenopalatine ganglion and thence to the lacrimal gland to produce tears.

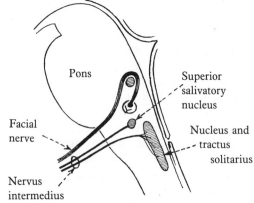

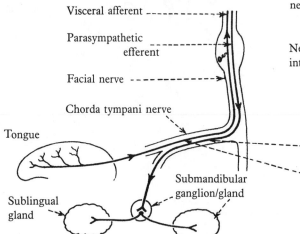

The chorda tympani nerve contains both parasympathetic efferent and visceral afferent fibres.

Parasympathetic fibres are responsible for salivation.

Visceral afferent fibres convey sensations of taste from the anterior two-thirds of the tongue. The geniculate ganglion contains the bipolar cell bodies of these afferent fibres.

Supranuclear control of facial muscles

The muscles in the lower face are controlled by the contralateral hemisphere, whereas those in the upper face receive control from both hemispheres (bilateral representation). Hence a lower motor neurone lesion paralyses all facial muscles on that side, but an upper motor neurone (supranuclear) lesion paralyses only the muscles in the lower half of the face on the opposite side.

Clinical examination of the facial nerve   (See page 16).

In addition to examining for facial weakness and taste impairment, also note whether the patient comments on reduced lacrimation or salivation on one side, or hyperacusis (exaggeration of sounds due to loss of the stapedius reflex).

Facial Weakness

LESION, LOCALISATION and CAUSE

Note the *distribution*:

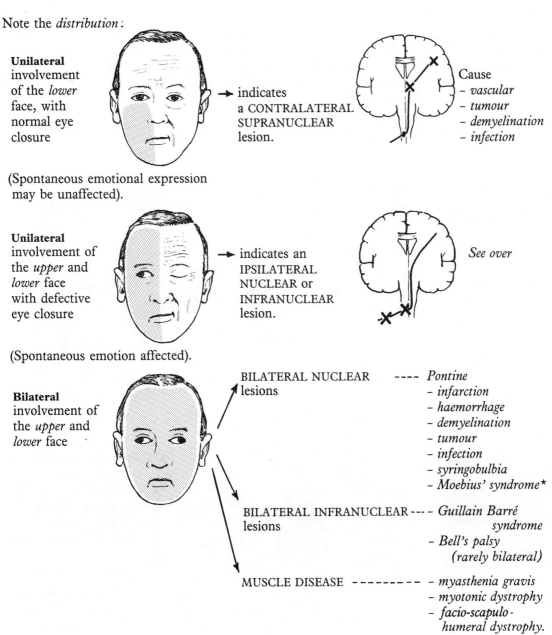

Unilateral involvement of the *lower* face, with normal eye closure

→ indicates a CONTRALATERAL SUPRANUCLEAR lesion.

Cause
- *vascular*
- *tumour*
- *demyelination*
- *infection*

(Spontaneous emotional expression may be unaffected).

Unilateral involvement of the *upper* and *lower* face with defective eye closure

→ indicates an IPSILATERAL NUCLEAR or INFRANUCLEAR lesion.

See over

(Spontaneous emotion affected).

Bilateral involvement of the *upper* and *lower* face

BILATERAL NUCLEAR lesions ---- *Pontine*
- *infarction*
- *haemorrhage*
- *demyelination*
- *tumour*
- *infection*
- *syringobulbia*
- *Moebius' syndrome*★

BILATERAL INFRANUCLEAR lesions ---- *Guillain Barré syndrome*
- *Bell's palsy (rarely bilateral)*

MUSCLE DISEASE -------- *myasthenia gravis*
- *myotonic dystrophy*
- *facio-scapulo-humeral dystrophy.*

★Moebius' syndrome: a congenital failure of the development of the facial and abducens nuclei (bilateral).

Facial Weakness

NUCLEAR / INFRANUCLEAR LESIONS.

The following features (if present) help in lesion location:

– VI nerve palsy → PONS
– contralateral   – *vascular*
    limb weakness   – *demyelination*
       – *tumour*
       – *encephalitis*
       – *syringobulbia*
       – *motor neurone*
         disease

– V,VIII,(IX,X,XI) → CEREBELLO-PONTINE
   nerve palsies.   ANGLE or INTERNAL
– loss of taste, salivation.   AUDITORY MEATUS
   and lacrimation   – *acoustic tumours*
– hyperacusis   – *meningioma*
       – *epidermoid*
       – *glomus jugulare*
         tumour

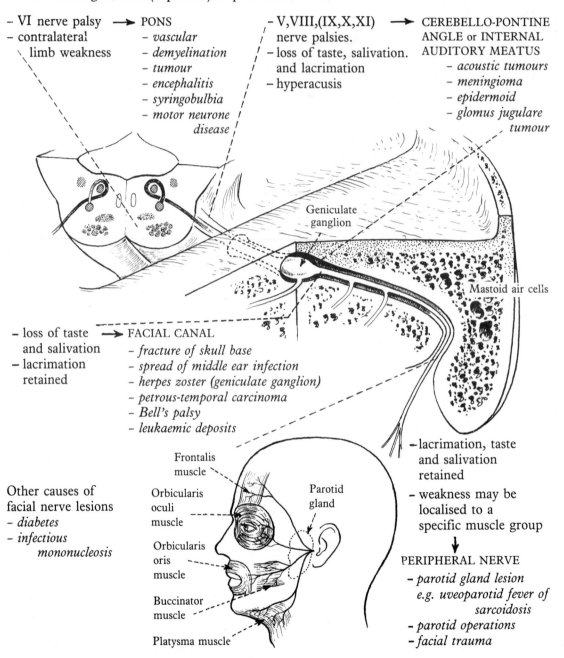

Geniculate ganglion

Mastoid air cells

– loss of taste → FACIAL CANAL
   and salivation   – *fracture of skull base*
– lacrimation   – *spread of middle ear infection*
   retained   – *herpes zoster (geniculate ganglion)*
       – *petrous-temporal carcinoma*
       – *Bell's palsy*
       – *leukaemic deposits*

– lacrimation, taste
   and salivation
   retained
– weakness may be
   localised to a
   specific muscle group
       ↓
PERIPHERAL NERVE
   – *parotid gland lesion*
     e.g. uveoparotid fever of
           sarcoidosis
   – *parotid operations*
   – *facial trauma*

Other causes of
facial nerve lesions
– *diabetes*
– *infectious*
    mononucleosis

Frontalis muscle

Orbicularis oculi muscle

Parotid gland

Orbicularis oris muscle

Buccinator muscle

Platysma muscle

Bell's Palsy

Bell's palsy is an acute paralysis of the face related to 'inflammation' and swelling of the facial nerve within the facial canal or at the stylomastoid foramen. It is usually unilateral, rarely bilateral, and may occur repetitively. In some, a family history of the condition is evident.

Aetiology: – unknown, but most suggest a viral origin, possibly herpes simplex; epidemics of Bell's palsy occur sporadically.

Symptoms: – pain of variable intensity behind an ear precedes weakness, which develops over a 48 hour period.

    Impairment of taste, hyperacusis and salivation depend on the extent of inflammation and will be lost in more severe cases. Lacrimation is seldom affected.

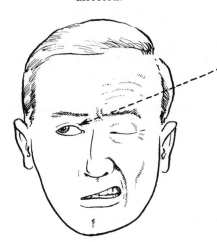

On attempting to close the eyes and show the teeth, the one eye does not close and the eyeball rotates upwards and outwards – Bell's phenomenon (normal eyeball movement on eye closure).

Treatment:

    During the acute stage protect the exposed eye during sleep.

    Prednisolone given in high dosage in the acute stage (40–60 mg per day for 5 days) may reduce inflammation, but there is no conclusive evidence of benefit.

Prognosis:

    Most patients (80%) recover in 4–8 weeks. In the remainder, residual facial asymmetry may require corrective surgery.

    Occasionally aberrant reinnervation – jaw winking (winking the eye when chewing/speaking) or lacrimation while eating may occur.

Other Facial Nerve Disorders

RAMSAY HUNT SYNDROME

Herpes zoster infection of the geniculate (facial) ganglion causes sudden severe facial weakness with a typical zoster vesicular eruption within the external auditory meatus. Pain is a major feature and may precede the facial weakness, and serosanguinous fluid may discharge from the ear.

Deafness may result from VIII involvement. Occasionally, other cranial nerves from V–XII are also affected.

Treatment:

Antiviral agents (acyclovir) may help, but benefits are uncertain.

HEMIFACIAL SPASM

This condition is characterised by unilateral spasms beginning in the orbicularis oculi and spreading to involve other facial muscles.

Onset usually occurs in middle to old age and women are preferentially affected.

The aetiology remains unknown but 'irritation' from an adjacent blood vessel (or from a tumour) may cause demyelination and 'short-circuiting' within the nerve. Occasionally hemifacial spasm follows a Bell's palsy.

The clinician must distinguish hemifacial spasm from milder habit spasms or tics which tend to be familial, and also from 'focal' seizures selectively affecting the face.

Progression may eventually result in facial paralysis.

Investigations:

A CT scan of the posterior fossa excludes the presence of a cerebellar pontine angle lesion.

Treatment:

Drugs: – Anxiolytics and carbamazopine may produce some benefit but are of no lasting value.

Surgery: – Posterior fossa exploration and microvascular decompression i.e. dissecting blood vessels off the facial nerve, gives excellent results, but carries the risk of producing deafness and rarely brainstem damage. Alternative, less successful treatments include phenol injection or partial section of the facial nerve; these methods inevitably cause some facial weakness.

Deafness, Tinnitus and Vertigo

Deafness, tinnitus and vertigo result from disorders affecting the auditory and vestibular apparatus or their central connections transmitted through the VIII cranial nerve.

MECHANISMS of AUDITORY and VESTIBULAR FUNCTION

Auditory function: the cochlea converts sound waves into action potentials in cochlear neurones. Sound waves are transmitted by the tympanic membrane and the ossicles to the oval window, setting up waves in the perilymph of the cochlea. The action of the waves on the spiral organ (of Corti) generates action potentials in the cochlear division of the VIII cranial nerve.

Vestibular function: the vestibular system responds to rotational and linear acceleration (including gravity) and along with a visual and proprioceptive input maintains equilibrium and body orientation in space. Inertia of the endolymph within the semicircular canals during rotational acceleration displaces the cupola, activates the hair cells and transmits action potentials to the vestibular division of the VIII cranial nerve. Linear acceleration results in displacement of the otoliths within the utricle or saccule. This distorts the hair cells and increases or decreases the frequency of action potentials in the vestibular division of the VIII cranial nerve.

CENTRAL CONNECTIONS

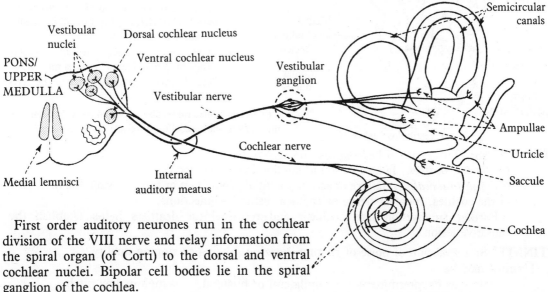

First order auditory neurones run in the cochlear division of the VIII nerve and relay information from the spiral organ (of Corti) to the dorsal and ventral cochlear nuclei. Bipolar cell bodies lie in the spiral ganglion of the cochlea.

First order vestibular neurones lie in the vestibular division of the VIII nerve and relay information from the utricle, saccule and semicircular canals to the vestibular nuclei (superior, inferior, medial and lateral). Bipolar cell bodies lie in the vestibular ganglion.

The cochlear (acoustic) and vestibular divisions travel together through the petrous bone to the internal auditory meatus where they emerge to pass through the subarachnoid space in the cerebellopontine angle, each entering the brain stem separately at the pontomedullary junction.

159

Deafness, Tinnitus and Vertigo

CENTRAL CONNECTIONS *(continued)*

Auditory:

From the cochlear nucleus, second order neurones either pass upwards in the lateral lemniscus to the ipsilateral inferior colliculus or decussate in the trapezoid body and pass up in the lateral lemniscus to the contralateral inferior colliculus.

Third order neurones from the inferior colliculus on each side run to the medial geniculate body on both sides.

Fourth order neurones pass through the internal capsule and auditory radiation to the auditory cortex.

The bilateral nature of the connections ensures that a unilateral central lesion will not result in lateralised hearing loss.

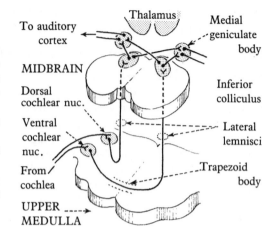

Vestibular:

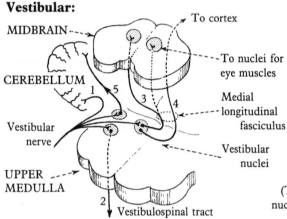

1. Directly to cerebellum.
2. Second order neurones arise in the vestibular nucleus and descend in the ipsilateral vestibulospinal tract.
3. Second order neurones project to the oculomotor nuclei (III, IV, VI) through the medial longitudinal fasciculus.
4. Second order neurones project to the cortex (temporal lobe). The pathway is unclear.
5. Second order neurones project to the cerebellum.

(There is a bilateral feedback loop to the vestibular nuclei from the cerebellum through the fastigial nucleus.)

DEAFNESS: Two types of hearing loss are recognised:
1. *Conductive deafness:* failure of sound conduction to the cochlea.
2. *Sensorineural deafness:* failure of action potential production or transmission due to disease of the cochlea, cochlear nerve or cochlear central connections.

   Further subdivision into cochlear and retrocochlear deafness helps establish the causative lesion.

TINNITUS: a sensation of noise of ringing, buzzing, hissing or singing quality.
Tinnitus may be:
   – continuous or intermittent.   – unilateral or bilateral.   – high or low pitch.

As a rule, when hearing loss is accompanied by tinnitus, conductive deafness is associated with low pitch tinnitus – sensorineural deafness is associated with high pitch tinnitus, except Meniere's disease where tinnitus is low pitch.

VERTIGO: an illusion of movement due to disturbed orientation of the body in space.
The sufferer may sense that the environment is moving. Vertigo may result from disease of the labyrinth, vestibular nerve or their central connections.

160

Deafness, Tinnitus and Vertigo

Clinical examination:

Examination of the external auditory meatus, tympanic membrane and eye movements (for nystagmus) and Weber's and Rinne's tests provide valuable information, but more detailed neuro-otological tests (page 58) are usually required to determine the exact nature of the auditory or vestibular dysfunction and to locate the lesion site. The results of these tests may indicate the need for further investigation (e.g. CT scan),

Causes of deafness:

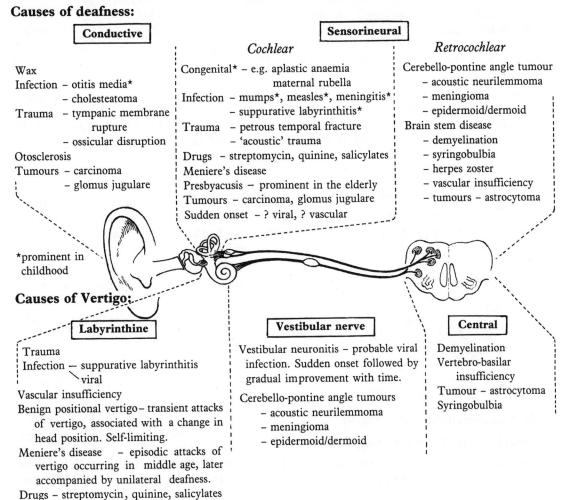

Conductive

Wax
Infection – otitis media*
    – cholesteatoma
Trauma – tympanic membrane rupture
    – ossicular disruption
Otosclerosis
Tumours – carcinoma
    – glomus jugulare

Sensorineural

Cochlear

Congenital* – e.g. aplastic anaemia
    maternal rubella
Infection – mumps*, measles*, meningitis*
    – suppurative labyrinthitis*
Trauma – petrous temporal fracture
    – 'acoustic' trauma
Drugs – streptomycin, quinine, salicylates
Meniere's disease
Presbyacusis – prominent in the elderly
Tumours – carcinoma, glomus jugulare
Sudden onset – ? viral, ? vascular

Retrocochlear

Cerebello-pontine angle tumour
    – acoustic neurilemmoma
    – meningioma
    – epidermoid/dermoid
Brain stem disease
    – demyelination
    – syringobulbia
    – herpes zoster
    – vascular insufficiency
    – tumours – astrocytoma

*prominent in childhood

Causes of Vertigo:

Labyrinthine

Trauma
Infection – suppurative labyrinthitis
    viral
Vascular insufficiency
Benign positional vertigo – transient attacks of vertigo, associated with a change in head position. Self-limiting.
Meniere's disease – episodic attacks of vertigo occurring in middle age, later accompanied by unilateral deafness.
Drugs – streptomycin, quinine, salicylates

Vestibular nerve

Vestibular neuronitis – probable viral infection. Sudden onset followed by gradual improvement with time.

Cerebello-pontine angle tumours
    – acoustic neurilemmoma
    – meningioma
    – epidermoid/dermoid

Central

Demyelination
Vertebro-basilar insufficiency
Tumour – astrocytoma
Syringobulbia

Causes of Tinnitus

Any lesion causing deafness may also cause tinnitus. Occasionally patients perceive a vibratory noise inside the head, transmitted from an arterio-venous malformation or carotid stenosis.

In addition, patients with non-specific disease e.g. anaemia, fever, hypertension occasionally complain of tinnitus.

Disorders of the Lower Cranial Nerves

The NINTH (GLOSSOPHARYNGEAL) CRANIAL NERVE

This is a mixed nerve with motor, sensory and parasympathetic functions.

1. Motor fibres to stylopharyngeus muscle arise in the nucleus ambiguus.
2. Preganglionic parasympathetic fibres arise in the inferior salivatory nucleus and pass to the otic ganglion. From there postganglionic fibres innervate the parotid gland.
3. General somatic sensory fibres innervate the area of skin behind the ear, pass to the superior ganglion and end in the nucleus and tract of the trigeminal nerve.
4. Sensory fibres supply the posterior part of the tongue (taste), pharynx, eustachian tube and carotid body/sinus and terminate centrally in the nucleus solitarius. The cell bodies lie in the inferior ganglion.

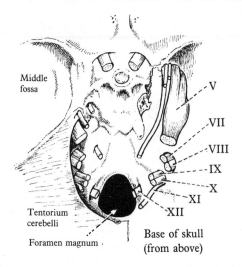

The IX nerve emerges as 5 or 6 rootlets from the medulla, dorsal to the olivary nucleus and passes with the vagus and accessory nerves through the jugular foramen in the neck.

Within the neck the nerve lies in close proximity to the internal carotid artery and internal jugular vein.

The superior and inferior ganglia lie in the jugular foramen, the otic ganglion in the neck below the foramen ovale.

Clinical examination – see page 18.

Disorders of the Glossopharyngeal Nerve

Glossopharyngeal palsy from either medullary or nerve root lesions does not occur in isolation. When associated with X and XI cranial nerve lesions, this consitutes the *jugular foramen syndrome.* Lesions producing this syndrome are listed on page 166.

GLOSSOPHARYNGEAL NEURALGIA

Short, sharp, lancinating attacks of pain, identical to trigeminal neuralgia in nature but affecting the posterior part of the pharynx or tonsillar area. The pain often radiates towards the ear and is triggered by swallowing. As with trigeminal neuralgia, carbamazepine often provides effective relief – if not, intracranial section of the IX nerve roots gives good results.

162

Disorders of the Lower Cranial Nerves

The TENTH (VAGUS) CRANIAL NERVE

This is a mixed nerve with motor, sensory and parasympathetic functions.

The central connections are complex though similar to those of the glossopharyngeal nerve.

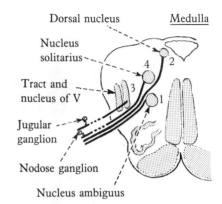

1. Motor fibres supplying the pharynx, soft palate and larynx arise in the nucleus ambiguus.
2. Preganglionic parasympathetic fibres arise in the dorsal motor nucleus. Postganglionic fibres supply the thoracic and abdominal viscera.
3. Afferent fibres from the pharynx, larynx and external auditory meatus have cell bodies in the jugular ganglion and end in the nucleus and tract of the trigeminal nerve.
4. Afferent fibres from abdominal and thoracic viscera have cell bodies in the nodose ganglion and end in the nucleus solitarius. Taste perception in the pharynx ends similarly.

The nerve emerges from the brain stem as a series of converging rootlets. It exits from the cranial cavity by the jugular foramen where both ganglia lie.

Extracranial branches:

Motor and sensory supply to the pharynx.

Superior laryngeal branch of the laryngeal muscles.

Recurrent laryngeal branch.

Supply to thoracic and abdominal viscera.

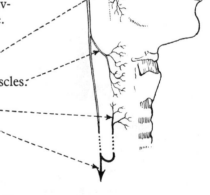

Disorders of the Vagus Nerve cause:

Palatal weakness
- Unilateral – minimal symptoms.
- Bilateral – nasal regurgitation of fluid, nasal quality of speech.

Pharyngeal weakness
Pharyngeal muscles are represented by the middle part of the nucleus ambiguus.
Unilateral – pharyngeal wall droops on the affected side.
Bilateral – marked dysphagia.

Laryngeal weakness
Motor fibres arise in the lowest part of the nucleus ambiguus.
Fibres to *tensors of the vocal cords* pass in *superior laryngeal nerves*.
Fibres to *adductors and abductors of the vocal cords* are supplied by the *recurrent laryngeal nerves*.

Disorders of the Lower Cranial Nerves

Clinical examination – see page 18.

Direct examination of the vocal cords helps identification of the lesion site.

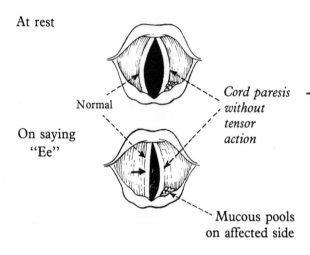

At rest

Normal

On saying "Ee"

Cord paresis without tensor action

Mucous pools on affected side

→ Vagus nerve lesion above the origin of the superior and recurrent laryngeal nerves.

Bilateral damage at this level causes bilateral cord paresis. The cough is weak. Pharyngeal and palatal involvement cause marked dysphagia and nasal regurgitation. Breathlessness and stridor do not occur.

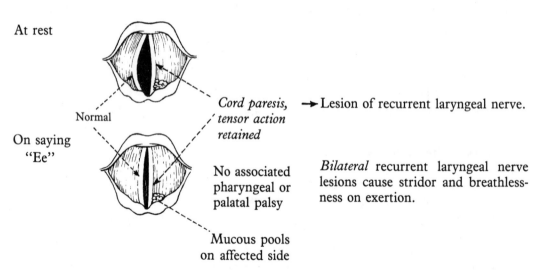

At rest

Normal

On saying "Ee"

Cord paresis, tensor action retained

No associated pharyngeal or palatal palsy

Mucous pools on affected side

→ Lesion of recurrent laryngeal nerve.

Bilateral recurrent laryngeal nerve lesions cause stridor and breathlessness on exertion.

Disorders of the Lower Cranial Nerves

The ELEVENTH (ACCESSORY) CRANIAL NERVE

This is purely a motor nerve supplying the sternomastoid and trapezius muscles.

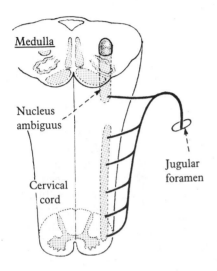

The cranial portion of the accessory nerve arises from the lowest part of the nucleus ambiguus in the medulla.

The spinal part arises in the ventral grey matter of the upper five cervical segments, ascends alongside the spinal cord and passes through the foramen magnum. After joining with the cranial portion it exits as the accessory nerve through the jugular foramen.

The *supranuclear connections* act on the ipsilateral sternomastoid (turning the head to the contralateral side) and on the contralateral trapezius. This results in:
– head turning away from the relevant hemisphere during a seizure.
– head turning towards the relevant hemisphere with cerebral infarction.

Clinical examination – see page 18.

The TWELFTH (HYPOGLOSSAL) CRANIAL NERVE

This is a purely motor nerve which supplies the intrinsic muscles of the tongue.

The nucleus lies in the floor of the IV ventricle and fibres pass ventrally to leave the brain stem lateral to the pyramidal tract.

Since each nucleus is bilaterally innervated, a unilateral supranuclear lesion will not produce signs or symptoms. A bilateral supranuclear lesion results in a thin pointed (spastic) tongue which cannot be protruded.

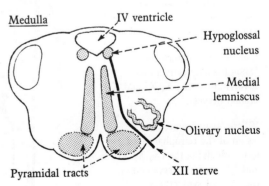

A lesion of the hypoglossal nerve results in atrophy and deviation of the tongue to the weak side.

Causes of Lower Cranial Nerve Lesions

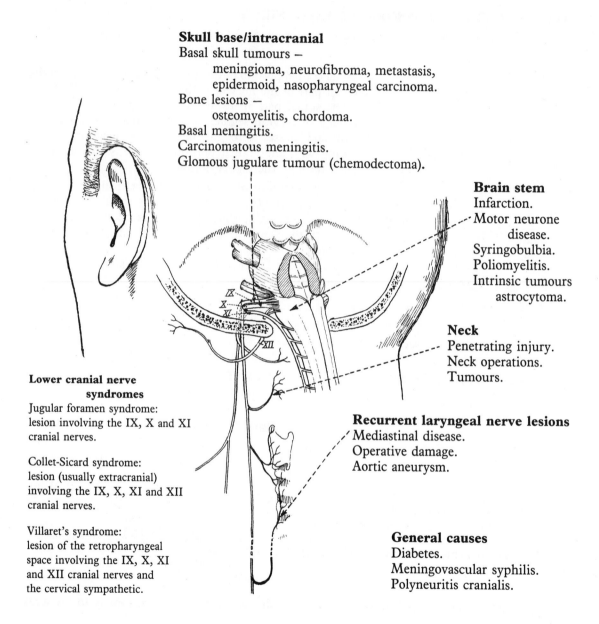

Skull base/intracranial
Basal skull tumours –
      meningioma, neurofibroma, metastasis,
      epidermoid, nasopharyngeal carcinoma.
Bone lesions –
      osteomyelitis, chordoma.
Basal meningitis.
Carcinomatous meningitis.
Glomous jugulare tumour (chemodectoma).

Brain stem
Infarction.
Motor neurone
    disease.
Syringobulbia.
Poliomyelitis.
Intrinsic tumours
    astrocytoma.

Neck
Penetrating injury.
Neck operations.
Tumours.

Lower cranial nerve
    syndromes
Jugular foramen syndrome:
lesion involving the IX, X and XI
cranial nerves.

Collet-Sicard syndrome:
lesion (usually extracranial)
involving the IX, X, XI and XII
cranial nerves.

Villaret's syndrome:
lesion of the retropharyngeal
space involving the IX, X, XI
and XII cranial nerves and
the cervical sympathetic.

Recurrent laryngeal nerve lesions
Mediastinal disease.
Operative damage.
Aortic aneurysm.

General causes
Diabetes.
Meningovascular syphilis.
Polyneuritis cranialis.

Polyneuritis cranialis
  Multiple cranial nerve palsies of unknown aetiology which spontaneously remit. The diagnosis is dependent upon exclusion of other possible causes. Occasionally underlying systemic illness such as lymphoma or sarcoidosis is responsible.

Cerebellar Dysfunction

Anatomy:

The cerebellum lies in the posterior fossa, posterior to the brain stem, separated from the cerebrum above by the tentorium cerebelli.

The cerebellum consists of 2 laterally placed hemispheres and the midline structure – the vermis.

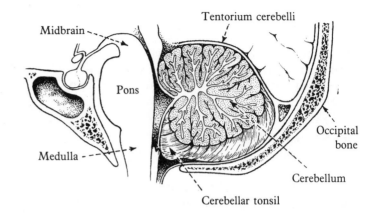

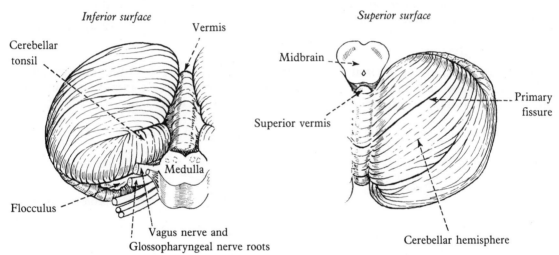

Three major phylogenetic subdivisions of the cerebellum are recognised, although of little clinical value.

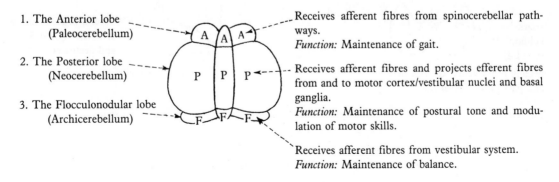

1. The Anterior lobe (Paleocerebellum)

Receives afferent fibres from spinocerebellar pathways.
Function: Maintenance of gait.

2. The Posterior lobe (Neocerebellum)

Receives afferent fibres and projects efferent fibres from and to motor cortex/vestibular nuclei and basal ganglia.
Function: Maintenance of postural tone and modulation of motor skills.

3. The Flocculonodular lobe (Archicerebellum)

Receives afferent fibres from vestibular system.
Function: Maintenance of balance.

Cerebellar Dysfunction

The cerebellar cortex is made up of 3 cell layers. The middle or Purkinje layer contains Purkinje cells. These are the only neurones capable of transmitting efferent impulses. Deep within the cerebellar hemispheres in the roof of the 4th ventricle, lie 4 paired nuclei separated by white matter from the cortex.

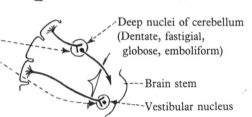

The Efferent System

The Purkinje cells give rise to all efferent axons. These pass either to the deep nuclei of the cerebellum and thence to the brain stem, or to the vestibular nuclei of the brain stem. From there fibres relay back to the cerebral cortex and thalamus, or project into the spinal cord, influencing motor control.

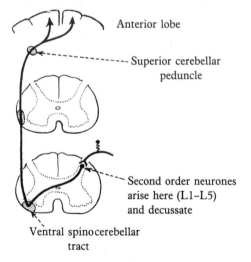

The Afferent System

Connections between the vestibular system and the cerebellum are described on page 160.

The spinocerebellar pathways form a major afferent input. These transmit 'subconscious' proprioception from muscles, joints and skin – especially of the lower limbs.

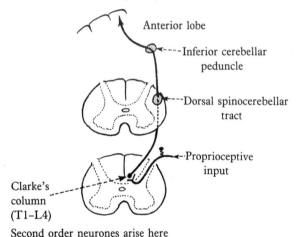

The Dorsal Spinocerebellar Tract

Anterior lobe

Inferior cerebellar peduncle

Dorsal spinocerebellar tract

Proprioceptive input

Clarke's column (T1–L4)

Second order neurones arise here and pass to the dorsal tract.

The Ventral Spinocerebellar Tract

Anterior lobe

Superior cerebellar peduncle

Second order neurones arise here (L1–L5) and decussate

Ventral spinocerebellar tract

The Cerebellar Peduncles: Three peduncles connect the cerebellum to the brain stem:

Superior peduncle	– afferent and efferent fibres.
Middle peduncle	– afferent fibres only.
Inferior peduncle	– afferent and efferent fibres.

Symptoms and Signs of Cerebellar Dysfunction

The close relationship of structures within the posterior fossa makes the identification of exclusively cerebellar symptoms and signs difficult. Disease of the brain stem and its connections may produce identical results.

Damage to midline structures – vermis (and flocculonodular lobe).

Results in: disturbance of equilibrium with unsteadiness on standing, walking and even sitting (truncal ataxia). The patient's gait is broad based and reeling. Eye closure does not affect balance (see Romberg's test). Tests of vestibular function e.g. calorics, may be impaired.

Damage to hemisphere structures – always produces signs *ipsilateral to the side of the lesion.*

Results in: a loss of the normal capacity to modulate fine voluntary movements. Errors or inaccuracies cannot be corrected. The patient complains of impaired limb coordination and certain signs are recognised:

Ataxia of extremities with unsteadiness of gait towards the side of the lesion.

Dysmetria: A breakdown of movement with the patient 'overshooting' the target when performing a specific motor task e.g. finger-to-nose test.

Dysdiadochokinesia: A failure to perform a rapid alternating movement.

Intention tremor: A tremor which increases as the limb approaches its target.

Muscle hypotonicity:

Manifestations: 'Rebound' on displacing the outstretched arm.

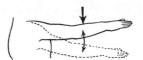

'Pendular' reflexes
– leg swings backwards and forwards when the knee jerk is elicited.

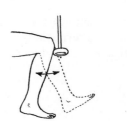

Eye movements:

Nystagmus results from disease affecting cerebellar connections to the vestibular nuclei.

In unilateral disease, amplitude and rate increase when looking towards the diseased side.

Other ocular signs may occur e.g. ocular dysmetria – an 'overshoot' when the eyes voluntarily fixate.

Symptoms and Signs of Cerebellar Dysfunction

Disturbance of Speech:
Scanning dysarthria may occur with speech occasionally delivered with sudden unexpected force – *explosive speech*. Whether dysarthria results from hemisphere or midline vermis disease remains debatable.

Dysarthria, like nystagmus, is an inconsistent finding in cerebellar disease.

Titubation:
Titubation is a rhythmic 'nodding' tremor of the head from side to side or to and fro, usually associated with distal limb tremor. It appears to be of little localising value.

Head tilt:
Abnormal head tilt suggests a lesion of the anterior vermis. Note that a IV (trochlear) cranial nerve palsy and tonsillar herniation also produce this abnormal posture.

Involuntary movements:
Myoclonic jerks and choreiform involuntary movements occur with extensive cerebellar disease involving the deep nuclei.

ASSOCIATED NON-CEREBELLAR SIGNS and SYMPTOMS   These arise from:

- obstructive hydrocephalus.
- cranial nerve involvement.
- brain stem involvement.

(Extensor spasms from brain stem damage may be wrongly described as 'cerebellar fits'.)

Classification of Cerebellar Dysfunction

The following disorders are dealt with in their specific sections.

Developmental
- agenesis.
- Dandy-Walker malformation.
- Arnold-Chiari malformations.
- Von Hippel Lindau disease.

Demyelinative
- multiple sclerosis.

Degenerative
- ataxia telangiectasia.
- Friedreich's ataxia, etc.

Neoplastic
- astrocytoma, medulloblastoma, haemangioblastoma, metastasis.
- non-metastatic cerebellar degeneration.

Infectious
- abscess formation.
- acute cerebellitis.
- acute disseminated encephalomyelitis.
- Guillain Barré variant.

Metabolic
- myxoedema.
- non-metastatic manifestation of malignancy.
- alcohol.
- inborn disorders of metabolism.

Vascular
- cerebellar haemorrhage.
- cerebellar infarction.

Nystagmus

Nystagmus is defined as an involuntary 'to and fro' movement of the eyes in a horizontal, vertical, rotatory or mixed direction. The presence and characteristics of such movements help to localise the site of neurological disease.

Nystagmus may be *pendular* – equal velocity and amplitude in all directions;

or *jerk* – with a fast phase (specifying the direction) and a slow phase.

The normal maintenance of ocular posture and alignment of the eyes with the environment depends upon....

....Retinal input Cerebral cortex

....Labyrinthine input Central connections in brain stem with vestibular nuclei/cerebellum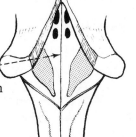

Nystagmus may result from:
- Retinal disease,
- Labyrinthine disease or
- Disorders affecting the cerebellum or a substantial portion of the brain stem.

Examination for Nystagmus

'Nystagmoid' movements of the eyes are present in many people at extremes of gaze. Nystagmus present with the eyes deviated less than 30° from the midline is abnormal.

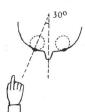

When nystagmus is present only with the eyes deviated to one side – *1st degree nystagmus.*

With eyes deviated to one side and in the midline position also – *2nd degree nystagmus.*

When present in all directions of gaze – *3rd degree nystagmus.*

If nystagmus is detected, note the type (jerk or pendular), direction (of fast phase) and degree.

Nystagmus suppressed by visual fixation may appear in darkness, but this requires specialised techniques (electronystagmography – see page 60) to demonstrate.

RETINAL or OCULAR Nystagmus

Physiological: following moving objects beyond the limits of gaze – Opticokinetic nystagmus.

Pathological : occurs when vision is defective. Fixation is impaired and the eyes vainly search.

Nystagmus is
Rapid.
Pendular (lacks slow and fast phase).
Increased when looking to sides.
Persistent throughout lifetime.

Occurs in *congenital cataract, congenital macular defect, albinism.*

Nystagmus

VESTIBULAR Nystagmus

Nystagmus arises from:

– natural stimulation of the vestibular apparatus – rotational or linear acceleration.

– artificially removing or increasing the stimulus from one labyrinth (e.g. caloric testing).

– damage to vestibular apparatus or the
vestibular nerve.

} creates an imbalance between each side resulting in a slow drift of the eyes towards the
damaged side (or side with the reduction in
stimulus) followed by a fast compensatory
movement to the opposite side.

Physiological:

(i) Rotational acceleration produces nystagmus in the plane of rotation.

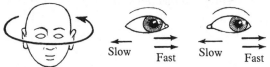

Slow Fast Slow Fast

Slow phase in a direction tending
to maintain the visual image.
Fast phase in the opposite direction.

(ii) Caloric testing sets up convection currents in the lateral semicircular canal producing a
horizontal nystagmus (see page 60).

Pathological:

Damage to labyrinth or vestibular nerve –

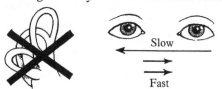

Slow

Fast

| Slow phase to side of lesion. |
| Quick or fast phase to normal side. |
| Rotatory component often present. |
| Turning eyes away from the side of the lesion in-creases amplitude but does not change direction of nystagmus. |
| In severe cases, the nystagmus is 3rd degree and gradually settles to 1st degree with recovery. |
| Enhanced by loss of ocular fixation. |
| Vertigo accompanies nystagmus. |

Often associated with tinnitus and
hearing loss. Vertigo and nystagmus
settle simultaneously.

Occurs in acute labyrinthine disease — *Ménière's disease, vestibular neuronitis, vascular disease.*

POSITIONAL NYSTAGMUS: this may occur in labyrinthine disease in association with vertigo
when the patient assumes a certain posture.

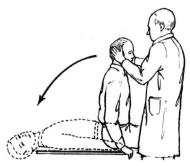

To elicit, suddenly reposition the patient

| After a delay of several seconds, nystagmus develops often with a rotatory component. With repeated testing, the nystagmus fatigues. |

Nystagmus

CENTRAL NERVOUS SYSTEM Nystagmus

Central nystagmus arises from damage to the central vestibular connections in the vestibular nuclei and brain stem. The nystagmus may be horizontal, vertical, rotatory or dissociated (present in one eye only).

> The direction (fast phase) is determined by direction of gaze (multidirectional).
> Vertigo is seldom present.
> Signs of other nuclear or tract involvement in brain stem should be evident.

Central nystagmus occurs in *vascular disease, demyelination, neoplasms, nutritional disease (Wernicke's encephalopathy) and drug toxicity e.g. Phenytoin.*

Posterior fossa lesions may produce *positional nystagmus*. This may be distinguished from labyrinthine disease by:

> Absence of delay before onset, lack of fatiguing with repetitive testing, and a tendency to occur with any rather than one specific head movement.

Although nystagmus often occurs in cerebellar disease, the rôle of the cerebellum in its production remains unclear. The fast phase tends to occur to the side of the cerebellar damage (i.e. the opposite of labyrinthine disease).

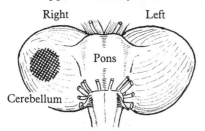

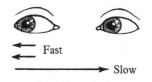

Rebound nystagmus occurs where the eyes 'overshoot' on return to the midline.

DISSOCIATE Nystagmus (Ataxic nystagmus or internuclear ophthalmoplegia)

The median longitudinal fasciculus links, among other structures, the innervation of the lateral rectus with the contralateral medial rectus muscle in order to coordinate horizontal gaze. A lesion of this fasciculus will cause *dissociate nystagmus.*

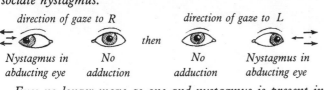

Eyes no longer move as one and nystagmus is present in one eye but not the other.

N.B. Dissociate nystagmus differs from a bilateral III nerve or nuclear lesion in that the pupil is not affected and when testing eye movements individually, some adduction occurs.

Nystagmus

OTHER VARIETIES OF CENTRAL NERVOUS SYSTEM NYSTAGMUS

1. *Downbeat nystagmus*   Occurs with lesions around the aqueduct of Sylvius or cervicomedullary junction. Fast phase is downwards (downbeating nystagmus).

2. *Convergence nystagmus*   Occurs with lesions in upper midbrain region.

3. *See-saw nystagmus*   One eye intorts and moves up while the other extorts and moves down. Occurs with sellar or parasellar mass lesions.

A group of confusing terms are used to describe abnormal, involuntary eye movements seen in cerebellar/brain stem disease:

Ocular bobbing — fast drift downwards, slow drift upwards; seen with large pontine lesions. (Horizontal eye movements are absent.)

Opsoclonus —— rapid conjugate jerks of eyes; made worse by movement. The movements are random.

Oscillopsia is a term used to describe the patient's awareness of jumping of the environment as a consequence of rapid jerking eye movements.

CONGENITAL Nystagmus

This is a mixed pendular/jerk nystagmus present from birth. A family history may be present. Recognition is important to obviate unnecessary investigations.

Tremor

Tremor is commonly encountered in clinical practice; two types are recognised:

1. Physiological tremor
2. Pathological tremor.

PHYSIOLOGICAL TREMOR: a fine, rapid (10–14 per sec.) rhythmical oscillation of part of the body, often not visible to the naked eye and worsening under stress. The basis of 'normal' tremor is poorly understood.

PATHOLOGICAL TREMOR: characterised by its selective distribution e.g. distal or proximal limb muscle groups, trunk or face, a slower rate (4–6 per sec) and its disappearance during sleep.

Diagnosis depends on examination of the character of the tremor as well as the presence of other specific features.

Note the presence of tremor:

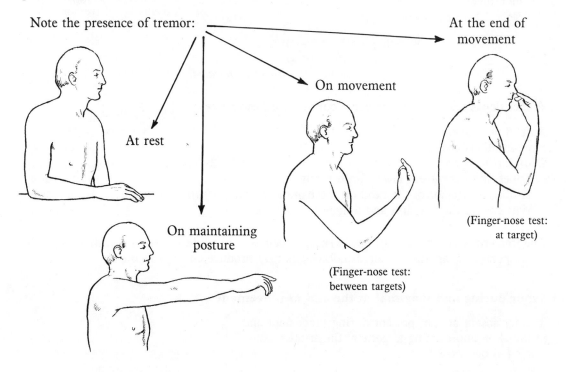

At rest

On maintaining posture

On movement

(Finger-nose test: between targets)

At the end of movement

(Finger-nose test: at target)

Observe:
- the *rate* (slow, <5 per sec), (rapid, >5 per sec).
- the *amplitude* (fine or coarse).
- the *distribution:* face, head, trunk;
  limbs – distal, proximal.

175

Tremor

Characteristics of Pathological Tremor

Tremor at rest

'Pill-rolling' tremor, decreasing
        with movement.
Rate: 3–7 per second.
Amplitude: coarse.
Distribution: distal limbs.

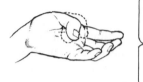

PARKINSONIAN TREMOR

Tremor on maintaining posture and throughout range of movement

Tremor absent at rest, when the limb is relaxed, but present on maintaining a fixed posture and during movement.
Rate: 10–14 per second.

POSTURAL TREMOR
Probably an exaggeration of physiological tremor.

Seen in   – *thyrotoxicosis,*
           – *liver disease,*
           – *drug* and *alcohol withdrawal.*

A specific type of postural tremor occurs with a slower rate.

Occurs with:

Rate: 8 per second.
Slow insidious onset.
Distribution:
    Upper limbs involved, lower limbs rarely.
    Titubation (tremor of the head on the trunk) present.
    May involve the jaw, lips and tongue.

FAMILIAL TREMOR   – Mendelian
                     dominant.
ESSENTIAL TREMOR – no family
                     history.
SENILE TREMOR   – develops
                     in old age.

The tremor may progress until handwriting becomes impossible and feeding difficult. Alcohol may temporarily abort the tremor; beta blockers may produce an improvement.

Tremor during and maximal at the end of movement

Tremor absent at rest; present during movement and maximal on approaching target e.g. finger-nose test.
Rate: 4–6 per second.
Amplitude: coarse.
Distribution: Proximal and distal.
            Titubation may occur.

CEREBELLAR TREMOR
('Intention tremor')

Extremely severe tremor – sufficient to interrupt movement and throw patient off balance.

MIDBRAIN TREMOR
due to disease involving the cerebellar/red nucleus connections e.g. *multiple sclerosis.*

Myoclonus

Myoclonus is a shock-like contraction of muscles which occurs irregularly and asymmetrically.Such jerks occur repetitively in the same muscle groups and range from a flicker in a single muscle to contraction in a group of muscles sufficient to displace the affected limb.

Pathophysiology:

The precise nature of myoclonus remains unclear. Several forms exist, some clearly related to epilepsy; others may be associated with damage to inhibitory mechanisms in the brainstem reticular formation. Myoclonus may result from pathological changes affecting a variety of different sites including the motor cortex, cerebellum and spinal cord.

Clinical features:

Myoclonic movements when repetitive vary in frequency between 5–60/minute. The muscles of the face, oral cavity and limbs are preferentially affected. The movements disappear during sleep and may be accentuated or precipitated by visual, auditory or tactile stimulation. Repetitive stimulation may result in a crescendo of myoclonus which resembles a seizure.

Causes:

Myoclonus occurs in many rare disorders of the nervous system. Three groups of disorder are recognised:

Progressive myoclonus

Familial disorders:
- Lafora body disease.
- Tay Sach's disease.
- Gaucher's disease.
- Ramsay Hunt syndrome.
- Benign polymyoclonus.

Degenerative disease:
- Subacute sclerosing panencephalitis.
- Alzheimer's disease.
- Creutzfeldt-Jacob disease.

Epileptic disorders in which myoclonus occurs.

Hypsarrhythmia.
Generalised seizures:
- associated with petit mal.
- during prodrome of grand mal.
- photosensitive myoclonus.

Lennox Gastaut syndrome.
  (atypical petit mal, drop attacks and mental retardation).

Metabolic disease associated with transient myoclonus:
- Hyponatraemia.
- Hypocalcaemia.
- Renal, hypoxic, hepatic encephalopathy.

Palatal myoclonus – an unusual myoclonic disorder with rapid regular movements of the soft palate and occasionally of the pharyngeal and facial musculature. This disorder is associated with degenerative changes in the olivary and dentate nuclei.

Treatment:
Benzodiazepine drugs such as clonazepam may suppress myoclonic movements.

Disorders of Stance and Gait

The normal gait is characterised by an erect posture, moderately sized steps and the medial malleoli of the tibia 'tracing' a straight line.

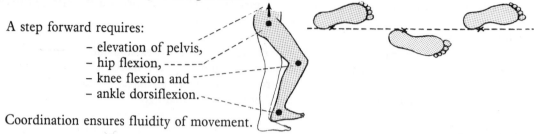

A step forward requires:

- elevation of pelvis,
- hip flexion,
- knee flexion and
- ankle dorsiflexion.

Coordination ensures fluidity of movement.

Antigravity reflexes maintain the erect posture. They depend upon spinal cord and brain stem connections to produce extension.

Assessment of Stance and Gait

In a patient complaining of disturbance of walking, careful assessment indicates the likely site of the causative lesion.

Watch the patient:
- walking
- performing *tandem gait* – heel to toe walking,
- standing with heels together with (a) eyes open, (b) eyes closed – this (Romberg's test) distinguishes cerebellar from sensory ataxia.

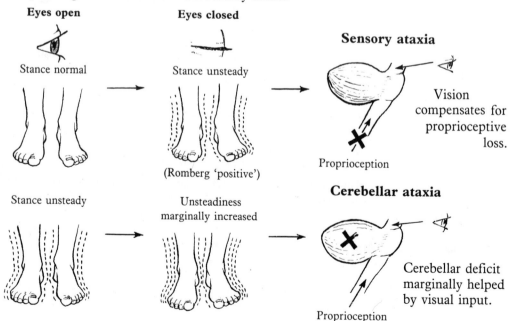

Specific Disorders of Stance and Gait

ATAXIC GAIT

1. Cerebellar   The feet are separated widely when
standing or walking.
Steps are jerky and unsure, varying in size.
The trunk sways forwards.

In mild cases: Tandem gait (heel-toe walking) is impaired;
the patient falling to one or both sides.

2. Sensory

Disturbed conscious or unconscious proprioception due to interruption of afferents in peripheral nerves or spinal cord (posterior columns, spinocerebellar tracts).

The gait appears normal when the eyes are open although the feet usually 'stamp' on the ground. Examination reveals a positive Romberg's test and impaired joint position sensation.

HEMIPLEGIC GAIT

The leg is extended and the toes forced downwards.
When walking, abduction and circumduction at the hip prevent the toes from catching on the ground.

In paraplegia, strong adduction at the hips can produce a scissor-like posture of the lower limbs.

Hemiplegic gait.

PARKINSONIAN (Festinating) GAIT

The patient adopts a flexed, stooping posture. To initiate walking, he leans forwards and then hurries (festinates) to 'catch up' on himself. The steps are short and shuffling.

STEPPAGE GAIT

Weakness of pretibial and peroneal muscles produces this gait disorder. The patient lifts the affected leg high so that the toes clear the ground.

When bilateral, it resembles a high-stepping horse.

MYOPATHIC (Waddling) GAIT

Characteristic of muscle disease.
Trunk and pelvic muscle weakness result in a sway-back, pot-bellied appearance with difficulty in pelvic 'fixation' when walking.

FRONTAL LOBE GAIT

Disturbance of connections between frontal cortex, basal ganglia and cerebellum produces this characteristic disturbance. The gait is wide based (feet wide apart). Initiation is difficult, the feet often seem 'stuck' to the floor. There is a tendency to fall backwards. Power and sensation are normal.

SENILE GAIT

With age, patients adopt a posture of flexion with a short steppage gait (marche à petit pas). A similar gait disturbance occurs with diffuse vascular disease.

HYSTERICAL GAIT

Characterised by its bizarre nature.
Numerous variations are seen. The hallmark is inconsistency supported by the lack of neurological signs. Close observation is essential.

Limb Weakness

Limb weakness results from damage to the MOTOR SYSTEM at any level from the motor cortex to muscle.

ANATOMY

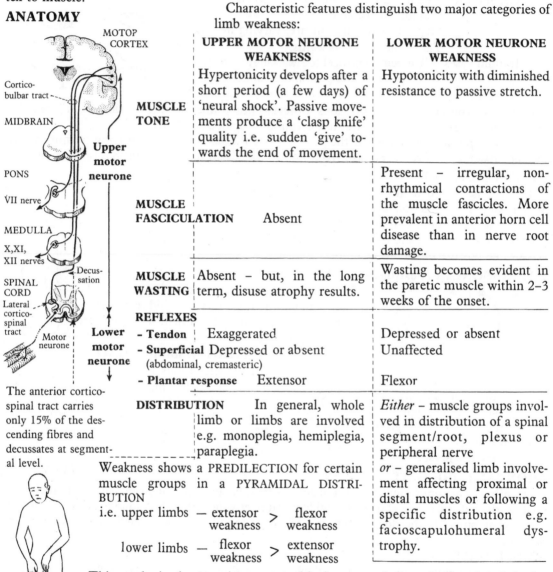

MOTOR CORTEX

Cortico-bulbar tract

MIDBRAIN

PONS

VII nerve

MEDULLA

X,XI, XII nerves

SPINAL CORD

Lateral cortico-spinal tract

Decussation

Upper motor neurone

Motor neurone

Lower motor neurone

The anterior cortico-spinal tract carries only 15% of the descending fibres and decussates at segmental level.

Characteristic features distinguish two major categories of limb weakness:

	UPPER MOTOR NEURONE WEAKNESS	LOWER MOTOR NEURONE WEAKNESS
MUSCLE TONE	Hypertonicity develops after a short period (a few days) of 'neural shock'. Passive movements produce a 'clasp knife' quality i.e. sudden 'give' towards the end of movement.	Hypotonicity with diminished resistance to passive stretch.
MUSCLE FASCICULATION	Absent	Present – irregular, non-rhythmical contractions of the muscle fascicles. More prevalent in anterior horn cell disease than in nerve root damage.
MUSCLE WASTING	Absent – but, in the long term, disuse atrophy results.	Wasting becomes evident in the paretic muscle within 2–3 weeks of the onset.
REFLEXES		
– **Tendon**	Exaggerated	Depressed or absent
– **Superficial** (abdominal, cremasteric)	Depressed or absent	Unaffected
– **Plantar response**	Extensor	Flexor
DISTRIBUTION	In general, whole limb or limbs are involved e.g. monoplegia, hemiplegia, paraplegia.	*Either* – muscle groups involved in distribution of a spinal segment/root, plexus or peripheral nerve *or* – generalised limb involvement affecting proximal or distal muscles or following a specific distribution e.g. facioscapulohumeral dystrophy.

Weakness shows a PREDILECTION for certain muscle groups in a PYRAMIDAL DISTRIBUTION

i.e. upper limbs — extensor weakness > flexor weakness

lower limbs — flexor weakness > extensor weakness

This results in the *'spastic' posture* with the arm and the wrist flexed and the leg extended. In upper motor neurone lesions, SKILLED movements are always more affected than unskilled movements.

NB *Dual innervation* from each hemisphere results in sparing of the upper face, muscles of mastication, the palate and tongue with unilateral upper motor neurone lesion.

Limb Weakness

LESION LOCALISATION

The foregoing clinical features readily distinguish weakness of an upper motor neurone, lower motor neurone or mixed pattern. Combining these findings with other neurological signs enables localisation of the lesion site.

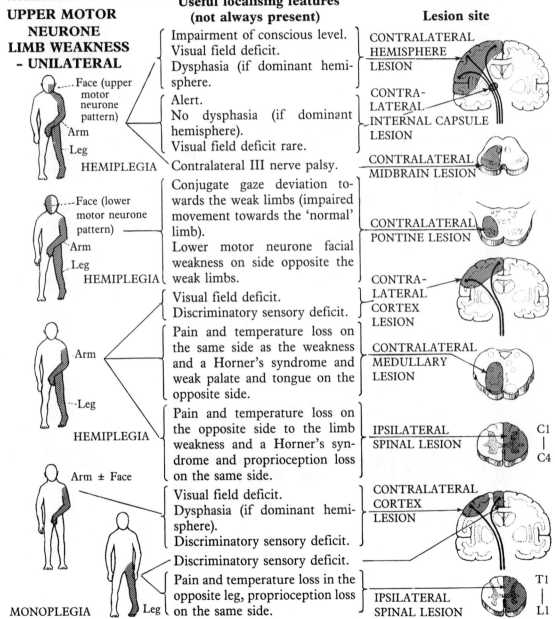

	Useful localising features (not always present)	Lesion site
UPPER MOTOR NEURONE LIMB WEAKNESS – UNILATERAL Face (upper motor neurone pattern) Arm Leg HEMIPLEGIA	Impairment of conscious level. Visual field deficit. Dysphasia (if dominant hemisphere.	CONTRALATERAL HEMISPHERE LESION
	Alert. No dysphasia (if dominant hemisphere). Visual field deficit rare.	CONTRALATERAL INTERNAL CAPSULE LESION
	Contralateral III nerve palsy.	CONTRALATERAL MIDBRAIN LESION
Face (lower motor neurone pattern) Arm Leg HEMIPLEGIA	Conjugate gaze deviation towards the weak limbs (impaired movement towards the 'normal' limb). Lower motor neurone facial weakness on side opposite the weak limbs.	CONTRALATERAL PONTINE LESION
Arm Leg HEMIPLEGIA	Visual field deficit. Discriminatory sensory deficit.	CONTRALATERAL CORTEX LESION
	Pain and temperature loss on the same side as the weakness and a Horner's syndrome and weak palate and tongue on the opposite side.	CONTRALATERAL MEDULLARY LESION
	Pain and temperature loss on the opposite side to the limb weakness and a Horner's syndrome and proprioception loss on the same side.	IPSILATERAL SPINAL LESION C1–C4
Arm ± Face	Visual field deficit. Dysphasia (if dominant hemisphere). Discriminatory sensory deficit.	CONTRALATERAL CORTEX LESION
MONOPLEGIA Leg	Discriminatory sensory deficit. Pain and temperature loss in the opposite leg, proprioception loss on the same side.	IPSILATERAL SPINAL LESION T1–L1

Limb Weakness

UPPER MOTOR
NEURONE
LIMB WEAKNESS
– BILATERAL

Useful localising features
(not always present)

Lesion site

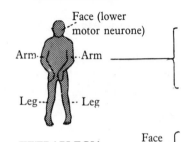

Face (lower
motor neurone)

Arm — Arm

Leg — Leg

Facial movements lost but vertical eye movements retained – 'locked-in syndrome'.

BILATERAL
PONTINE LESION

TETRAPLEGIA
(syn. QUADRA-
PARESIS)

Both arms

Both legs

Face
spared

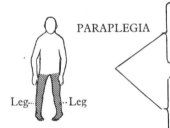

Facial movements retained, but no tongue or palate movement or speech – a variant of the 'locked-in' syndrome.

BILATERAL
MEDULLARY
LESION

Ventilatory support or diaphragmatic respiration (no cranial nerve lesion).

BILATERAL
CERVICAL
SPINE
LESION

C1
|
C4

PARAPLEGIA

Leg — Leg

Discriminatory sensory loss.
'Frontal' incontinence.
(pain and temperature sensation intact).

'Sensory level' – impairment or loss of *all* sensory modalities. Hesitancy of micturition or acute urinary retention.

BILATERAL
THORACIC
SPINE
LESION

T2
|
L1

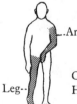

Arm

Leg

CRUCIATE
HEMIPLEGIA

Weakness of the palate and tongue on the side of the arm weakness.

MEDULLARY
LESION
(below
'arm' fibre
decussation
above 'leg' fibre
decussation)

'leg' fibres

'arm' fibres

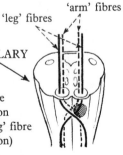

Limb Weakness

MIXED UPPER and LOWER MOTOR NEURONE WEAKNESS – UNILATERAL or BILATERAL

Useful localising features (not always present)

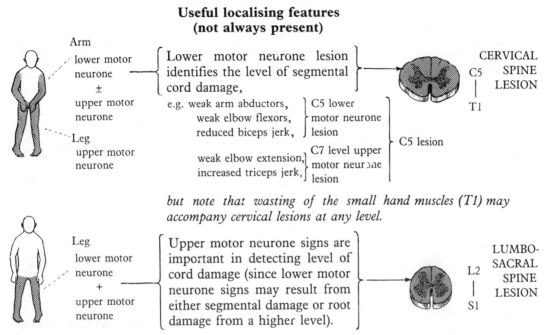

Arm
lower motor neurone
±
upper motor neurone

Leg
upper motor neurone

Lower motor neurone lesion identifies the level of segmental cord damage,

e.g. weak arm abductors, weak elbow flexors, reduced biceps jerk, } C5 lower motor neurone lesion

weak elbow extension, increased triceps jerk, } C7 level upper motor neurone lesion

} C5 lesion

CERVICAL SPINE LESION

C5
|
T1

but note that wasting of the small hand muscles (T1) may accompany cervical lesions at any level.

Leg
lower motor neurone
+
upper motor neurone

Upper motor neurone signs are important in detecting level of cord damage (since lower motor neurone signs may result from either segmental damage or root damage from a higher level).

LUMBO-SACRAL SPINE LESION

L2
|
S1

NB. Dual lesions e.g. cervical + lumbar spondylosis may cause mixed (umn and lmn) signs in both arm and leg.

LOWER MOTOR NEURONE LIMB WEAKNESS – UNILATERAL or BILATERAL

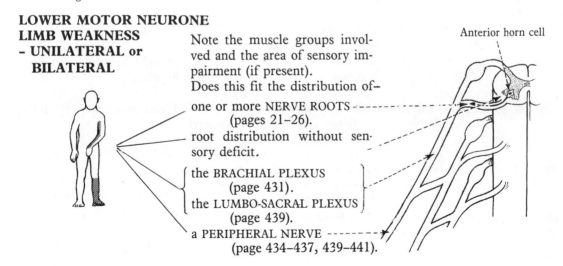

Note the muscle groups involved and the area of sensory impairment (if present).
Does this fit the distribution of–

one or more NERVE ROOTS (pages 21–26).

root distribution without sensory deficit.

the BRACHIAL PLEXUS (page 431).
the LUMBO-SACRAL PLEXUS (page 439).

a PERIPHERAL NERVE (page 434–437, 439–441).

Anterior horn cell

Limb Weakness

**LOWER MOTOR NEURONE
LIMB WEAKNESS
– BILATERAL** *(continued)*

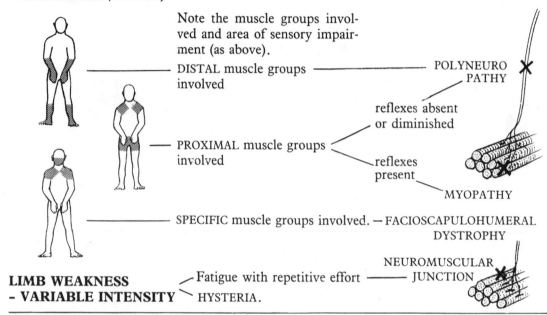

Note the muscle groups involved and area of sensory impairment (as above).

DISTAL muscle groups involved ————— POLYNEUROPATHY

PROXIMAL muscle groups involved

reflexes absent or diminished

reflexes present ——— MYOPATHY

SPECIFIC muscle groups involved. — FACIOSCAPULOHUMERAL DYSTROPHY

NEUROMUSCULAR JUNCTION

**LIMB WEAKNESS
– VARIABLE INTENSITY**
- Fatigue with repetitive effort
- HYSTERIA.

LESION SITE	DIFFERENTIAL DIAGNOSIS	PRELIMINARY INVESTIGATIONS
Cerebral hemispheres, midbrain, pons, medulla	– *Vascular* – *Tumour* – *Infection*	CT scan.
	– *Demyelination*	Visual evoked potentials. CSF oligoclonal bands.
Spinal cord	– *Demyelination* – *Spondylosis/Disc disease* – *Tumour* – *Infection* – *Vascular*	Straight X-ray, Myelography.
Anterior horn cell (± spinal cord)	– *Motor neurone disease* *(progressive muscular atrophy)*	Electromyography (EMG).
Nerve roots	– *Spondylosis/Disc disease* – *Tumour*	Myelography.
Plexus/Peripheral nerves	– *Peripheral neuropathy* – *Trauma* – *Tumour infiltration*	EMG, Nerve conduction studies.
N.muscular junction	– *Myasthenia gravis*	EMG, Tensilon test.
Muscle	– *Myopathy* – *Dystrophy*	EMG, Muscle biopsy.

184

Sensory Impairment

ANATOMY and PHYSIOLOGY

The sensory system relays information from both the external and the internal environment.

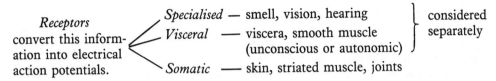

Receptors convert this information into electrical action potentials.

- *Specialised* — smell, vision, hearing ⎫ considered
- *Visceral* — viscera, smooth muscle (unconscious or autonomic) ⎬ separately
- *Somatic* — skin, striated muscle, joints

Cutaneous receptors consist of several types –

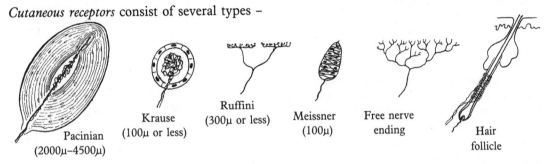

Pacinian (2000μ–4500μ)   Krause (100μ or less)   Ruffini (300μ or less)   Meissner (100μ)   Free nerve ending   Hair follicle

Considerable functional overlap exists. All appear to respond to touch yet some specificity occurs:
Ruffini – warmth.
Krause – cold.
Pacinian – pressure and vibration.

Repetitive stimulation of most receptors results in a reduction in the action potential frequency – ADAPTATION.

CENTRAL CONNECTIONS

Sensory neurones (bipolar cells) relay information to the spinal cord via the dorsal root to the dorsal root entry zone. The anatomical and physical characteristics of the neurones vary depending on the information they carry (see page 417), as do the central pathways:

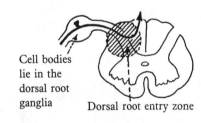

Cell bodies lie in the dorsal root ganglia   Dorsal root entry zone

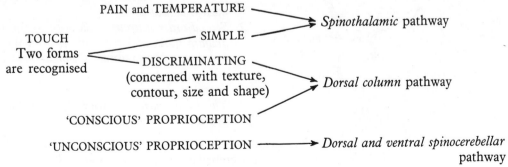

PAIN and TEMPERATURE ⟶ *Spinothalamic* pathway

TOUCH — Two forms are recognised
- SIMPLE ⟶ *Spinothalamic* pathway
- DISCRIMINATING (concerned with texture, contour, size and shape) ⟶ *Dorsal column* pathway

'CONSCIOUS' PROPRIOCEPTION ⟶ *Dorsal column* pathway

'UNCONSCIOUS' PROPRIOCEPTION ⟶ *Dorsal and ventral spinocerebellar* pathway

Sensory Impairment

SPINOTHALAMIC PATHWAY

1. Fibres enter the root entry zone and pass up or down for several segments in *Lissauer's* tract before terminating in the dorsal aspect of the dorsal horn.
2. *Second order neurones* synapse locally and cross the midline and run up the *spinothalamic* tract and *lateral lemniscus* to terminate in the posterolateral nucleus of the *thalamus*. Throughout its course, the fibres lie in a *somatotopic arrangement* with sacral fibres outermost. In the brain stem the lateral lemniscus gives off collateral branches to the *reticular formation,* which projects widely to the cerebral cortex and limbic system and is joined by fibres from the contralateral nucleus and tract of the trigeminal nerve.
3. From the thalamus, *third order neurones* project to the *parietal cortex*.

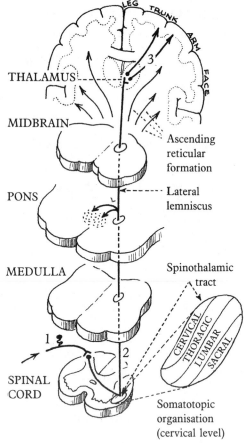

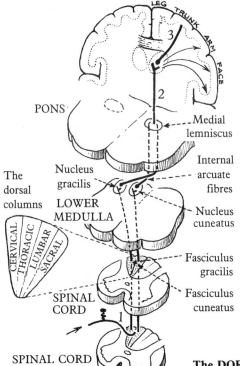

The DORSAL COLUMN PATHWAY

1. Fibres enter in the root entry zone and run upwards in the *dorsal columns* to the *lower medulla* where they terminate in the *nucleus gracilis* and *nucleus cuneatus*.
2. *Second order neurones* decussate as the *internal arcuate fibres* and pass upwards in the *medial lemniscus*. Maintaining a *somatotopic arrangement*, they terminate in the ventral posterolateral *thalamus*.
3. *Third order neurones* arise in the thalamus and project to the *parietal cortex*.

The DORSAL and VENTRAL SPINOCEREBELLAR PATHWAY: see Cerebellar dysfunction, page 168.

186

Sensory Impairment

EXAMINATION of the SENSORY SYSTEM: see page 22.

CLINICAL FEATURES

Sensory disturbance may result in:

           NEGATIVE symptoms: 'a loss of feeling',
                                           'a deadness'.
           POSITIVE symptoms: 'a pins and needles sensation',
                                           'a burning feeling'.

Lesions of the PERIPHERAL NERVES may produce 'negative' or 'positive' symptoms.

SPINOTHALAMIC TRACT lesions – seldom produce pain but usually a *lack of awareness of pain and temperature.*
 	
   This may result in:
   – trophic changes: cold,
                              blue extremities,
                              hair loss,
                              brittle nails.
 	
  –painless burns.
  – joint disruption (Charcot's joints)
	DORSAL COLUMN lesions – produce a *discriminatory type of sensory loss.*
	
	   – impaired two point discrimination.
	   – astereognosis (failure to discriminate
	        objects held in the hand).
	   – sensory ataxia
	        (disturbed proprioception).

Lesions of the PARIETAL CORTEX also produce a *discriminatory type of sensory loss.*

LESION LOCALISATION

The pattern of the sensory deficit aids lesion localisation.

Sensory Deficit	Useful localising features (if present)	Lesion Site
HEMISENSORY LOSS	'Discriminatory' sensory deficit. Sensory inattention (perceptual rivalry) Only minimal pain and temperature loss	LESION of CONTRALATERAL PARIETAL CORTEX
	or selective deficit in face, arm, trunk or leg.	SELECTIVE CORTICAL LESION
	Loss of all sensory modalities including pain and temperature in the face, arm, trunk and leg.	CONTRALATERAL THALAMIC LESION

Sensory Impairment

LESION LOCALISATION *(continued)*

Sensory Deficit	Useful localising features (if present)	Lesion Site

FACIAL SENSORY LOSS — HEMISENSORY LOSS

Loss of all modalities in the limbs (depending on the extent of the lesion.
Loss of pain and temperature on the opposite side of the face with or without 'muzzle' area sparing and a lateral gaze palsy towards that side.

CONTRALATERAL PONTINE LESION

(Ipsilateral to the facial sensory loss)

As above – but lateral gaze normal.
Weakness of palate and tongue on side opposite to the limb sensory deficit.

CONTRALATERAL MEDULLARY LESION

Loss of pain, temperature and light touch below a specific dermatome level (may spare sacral sensation).

CONTRALATERAL SPINOTHALAMIC TRACT LESION

(Partial spinothalamic tract lesion)

Loss of all modalities at one or several dermatome levels.

Loss of pain and temperature below a specific dermatome level.

Loss of proprioception and 'discriminatory' touch up to similar level and limb weakness.

BROWN-SEQUARD SYNDROME

(Partial cord lesion)

Bilateral loss of all modalities.
Bilateral leg weakness.

COMPLETE CORD LESION

'SUSPENDED' SENSORY LOSS

Bilateral loss of pain and temperature.
Preservation of proprioception and 'discriminatory' sensation.

CENTRAL CORD LESION

Sensory Impairment

LESION LOCALISATION *(continued)*

Loss of all sensory modalities in dermatome distribution.

DORSAL ROOT LESION

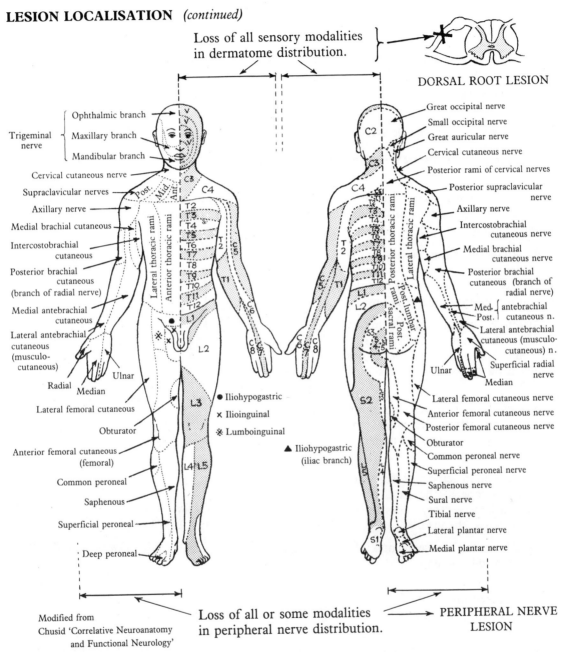

Trigeminal nerve
- Ophthalmic branch
- Maxillary branch
- Mandibular branch

Cervical cutaneous nerve

Supraclavicular nerves

Axillary nerve

Medial brachial cutaneous

Intercostobrachial cutaneous

Posterior brachial cutaneous (branch of radial nerve)

Medial antebrachial cutaneous

Lateral antebrachial cutaneous (musculo-cutaneous)

Radial   Ulnar
    Median

Lateral femoral cutaneous

Obturator

Anterior femoral cutaneous (femoral)

Common peroneal

Saphenous

Superficial peroneal

Deep peroneal

● Iliohypogastric
✕ Ilioinguinal
❋ Lumboinguinal

▲ Iliohypogastric (iliac branch)

Great occipital nerve
Small occipital nerve
Great auricular nerve
Cervical cutaneous nerve
Posterior rami of cervical nerves
Posterior supraclavicular nerve
Axillary nerve
Intercostobrachial cutaneous nerve
Medial brachial cutaneous nerve
Posterior brachial cutaneous (branch of radial nerve)
Med.⎫ antebrachial
Post.⎭ cutaneous n.
Lateral antebrachial cutaneous (musculo-cutaneous) n.
Superficial radial nerve
Ulnar
    Median
Lateral femoral cutaneous nerve
Anterior femoral cutaneous nerve
Posterior femoral cutaneous nerve
Obturator
Common peroneal nerve
Superficial peroneal nerve
Saphenous nerve
Sural nerve
Tibial nerve
Lateral plantar nerve
Medial plantar nerve

Modified from Chusid 'Correlative Neuroanatomy and Functional Neurology'

Loss of all or some modalities in peripheral nerve distribution.

PERIPHERAL NERVE LESION

DIFFERENTIAL DIAGNOSIS – as for limb weakness – page 184.

189

Pain

Peripheral receptors of pain – free nerve endings lying in skin or other organs – are the distal axons of sensory neurones. Such unmyelinated or only thinly myelinated axons are of small diameter. The termination and central connections of these axons are described on page 185.

The type of stimulus required to activate free endings varies e.g. in muscle – ischaemia, in abdominal viscera – distension.

Certain substances – bradykinins, prostaglandins, histamine may stimulate free nerve endings.

These substances are released in damaged tissue.

CONTROL of SENSORY (PAIN) INPUT

The Gate control theory

A relay system in the posterior horn of the spinal cord modifies pain input. This involves interneuronal connections within the tract of Lissauer and the substantia gelatinosa (a layer of the posterior horn).

An afferent impulse arriving at the posterior horn in *thick myelinated fibres* has an inhibitory effect in the region of the substantia gelatinosa.

An efferent impulse arriving in *thin myelinated or unmyelinated fibres* (i.e. transmitting pain) has an excitatory effect in the region of the substantia gelatinosa.

The interaction of these inhibitory or excitatory effects determines the activity of second order neurones of the spinothalamic pathway.

A reduction in activity of large sensory fibres 'opens' the gate. Stimulation of large sensory fibres theoretically 'closes' the gate.

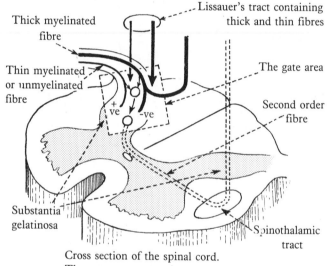

Cross section of the spinal cord.
The gate area connections.

In addition to these segmental influences, higher centres also control the gate region and form part of a feed-back loop.

Pain perception

The awareness of pain is brought about by projection from the thalamus to cerebral cortex. Personality, mood and neuroticism all influence the intensity of pain perception. Diffuse projections through Lissauer's tract and the reticular core of the spinal cord white matter to the reticular formation and limbic system probably contribute to the unpleasant, emotionally disturbing aspects of pain.

Pain

NEUROTRANSMITTER SUBSTANCES

Evidence based on both human and animal studies has shown that an endogenous system, lying within the central nervous system can induce a degree of analgesia. Electrical stimulation of certain sites such as the periaqueductal grey matter can inhibit pain perception.

Receptor sites for endogenous opiates have been found in the posterior horns and thalamus as well as at several other sites. The endogenous substances which bind to these sites are called *encephalins* or *endorphins*.

Substance P, a polypeptide, found predominantly around free nerve ending receptors and in the spinal cord posterior horns is the likely primary transmitter of pain.

DRUG TREATMENT

Sites of potential drug action.

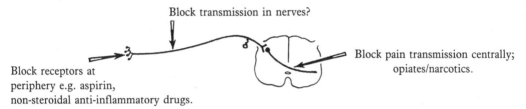

Block transmission in nerves?

Block receptors at periphery e.g. aspirin, non-steroidal anti-inflammatory drugs.

Block pain transmission centrally; opiates/narcotics.

Drug selection in pain treatment depends on the severity, cause and the expected duration of the pain;

i.e. *acute* pain – less than 2 weeks duration
e.g. post-operative,
post-traumatic,
renal colic.

chronic pain – *benign* origin e.g. post-herpetic neuralgia
phantom limb pain
chronic back pain.

– *malignant* origin.

(a) In acute pain drug therapy ranges from *mild analgesics* – aspirin, paracetamol to *narcotic agents* – morphine, heroin. *Tranquillisers* may also help.

(b) In chronic pain of benign origin, narcotics and sedatives must be avoided. In these patients, depression usually plays a rôle and the clinician must not underestimate the value of *antidepressants.*
Anticonvulsants – carbamazepine appears to benefit many patients although its mode of action in pain relief remains unknown.

(c) In chronic pain from terminal malignancy, patients often require *strong narcotics* – morphine, heroin. Frequent administration of small doses provides the greatest effect.

Pain – Treatment

CENTRAL TECHNIQUES:

STEREOTACTIC THALAMOTOMY: The spinoreticular system appears largely responsible for the unpleasant aspects of pain sensation. Stereotactic obliteration of the spinoreticular relay nuclei in the thalamus (page 369) may help patients with intractable pain from malignancy involving the head, neck or brachial plexus, sites where other methods of pain control are limited.

DEEP BRAIN STIMULATION: Stimulation of implanted electrodes inserted in the periventricular grey matter, sensory relay nucleus of the thalamus or internal capsule produces pain relief in some patients.
If successful, a radio-controlled stimulator is implanted subcutaneously. ----------

HYPOPHYSECTOMY: by transphenoidal excision ---------- or with radioactive yttrium benefits pain due to metastatic deposits. The mechanism of relief remains uncertain; this is not merely due to tumour regression.

MEDULLARY TRACTOTOMY: A radiofrequency heat lesion in a hand held or stereotactically implanted electrode inserted into the descending nucleus of the V nerve produces some facial and oral analgesia in patients with intractable pain from head or neck malignancy. The complication rate is high. Few use this method and then only as a last resort.

DORSAL ROOT ENTRY ZONE LESIONS:
Following cord exposure, multiple radio-frequency heat lesions of the dorsal root entry zone are produced with a hand held electrode. This may help deafferentation pain i.e. brachial plexus avulsion, post-herpetic neuralgia, but ipsilateral leg weakness is a major complication.

PERCUTANEOUS ANTEROLATERAL CORDOTOMY:

A percutaneous radiofrequency heat lesion of the spinothalamic tract now replaces open cordotomy. This produces pain relief in 90% of patients in the contralateral limbs. It is usually applicable in malignant states where simple methods of pain control have failed. Risks (ipsilateral limb weakness and respiratory difficulties) are small.

MYELOTOMY: Exposure of the cord and division of the decussating pain fibres produces pain relief on a temporary basis, restricting use to patients with terminal malignancy.

DORSAL COLUMN STIMULATION: Stimulation of electrodes inserted percutaneously into the epidural space may benefit patients with chronic pain, unresponsive to non-invasive techniques. A trial with exteriorised electrodes permits evaluation, prior to implanting a radio-controlled stimulator.

Pain – Treatment

PERIPHERAL TECHNIQUES

NERVE BLOCKS: Injections of agents into peripheral nerves or roots abolishes pain in the appropriate dermatome; motor and sympathetic function are also lost. Local anaesthetics produce a temporary effect; neurolytic agents e.g. phenol, alcohol, give permanent results.

– *Intraspinal* – phenol or hypertonic saline for chronic pain usually used in patients with terminal malignancy.

– *Epidural* – local anaesthetic produces temporary analgesia. Narcotic infusion appears useful for controlling postoperative pain and intractable pain in patients with terminal malignancy.

– *Sympathetic ganglion or trunk*
  – local anaesthetic or neurolytic agent often helps causalgic pain.

– *Paravertebral or peripheral nerve*
  – local anaesthetics may benefit temporary pain states e.g. fractured rib, but neurolytic agents often cause a painful neuritis.

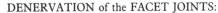

DORSAL RHIZOTOMY:
Division of the dorsal roots via a laminectomy has a high failure rate and provides only short lasting benefit. Now seldom performed.

ACUPUNCTURE:
Insertion and rotation of needles in specific cutaneous points appears to produce slight analgesia in acute pain. Long term results in chronic pain are disappointing. Although endorphin release occurs, the rôle of the placebo effect remains unclear.

DENERVATION of the FACET JOINTS:
A percutaneous radiofrequency heat lesion applied to the posterior ramus of the spinal nerves exiting from the intervertebral foramen, denervates the facet joints. A preliminary test injection of local anaesthetic serves as a useful diagnostic procedure.
This technique relieves facet joint pains in the majority of patients, but as the nerve regenerates, pain returns unless preventative measures are adopted.

TRANSCUTANEOUS ELECTRICAL NERVE STIMULATION (TENS):
Prolonged electrical stimulation over the affected site often alleviates pain of peripheral origin. This technique acts either by stimulating large diameter fibres, thus closing the 'gate' at the dorsal root entry zone or via higher centres.

Pain Syndromes

Pain is not primarily a pathological phenomenon but serves a protective function. Conditions with a pathological loss of pain perception exemplify this, resulting in frequent injuries, burns and subsequent mutilations e.g. syringomyelia, hereditary sensory neuropathy, congenital insensitivity to pain.

Pain may however be pathological – as a symptom of cancer, injury or other disease.

The following conditions produce characteristic pain syndromes.

CAUSALGIA

Causalgia is an incomplete peripheral nerve injury producing intense, continuous, burning pain. Touching the limb aggravates the pain, and the patient resents any interference or attempt at limb mobilisation. The skin becomes red, warm and swollen.

Theoretical mechanism

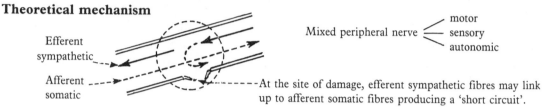

Causalgia only occurs with damage to peripheral nerves containing a large number of sympathetic fibres, and responds in part to sympathetic blockade (pharmacological or surgical).

POST-HERPETIC NEURALGIA

Following activation of a latent infection with varicella zoster virus lying dormant in the dorsal root or gasserian ganglion, the patient develops a burning, constant pain with severe, sharp paroxysmal twinges over the area supplied by the affected sensory neurones. Touch exacerbates the pain. Thick myelinated fibres are preferentially damaged, possibly opening the 'gate'.

Treatment of post-herpetic neuralgia is particularly difficult. Carbamazepine and/or antidepressants may help. Ethylchloride spray over the affected area provides temporary relief and percutaneous cordotomy benefits some patients. Dorsal root entry zone lesions in this condition await evaluation.

THALAMIC PAIN

Thalamic stimulation may produce or abolish pain depending upon the electrode site. A vascular accident which involves the inhibitory portion of the thalamus may result in pain – the thalamic syndrome – described by Déjèrine and Roussy (the Déjèrine-Roussy Syndrome).

Clinical features Hemianaesthesia at onset precedes the development of pain contralateral to the lesion. The pain is burning and diffuse, and exacerbated by the touch of clothing.

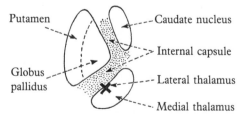

Drug treatment gives poor results. A stereotactic procedure although increasing the sensory deficit may help.

Paradoxically the thalamic syndrome may occur following a thalamic stereotactic procedure for movement disorders.

Pain Syndromes

PHANTOM LIMB PAIN

Following amputation of a limb, 10% of patients develop pain with a continuous persistent burning quality, caused by neuroma formation in the stump. The patient 'feels' the pain arising from some point on the missing limb (the pain input projects through pathways which retain the topographical image of the absent limb).

Treatment: as for post-herpetic neuralgia: – no specific treatment.

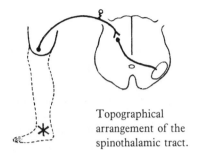

Topographical arrangement of the spinothalamic tract.

VISCERAL and REFERRED PAIN

Deep visceral pain is dull and boring; it is the consequence of distension or traction on free nerve endings.

Referred pain of a dull quality relates to a specific area of the body surface – often hypersensitive to touch.

The basis of referred pain

The visceral afferents converge upon the same cells in the posterior horns as the somatic efferents. The patient 'projects' pain from the viscera to the area supplied by corresponding somatic afferent fibres.

A knowledge of the source of referred pain is important in diagnosis and treatment.

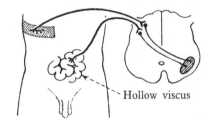

Hollow viscus

SITES OF REFERRED PAIN FROM SPECIFIC ORGANS

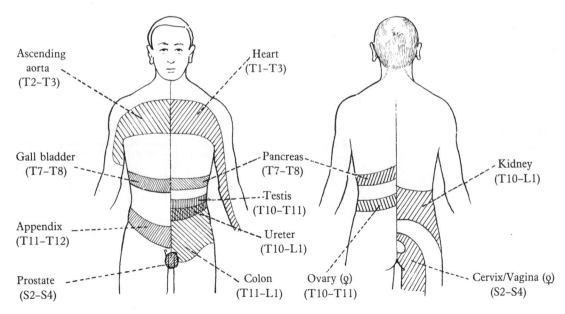

Ascending aorta (T2–T3)

Heart (T1–T3)

Gall bladder (T7–T8)

Pancreas (T7–T8)

Testis (T10–T11)

Kidney (T10–L1)

Appendix (T11–T12)

Ureter (T10–L1)

Prostate (S2–S4)

Colon (T11–L1)

Ovary (♀) (T10–T11)

Cervix/Vagina (♀) (S2–S4)

Limb Pain

Pain may arise from any anatomical structure within the limb. Each produces characteristic features:

BONE – diffuse, aching pain
± palpable mass.

JOINTS – pain localised to affected joint.
– tenderness on palpation.
– movements restricted and painful.
– wasting of surrounding muscles may follow.

MUSCLES – pain localised to specific muscle.
± wasting and weakness.
± palpable mass.

TENDONS – pain localised to swollen, tender tendon sheath.

BLOOD VESSELS – pain brought on by exertion (claudication), relieved by rest.
– pain at rest in pale, pulseless limb (occlusion).
– pain associated with paraesthesia and digital pallor (Raynaud's).

NERVE ROOT – pain increased by coughing or by movement
± associated neurological deficit.

PLEXUS or PERIPHERAL NERVE – burning pain
± sweating, cyanosis and oedema of extremity.
± associated neurological deficit.

Causes of Upper Limb Pain

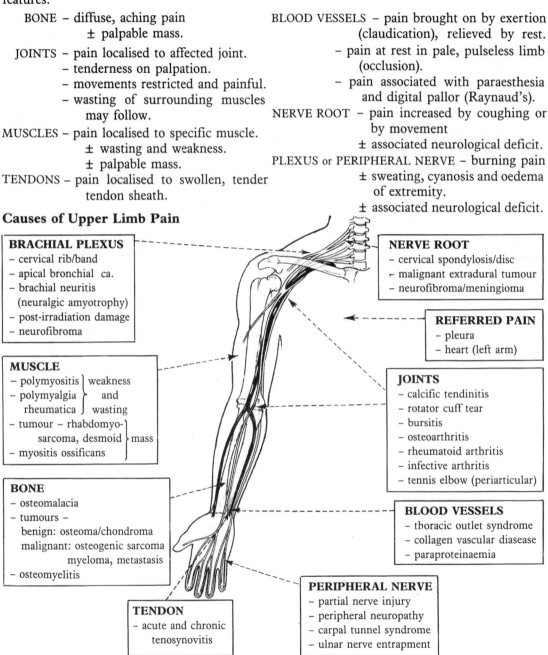

BRACHIAL PLEXUS
- cervical rib/band
- apical bronchial ca.
- brachial neuritis (neuralgic amyotrophy)
- post-irradiation damage
- neurofibroma

MUSCLE
- polymyositis ⎫ weakness
- polymyalgia ⎬ and
  rheumatica ⎭ wasting
- tumour – rhabdomyo- ⎫
  sarcoma, desmoid ⎬ mass
- myositis ossificans ⎭

BONE
- osteomalacia
- tumours –
  benign: osteoma/chondroma
  malignant: osteogenic sarcoma
      myeloma, metastasis
- osteomyelitis

TENDON
- acute and chronic tenosynovitis

NERVE ROOT
- cervical spondylosis/disc
- malignant extradural tumour
- neurofibroma/meningioma

REFERRED PAIN
- pleura
- heart (left arm)

JOINTS
- calcific tendinitis
- rotator cuff tear
- bursitis
- osteoarthritis
- rheumatoid arthritis
- infective arthritis
- tennis elbow (periarticular)

BLOOD VESSELS
- thoracic outlet syndrome
- collagen vascular diasease
- paraproteinaemia

PERIPHERAL NERVE
- partial nerve injury
- peripheral neuropathy
- carpal tunnel syndrome
- ulnar nerve entrapment

Limb Pain

Causes of Lower Limb Pain

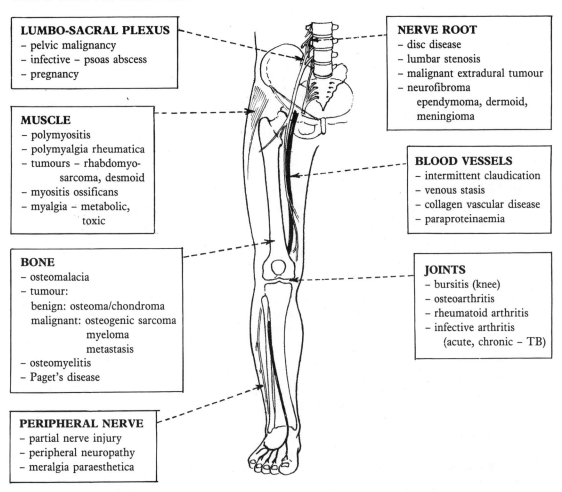

LUMBO-SACRAL PLEXUS
- pelvic malignancy
- infective – psoas abscess
- pregnancy

MUSCLE
- polymyositis
- polymyalgia rheumatica
- tumours – rhabdomyo-
        sarcoma, desmoid
- myositis ossificans
- myalgia – metabolic,
        toxic

BONE
- osteomalacia
- tumour:
    benign: osteoma/chondroma
    malignant: osteogenic sarcoma
                myeloma
                metastasis
- osteomyelitis
- Paget's disease

PERIPHERAL NERVE
- partial nerve injury
- peripheral neuropathy
- meralgia paraesthetica

NERVE ROOT
- disc disease
- lumbar stenosis
- malignant extradural tumour
- neurofibroma
        ependymoma, dermoid,
        meningioma

BLOOD VESSELS
- intermittent claudication
- venous stasis
- collagen vascular disease
- paraproteinaemia

JOINTS
- bursitis (knee)
- osteoarthritis
- rheumatoid arthritis
- infective arthritis
        (acute, chronic – TB)

Meralgia paraesthetica: burning, tingling pain over the outer aspect of the thigh, increased when standing or by walking, due to a localised neuritis of the lateral cutaneous nerve of the thigh. A patch of sensory impairment may be evident over the outer aspect of the thigh.

Ekbom's syndrome: (syn. Restless legs syndrome): intolerable tingling, burning sensation or pain in both legs, occurring only when sitting or lying down and relieved by walking; no associated neurological abnormality.

Investigation of limb pain depends on the suspected cause and may include straight X-rays, myelography, nerve conduction studies and EMG.

Muscle Pain

The basis of muscle pain is normally ischaemia. Reduction of blood flow results in the accumulation of prostaglandins, histamine, serotonin and other substances which, along with a fall in pH, probably stimulate free nerve ending receptors. Swelling of muscle fibres will similarly evoke pain.

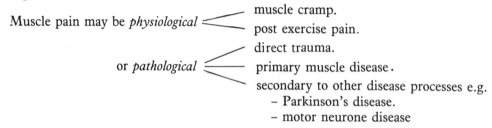

Muscle pain may be *physiological*
- muscle cramp.
- post exercise pain.

or *pathological*
- direct trauma.
- primary muscle disease.
- secondary to other disease processes e.g.
  - Parkinson's disease.
  - motor neurone disease

DISORDERS of MUSCLE RESULTING in PAIN

Pain occurs in conditions in which muscle fibres are actively damaged, or blood supply and metabolism are significantly impaired.

Inflammatory myopathies: (see page 458)

Polymyalgia rheumatica

Proximal severe shoulder girdle pain occurring in elderly people, often associated with giant cell arteritis. The ESR is elevated but EMG and muscle enzyme estimations are normal. Muscle biopsy shows loss of type II muscle fibres. Steroids produce a dramatic response.

DRUG INDUCED

Drugs – opiates, antimitotics (vincristine), cimetidine and clofibrate may cause severe pain and muscle tenderness, with elevated muscle enzymes and breakdown products (myoglobin) in the urine from extensive muscle necrosis. Recovery is usually complete. Alcohol abuse (binge drinking) can produce a similar picture.

IDIOPATHIC PAROXYSMAL MYOGLOBINURIA

Intermittent episodes of muscle cell damage with myoglobin in the urine, occurring spontaneously or precipitated by exercise. Drugs and alcohol should be excluded. Recovery between attacks is complete.

MALIGNANT HYPERPYREXIA

Characterised by a sudden rise in body temperature while undergoing a general anaesthetic, usually with halothane. Cardiac failure may result in death. In survivors, muscle pain due to extensive necrosis with myoglobinuria follows. Certain hereditary myopathic disorders e.g. myotonic dystrophy, central core disease, show a tendency to develop this severe problem.

DISORDERS of MUSCLE METABOLISM

The enzyme deficiency disorders (page 463) are characterised by the development of muscle pain following moderate exertion and relieved by rest.

Muscle Pain

METABOLIC BONE DISEASE

Osteomalacia (common in immigrants with dietary vit.D deficiency) causes muscle weakness, diffuse muscle pain and a waddling gait. Muscle wasting is absent and EMG and muscle enzymes are normal.

Muscle biopsy shows the same fibre type loss as seen in polymyalgia rheumatica.

Confirmation of diagnosis requires serum vit.D estimation. Osteomalacia secondary to renal disease, malabsorption syndrome, hyperparathyroidism and chronic anticonvulsant medication may produce a similar picture.

DIAGNOSTIC APPROACH to MUSCLE PAIN

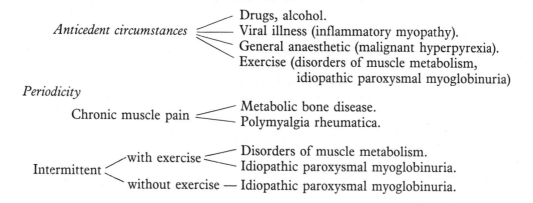

Anticedent circumstances
- Drugs, alcohol.
- Viral illness (inflammatory myopathy).
- General anaesthetic (malignant hyperpyrexia).
- Exercise (disorders of muscle metabolism, idiopathic paroxysmal myoglobinuria)

Periodicity

Chronic muscle pain
- Metabolic bone disease.
- Polymyalgia rheumatica.

Intermittent
- with exercise
  - Disorders of muscle metabolism.
  - Idiopathic paroxysmal myoglobinuria.
- without exercise — Idiopathic paroxysmal myoglobinuria.

A large number of patients referred with muscle pain remain undiagnosed even after extensive investigation.

Brain Death

The advent of improved intensive care facilities and more aggressive resuscitation techniques has led to an increase in numbers of patients with irreversible brain damage in which tissue oxygenation is maintained by a persistent heart beat and artificial ventilation.

In recent years, a Government working party has published guidelines for the diagnosis of brain death, which when fulfilled indicate that recovery is impossible. In these patients, organs may be removed for transplantation before discontinuing ventilation.

The tests are designed to detect failure of *brain stem* function but certain *preconditions* must first be met.

Preconditions:

Depressant drugs must not contribute towards the patient's clinical state – if in doubt allow an adequate time interval to elapse to eliminate any possible persistent effect.

Hypothermia must not be a primary cause – ensure that temperature is not less than 35°C.

Severe *metabolic* or *endocrine* disturbance must be excluded as a possible cause of the patient's condition.

The patient must be on a ventilator as a result of inadequate spontaneous respiration or respiratory arrest – if a neuromuscular blocking drug has been used, exclude a prolonged effect by observing a muscle twitch on nerve stimulation e.g. electrical stimulation of the median nerve should cause a thumb twitch.

The cause of the patient's condition must be established and this must be compatible with irreversible brain damage e.g. severe head injury, spontaneous intracerebral haematoma. *If in doubt, delay brain death testing.*

BRAIN DEATH TESTS

PUPIL
RESPONSE

CORNEAL REFLEX

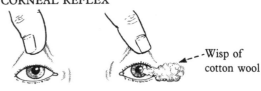

-Wisp of cotton wool

No pupil reaction to light.
N.B. Ensure light intensity is adequate.

No orbicularis oculi contraction in response to corneal stimulation.

VESTIBULO-OCULAR
REFLEX

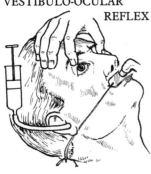

No eye movements occur when 50ml of iced water are slowly injected into the external meatus.
N.B. – Ensure that the external meatus is not occluded with wax or blood.
– Response is not normally expected for 20 seconds.
– Maximal response is obtained with the head raised 30° from the horizontal.

GAG REFLEX

Suction tube

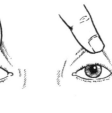

Bronchial stimulation (with a suction tube) fails to produce a 'gag' response.

Brain Death

MOTOR RESPONSE

No motor response in the face or in the muscles supplied by cranial nerves in response to a painful stimulus e.g. supraorbital pain.

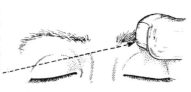

N.B. Limb responses are of no value in testing brain stem integrity. Movements can occur in response to limb or trunk stimulation in a patient with brain stem death but intact cord function, and be absent in a patient with an intact brain stem and spinal cord damage.

RESPIRATORY MOVEMENTS

No respiratory movements are observed when the patient is disconnected from the ventilator. During this test, anoxia is prevented by passing 6 litres O_2 per minute down the endotracheal tube. This should maintain adequate PO_2 levels for up to 10 minutes.

N.B. Ensure that apnoea is not a result of a low PCO_2 This should be greater than 6.65kPa (50mmHg).

Clinician's Status

Recommendations state that these tests should be carried out by two doctors, both with expertise in the field; one of consultant status, the other of consultant or senior registrar status. The doctors may carry out the tests individually or together.

Test Repetition and Timing

The test should be repeated but the interval should be left to the discretion of the clinician. The initial test may be performed within a few hours of the causal event, but in most instances is delayed for 12 – 24 hours, or longer if there is any doubt about the preconditions.

Timing of Death

Certification of death occurs when brain death is established i.e. at the time of the second test. Old concepts of death occurring at the time the heart ceases to beat are no longer applicable.

Supplementary Investigations

Electroencephalography (EEG) is of no value in diagnosing brain death. Some patients with the potential to recover show a 'flat' trace whereas, in others with irreversible brain stem damage, electrical activity can occasionally be recorded from the scalp electrodes.

Similarly, angiography or cerebral blood flow measurement are of no additional value to the clinical tests described above, provided the preconditions are fulfilled.

SECTION IV

Localised Neurological Disease
and its Management

A. Intracranial

Head Injury

INTRODUCTION

Many patients attend accident and emergency departments with head injury. Approximately 300 per 100,000 of the population per year require hospital admission; of these 9 per 100,000 die i.e. 5000 patients per year in Britain. Some of these deaths are inevitable, some are potentially preventable.

The principle causes of head injury include road traffic accidents, falls, assaults, injuries occurring at work, in the home and during sports. The relative frequency of each cause varies between different age groups and from place to place throughout the country.

Head injuries from road traffic accidents are most common in young males; alcohol is frequently involved. Road traffic accidents, although only constituting about 25% of all patients with head injury, are the cause of more serious injuries. This cause contributes to 60% of the deaths from head injury; of these, half die before reaching hospital.

Many measures have been introduced to reduce the incidence, such as seat belt and crash helmet legislation. Once a head injury has occurred, nothing can alter the impact damage. The aim of head injury management is to minimise damage arising from secondary complications.

PATHOLOGY

Brain damage occurs both at impact and as a result of the development of secondary complications.

Impact damage is of two types which may coexist:

1. CORTICAL CONTUSIONS and LACERATIONS.

These may occur under or opposite (contre-coup) the site of impact, but most commonly involve the frontal and temporal lobes. Contusions are usually multiple and may occur bilaterally. Multiple contusions do not in themselves contribute to depression of conscious level, but this may arise when bleeding into the contusions produces a space-occupying haematoma.

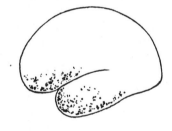

2. DIFFUSE WHITE MATTER LESIONS

This type of brain damage occurs as a result of mechanical shearing following deceleration, causing disruption and tearing of axons. Depending on the severity of injury it may cause immediate mild to severe depression of conscious level and even death.

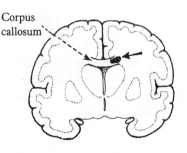

Corpus callosum

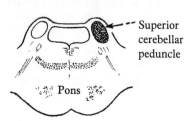

Superior cerebellar peduncle

Pons

The *macroscopic* appearance may appear entirely normal but in some patients coronal sections may reveal small intracerebral haematomas in the corpus callosum or in the superior cerebellar peduncle.

Head Injury

DIFFUSE WHITE MATTER LESIONS *(continued)*

Microscopic evidence of neuronal damage depends on the duration of survival and on the severity of the injury.   After a few days, retraction balls and microglial clusters are seen in the white matter.

 Retraction balls reflect axonal damage.   Note only axons in one plane are involved, indicating the direction of the 'shear'.

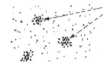 Microglial clusters (hypertrophied microglia) are found diffusely throughout the white matter.

If the patient survives 5 weeks or more after injury then appropriate staining demonstrates Wallerian degeneration of the long tracts and white matter of the cerebral hemispheres. Even a minor injury causing a transient loss of consciousness produces some neuronal damage. Since neuronal regeneration cannot occur, the effects of repeated minor injury are cumulative.

Secondary brain damage may occur at any time after the initial impact. Impact damage is unavoidable but secondary brain damage caused by haematoma, brain swelling, brain shift, ischaemia and infection may be preventable and this must be the aim of head injury management.

1. INTRACRANIAL HAEMATOMA

Intracranial bleeding may occur either outside (extradural) or within the dura (intradural).

Intradural lesions usually consist of a mixture of both subdural and intracerebral haematomas although pure subdurals occur in a proportion. Brain damage is caused directly or indirectly as a result of tentorial or tonsillar herniation.

Incidence of Haematoma	
Extradural ——————— 16%	
Intradural:	
Pure subdural —— 22%	
Intracerebral	
± subdural —— 54%	
Extra- + Intradural — 8%	

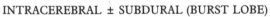

EXTRADURAL

A skull fracture tearing the middle meningeal vessels bleeds into the extradural space. This usually occurs in the temporal or temporoparietal region.

Occasionally extradural haematomas are caused by a ruptured sagittal or transverse sinus.

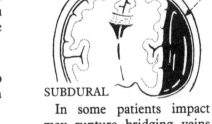

INTRACEREBRAL ± SUBDURAL (BURST LOBE)

Contusions in the frontal and temporal lobes often lead to bleeding into the brain substance, usually associated with an overlying subdural haematoma.

'Burst lobe' is a term sometimes used to describe the appearance of intracerebral haematoma mixed with necrotic brain tissue, rupturing out into the subdural space.

SUBDURAL

In some patients impact may rupture bridging veins from the cortical surface to the venous sinuses producing a pure subdural haematoma with no evidence of underlying cortical contusion or laceration.

206

Head Injury

Secondary brain damage *(continued)*

2. CEREBRAL SWELLING

This may occur with or without intracranial haematoma. It results from either vascular engorgement or an increase in extra- or intracellular fluid, the exact causative mechanisms in different injuries remaining unknown.

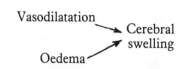

Vasodilatation → Cerebral swelling
Oedema → Cerebral swelling

3. TENTORIAL/TONSILLAR HERNIATION (syn. 'cone')

It is unlikely that high intracranial pressure alone directly damages neuronal tissue, but brain damage occurs as a result of tonsillar or tentorial herniation (see page 76). A progressive increase in intracranial pressure due to a supratentorial haematoma initially produces midline shift. Herniation of the medial temporal lobe through the tentorial hiatus follows *(lateral tentorial herniation)*, causing midbrain compression and damage. Uncontrolled lateral tentorial herniation or diffuse bilateral hemispheric swelling will result in *central tentorial herniation*. Herniation of the cerebellar tonsils through the foramen magnum *(tonsillar herniation)* and concomitant lower brain stem compression may follow central tentorial herniation or may result from the infrequently occurring traumatic posterior fossa haematoma.

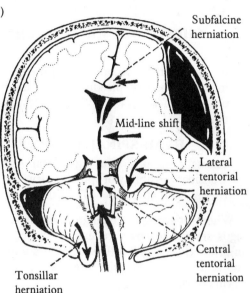

Subfalcine herniation
Mid-line shift
Lateral tentorial herniation
Central tentorial herniation
Tonsillar herniation

4. CEREBRAL ISCHAEMIA

Cerebral ischaemia commonly occurs after severe head injury and is caused by either hypoxia or impaired cerebral perfusion. In the normal subject, a fall in blood pressure does not produce a drop in cerebral perfusion since 'autoregulation' results in cerebral vasodilatation. After head injury, however, autoregulation is often defective and hypotension may have more drastic effects.

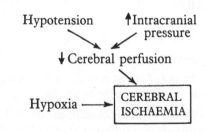

Hypotension ↓Cerebral perfusion ↑Intracranial pressure
Hypoxia → CEREBRAL ISCHAEMIA

5. INFECTION

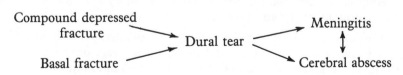

Compound depressed fracture → Dural tear → Meningitis
Basal fracture → Dural tear → Cerebral abscess
Meningitis ↕ Cerebral abscess

The presence of a dural tear provides a potential route for infection. This seldom occurs within 48 hours of injury and may develop after several months or years

Head Injury – Clinical Assessment

MULTIPLE INJURY – PRIORITIES OF ASSESSMENT

Patients admitted in coma with multiple injuries require urgent care and the clinician must be aware of the priorities of assessment and management.

AIRWAY

Check for obstruction and use oropharyngeal airway or endotracheal tube. ⟶

BREATHING

Administer oxygen and check respiratory movements are adequate; if not, ventilate.

↓

CHEST/ABDOMINAL INJURY

Examine chest for possible flail segment or haemo/pneumothorax. Examine abdomen for possible bleeding; if in doubt, use peritoneal lavage. (X-ray chest and abdomen.) ⟵

CIRCULATION

Check pulse and blood pressure. If patient is hypotensive, replace blood loss with plasma substitute followed by whole blood when available.

↓

HEAD/SPINAL INJURY

Assess conscious level and focal signs. Consider possibility of spinal injury. (X-ray skull and spine. CT scan.) ⟶

LIMB INJURY

Examine limbs for lacerations and fractures. (X-ray).

When intracranial haematoma is suspected a CT scan is essential, especially before clinical signs are masked by a general anaesthetic required for the management of limb or abdominal injuries. However, if difficulty occurs in maintaining blood pressure, then urgent laparotomy or thoracotomy would take precedence over further investigation of a possible intracranial haematoma.

HEAD INJURY – ASSESSMENT

Some patients may describe the events leading to and following head injury, but often the doctor depends on descriptions from witnesses.

Points to determine:

Period of loss of consciousness: Relates to severity of diffuse brain damage and may range from a few seconds to several weeks.

Period of post-traumatic amnesia: This is the period of permanent amnesia occurring after head injury. It also reflects the severity of damage and in severe injuries may last several weeks. (Period of retrograde amnesia i.e. amnesia for events before the injury is of less value since it bears no relation to the severity of injury and may improve with time.)

Cause and circumstances of the injury: The patient may collapse, or crash his vehicle as a result of some preceding intracranial event e.g. subarachnoid haemorrhage or epileptic seizure. The more 'violent' the injury, the greater the risk of associated extracranial injuries.

Presence of headache and vomiting: These are common symptoms after head injury. If they persist, the possibility of intracranial haemorrhage must be considered.

Head Injury – Clinical Assessment

EXAMINATION

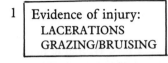

1 | Evidence of injury:
LACERATIONS
GRAZING/BRUISING

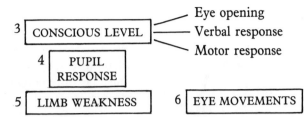

3 | CONSCIOUS LEVEL — Eye opening
— Verbal response
— Motor response

4 | PUPIL RESPONSE

2 | BASAL FRACTURE SIGNS

5 | LIMB WEAKNESS

6 | EYE MOVEMENTS

1. LACERATIONS and BRUISING

The presence of these features confirm the occurrence of a head injury, but traumatic intracranial haematoma can occur in patients with no external evidence of injury.

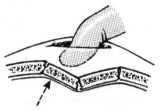

Always explore deep lacerations with a gloved finger for evidence of a *depressed fracture.*

Beware of falling into the trap of diagnosing a depressed fracture when only scalp haematoma is present.

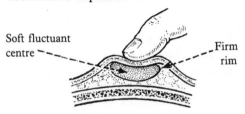

Soft fluctuant centre ---

Firm rim

Consider the possibility of an extension injury to the cervical spine if frontal laceration or bruising is present.

2. BASAL SKULL FRACTURE

Clinical features indicate the presence of a basal skull fracture which may not be evident on routine skull X-ray or even on specific views of the skull base. If present, a potential route of infection exists with the concomitant risk of meningitis.

ANTERIOR FOSSA FRACTURE

CSF rhinorrhoea

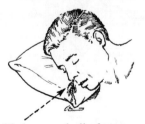

If the nasal discharge contains glucose, then the fluid is CSF rather than mucin.

Bilateral periorbital haematoma

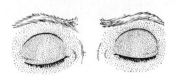

Bruising limited to the orbital margins indicates blood tracking from behind.

Subconjunctival haemorrhage

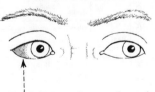

Bruising under conjunctiva extending to posterior limits of the sclera indicates blood tracking from orbital cavity.

Head Injury – Clinical Assessment

Basal skull fracture *(continued)*

PETROUS FRACTURE

Bleeding from the external auditory meatus or CSF otorrhoea.

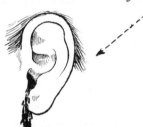

Blood or CSF leaking through a torn tympanic membrane must be differentiated from a laceration of the external meatus.

Battle's sign.

Bruising over the mastoid may take 24–48 hours to develop.

Patients with signs of basal fracture require prophylactic antibiotic treatment for at least seven days or if a CSF leak is present for seven days after this has stopped.

3. CONSCIOUS LEVEL

Assess patient's conscious level in terms of *eye opening, verbal* and *motor response* on admission (see page 6) and record at regular intervals thereafter. An observation chart incorporating these features is essential and clearly shows the trend in the patient's condition. Deterioration in conscious level indicates the need for immediate investigation and action where appropriate.

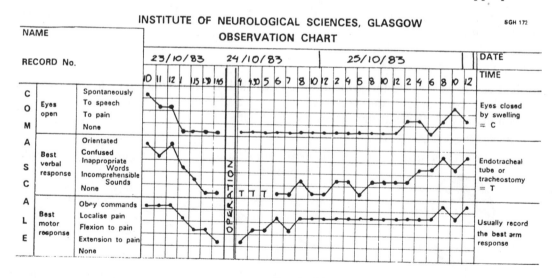

Reproduced by permission of the Nursing Times.

Head Injury – Clinical Assessment

4. PUPIL RESPONSE

The light reflex (page 129) tests optic (II) and oculomotor (III) nerve function. Although II nerve dysfunction after head injury is important to record and may result in permanent visual impairment, it is the III nerve function which is the most useful indicator of an expanding intracranial lesion. Herniation of the medial temporal lobe through the tentorial hiatus directly damages the III nerve resulting in pupil dilatation with impaired or absent reaction to light. The *pupil dilates on the side of the expanding lesion* and is an important localising sign. With a further increase in intracranial pressure, bilateral III nerve palsies may occur.

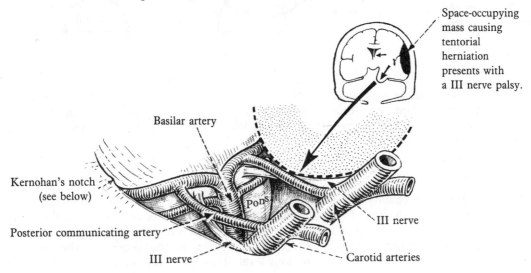

Space-occupying mass causing tentorial herniation presents with a III nerve palsy.

Basilar artery

Kernohan's notch (see below)

Posterior communicating artery

Pons

III nerve

III nerve

Carotid arteries

5. LIMB WEAKNESS

Determine limb weakness by comparing the response in each limb to painful stimuli (page 31). Hemiparesis or hemiplegia usually occurs in the limbs contralateral to the side of the lesion but may also occur in the ipsilateral limbs. This is due to indentation of the contralateral cerebral peduncle by the edge of the tentorium cerebelli (Kernohan's notch). Limb deficits are therefore of limited value in localising the site of the lesion.

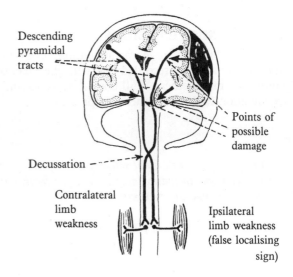

Descending pyramidal tracts

Points of possible damage

Decussation

Contralateral limb weakness

Ipsilateral limb weakness (false localising sign)

211

Head Injury – Clinical Assessment

6. EYE MOVEMENTS

The presence or absence of abnormal eye movements is of limited value in immediate management, but provides a useful prognostic guide.

Eye movements may occur spontaneously or can be elicited reflexly (page 31) by head rotation (oculocephalic reflex) or by caloric stimulation (oculovestibular reflex).

Spontaneous

Oculocephalic (Doll's eye) **reflex**

Oculovestibular reflex

Slow drift

Fast corrective phase

Iced water

Abnormal eye movements may result from:
brainstem dysfunction, damage to the nerves supplying the extraocular muscles or damage to the vestibular apparatus. Absent eye movements relate to low levels of responsiveness and indicate a gloomy prognosis.

VITAL SIGNS

At the beginning of the century, the eminent neurosurgeon Harvey Cushing noted that a rise in intracranial pressure led to a rise in blood pressure and a fall in pulse rate and produced abnormal respiratory patterns. In the past, much emphasis has been placed on close observation of these vital signs in patients with head injury. These changes, however, may not occur and when present are usually preceded by deterioration in conscious level. This last observation is therefore more relevant.

CRANIAL NERVE LESIONS

Basal skull fracture or extracranial injury can result in damage to the cranial nerves. Evidence of this damage must be recorded but, with the exception of a III nerve lesion, does not usually help immediate management. Full cranial nerve examination is difficult in the comatose patient and examination can await patient cooperation.

Clinical assessment cannot reliably distinguish the type or even the site of intracranial haematoma, but is invaluable in indicating the need for further investigation and in providing a base line against which any change can be compared.

Head Injury – Investigative Approach

In the Accident and Emergency Department

X-ray the skull if:

(plus cervical spine, chest, abdomen, pelvis and limbs if required)

– Conscious level is impaired at the time of examination or if the patient has lost consciousness at any time since the injury.
– Focal neurological signs are present.
– CSF leak from the nose (rhinorrhoea) or ear (otorrhoea).
– Penetrating injury is suspect.
– Significant scalp bruising or swelling.

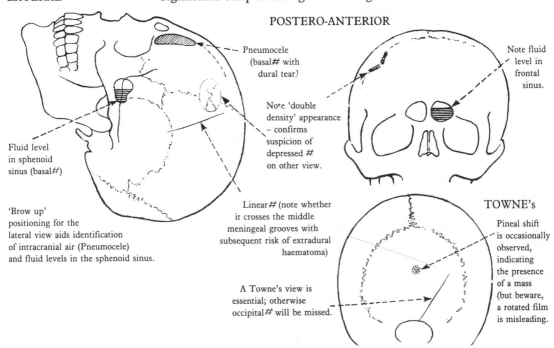

LATERAL

POSTERO-ANTERIOR

Pneumocele (basal # with dural tear)

Note fluid level in frontal sinus.

Note 'double density' appearance – confirms suspicion of depressed # on other view.

Fluid level in sphenoid sinus (basal #)

'Brow up' positioning for the lateral view aids identification of intracranial air (Pneumocele) and fluid levels in the sphenoid sinus.

Linear # (note whether it crosses the middle meningeal grooves with subsequent risk of extradural haematoma)

A Towne's view is essential; otherwise occipital # will be missed.

TOWNE's

Pineal shift is occasionally observed, indicating the presence of a mass (but beware, a rotated film is misleading.

Admission for observation

Patients at risk of developing secondary complications (e.g. intracranial haematoma) require admission, viz: patients with:

– a depressed conscious level (including confusion).
– focal neurological signs.
– a skull fracture (base or vault).
– transitory loss of consciousness or posttraumatic amnesia if unsupervised at home.

IF IN DOUBT, ADMIT.

Risk of intracranial haematoma (requiring removal) in adult attending A and E departments after head injury.		
No skull #	– orientated	1 in 6000
No skull #	– not orientated	1 in 120
Skull #	– orientated	1 in 32
Skull #	– not orientated	1 in 4

Adapted with permission Mendelow et al, BMJ ii, 1173–1176.

Head Injury – Investigative Approach

Neurosurgical referral/CT scan

IMMEDIATE	DELAYED

– Skull# with – confusion
            or focal neurological signs
            or epilepsy.
	– Persistent confusion or focal signs of
	   > 8 hours duration.

– Coma (with or without skull#)
    i.e. not obeying commands, no eye
    opening, no verbal response.
	– Depressed skull # (refer within 12
	   hours)

– Deterioration in level of consciousness
   (e.g. confused verbal response →
    no verbal response).
	– Persistent CSF leak of ⩾7 days
	   duration.

Transfer to the Neurosurgical Unit

Prior to the transfer, ensure that resuscitation is complete, and that more immediate problems have been dealt with (see page 208). If the patient's conscious level is deteriorating, an intravenous bolus infusion of 100 ml of 20% mannitol should 'buy time' by temporarily reducing the intracranial pressure.

CT scan in head injury

Scans must extend from the posterior fossa to the vertex, otherwise haematomas in these sites will be missed.

EXTRADURAL haematoma
– area of increased density, convex inwards. - - - - - - - - - -
Spread limited by dural adhesion to skull.

Mid-line shift with compression of ipsilateral ventricle.

SUBDURAL haematoma – area of increased density spreading around surface of cerebral hemisphere. - - - - -
Subdural haematomas become isodense with brain 10–20 days following injury and hypodense thereafter.

The contralateral ventricle often dilates due to obstruction at the foramen of Munro.

INTRACEREBRAL haematoma –
'BURST LOBE' (± subdural haematoma)
– appears as an irregular area of increased density (blood clot) surrounded by area of low density (oedematous brain).

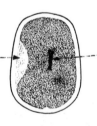

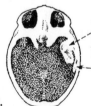

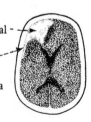

'Burst' temporal lobe

'Burst' frontal lobe

overlying subdural haematoma

Head Injury – Investigative Approach

CT scan in head injury *(continued)*

If *hydrocephalus* is present on the upper scan cuts, look carefully for a haematoma (extradural, subdural or intracerebral) in the posterior fossa, compressing and obstructing the fourth ventricle.

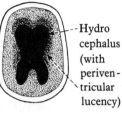

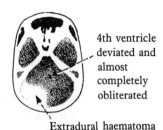

Hydro cephalus (with periven-tricular lucency)

4th ventricle deviated and almost completely obliterated

Extradural haematoma

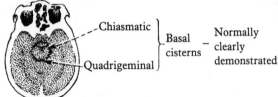

Chiasmatic

Quadrigeminal

Basal cisterns – Normally clearly demonstrated

When no significant intracranial haematoma exists, look for the basal cisterns. Obliteration indicates *raised intracranial pressure.*

With *diffuse shearing injuries* a small haematoma may be detected on CT scan in the corpus callosum or even in the superior cerebellar peduncle.

In some situations, when CT scanning is not available, ANGIOGRAPHY shows displacement of vessels and gives a useful guide to the haematoma site. Failing this, bilateral burr holes are placed in frontal, temporal and parietal sites; even in experienced hands however, this exploratory approach will miss 30% of intracranial haematomas.

Further investigation may be required to exclude other coincidental or contributory cause of the head injury e.g. drugs, alcohol, post-ictal state, encephalitis (causes of coma, see page 81).

Head Injury – Management

Management aims at preventing the development of secondary brain damage from intracranial haematoma, ischaemia, raised intracranial pressure with tentorial or tonsillar herniation and infection.

- Ensure the *airway is patent* and that *blood oxygenation is adequate. Intubation* is advised in patients 'flexing to pain' or worse. *Artificial ventilation* may be required if respiratory movements are depressed or lung function is impaired e.g. 'flail' segment, aspiration pneumonia, pulmonary contusion or fat emboli. Hypoxia can cause direct cerebral damage, but in addition causes vasodilatation resulting in an increase in cerebral blood volume with subsequent rise in ICP.

- A *space-occupying haematoma requires urgent evacuation* (see over). If the patient's conscious level is deteriorating, an initial or repeat i.v. bolus of mannitol (100 ml of 20%) is given.

- Scalp *lacerations* require cleaning, inspection to exclude an underlying depressed fracture and suturing.

- *Correct hypovolaemia* following blood loss – but avoid fluid overload as this may aggravate cerebral oedema. In adults, two litres/day of fluid is sufficient. Commence nasogastric fluids or oral fluids when feasible.

Head Injury – Management

— Administer *prophylactic antibiotics* (e.g. penicillin and sulphadimidine) if clinical findings suggest a basal fracture. If a CSF leak persists for more than 7 days, operation is required.

— *Anticonvulsants* (e.g. phenytoin) must be given intravenously if a seizure occurs; further seizures and in particular status epilepticus significantly increase the risk of cerebral anoxia.

— Consider *treatment of raised ICP*, when cerebral swelling occurs in the absence of a haematoma or in the post-operative period following removal of a haematoma (see below).

[*Steroids:* it is now well established that steroids, even in mega-dosage, are of no benefit in the management of the head injured patient.]

INTRACRANIAL HAEMATOMA

Most intracranial haematomas require urgent evacuation – as is evident from the patient's clinical state combined with the CT scan appearance of a space occupying mass.

Extradural haematoma

Using the CT scan the position of the extradural haematoma is accurately delineated and a 'horse shoe' craniotomy flap is turned over this area, allowing complete evacuation of the haematoma. For low temporal extradural haematomas, a 'question mark' flap may be more suitable. If patient deterioration is rapid, a burr hole positioned centrally over the haematoma may provide temporary relief, but this alone is inadequate to provide a satisfactory decompression.

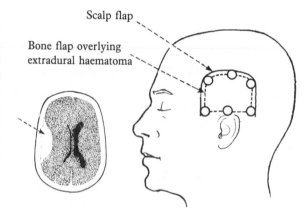

Scalp flap

Bone flap overlying extradural haematoma

Subdural/Intracerebral haematoma ('burst lobe')

Subdural and intracerebral haematomas usually arise from lacerations on the undersurface of the frontal and/or temporal lobes. Again the CT scan is useful in demonstrating the exact site. A 'question mark' flap permits good access to both frontal and temporal 'burst' lobes. The subdural collection is evacuated and any underlying intracerebral haematoma is removed along with necrotic brain.

N.B. Burr holes are insufficient to evacuate an acute subdural haematoma or to deal with any underlying cortical damage.

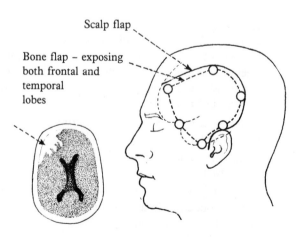

Scalp flap

Bone flap – exposing both frontal and temporal lobes

Head Injury – Management

Intracranial haematoma (continued)

Conservative management of traumatic intracranial haematomas

Not all patients with traumatic intracranial haematomas deteriorate. In some, the haematomas are small and clearly do not require evacuation. In others however, the decision to operate or not proves difficult e.g. the CT scan may reveal a moderate sized haematoma with minimal or no mass effect in a conscious but confused patient.

If conservative management is adopted, careful observation in a neurosurgical unit is essential. Any deterioration indicates the need for operation. In this group of patients, intracranial pressure monitoring may serve as a useful guide. An intracranial pressure of 30 mmHg or more suggests that haematoma evacuation is required as the likelihood of subsequent deterioration with continued conservative management would be high.

DIFFUSE BRAIN DAMAGE/NEGATIVE CT SCAN

A proportion of patients have no intracranial haematoma on CT scan or have only a small haematoma, clearly not causing any mass effect.

In these patients, coma or impairment of conscious level may be due to:

- *diffuse shearing injury*   – suspect if no improvement in conscious level since the impact.

- *cerebral ischaemic damage*
- *cerebral swelling*   suspect if deterioration is delayed – a patient who talks after
- *fat emboli*   impact does not have a significant shearing injury.
- *meningitis*

Several of these factors may coexist and may also contribute to brain damage in patients with intracranial haematoma.

The management principles outlined above apply; in particular it is essential to ensure that respiratory function is adequate.

Fat emboli usually occur 1 or 2 days after injury and may be related to fracture manipulation; deterioration of respiratory function usually accompanies cerebral damage and most patients require ventilation.

Meningitis may occur several days after injury in the presence of basal fractures, but this is rare when prophylactic antibiotics are given.

Cerebral swelling may occur at any time after injury and cause a rise in intracranial pressure.

Head Injury – Management

Treatment of raised intracranial pressure (ICP)

Treatment of raised intracranial pressure (in the absence of any identifiable cause e.g. haematoma or↑PCO_2) is a controversial topic in head injury management. Some believe that active reduction of an elevated ICP significantly reduces management mortality and morbidity. Others feel that if brain damage is severe enough to cause a rise in ICP, then artificially reducing the ICP to normal levels does not alter the extent of the damage, or improve outcome. In adults, there is as yet no conclusive evidence that active ICP reduction improves mortality or morbidity. In children, however, the pathogenesis of raised ICP may differ; some studies suggest that cerebral vasodilatation with a subsequent increase in cerebral blood volume is a major factor, rather than an increase in brain water content (cerebral oedema). If so, treatment of raised ICP may well benefit.

Patient selection: Consider patients with a 'flexion' motor response or worse (a response of 'localising' to pain signifies a milder degree of injury and spontaneous recovery is likely).

Insert a ventricular catheter and monitor ICP. If ICP is high (e.g.> 30 mmHg) this may be reduced by:

— *hyperventilation,* reducing the PCO_2 to 3.5kPa
— *repeated mannitol infusion*   } see page 79.
— *CSF drainage*

These artificial methods of ICP reduction are maintained until the level falls spontaneously to within normal limits. In many patients, this treatment fails to produce a sustained effect and the ICP returns to previous levels or continues to rise unabated until death ensues.

Repeat CT scanning
Indications:

Delayed deterioration in clinical state
or   } In patients with diffuse injury or following
Failure to improve after 48 hours   evacuation of an intracranial haematoma.

Occasionally, small areas of 'insignificant' contusion on an initial CT scan may develop into a space-occupying haematoma requiring evacuation. Following haematoma evacuation, recollection may occur in 5–10% of cases.

Depressed Skull Fracture

This injury is caused by a blow from a sharp object. Since diffuse 'deceleration' damage is minimal, patients seldom lose consciousness.

Simple depressed fracture (closed injury)

There is no overlying laceration and no risk of infection. Operation is not required except for cosmetic reasons. Removal of any bone spicules imbedded in brain tissue does not reverse neuronal damage.

Compound depressed fracture (open injury)

A scalp laceration is related to (but does not necessarily overly) the depressed bone segments. Failure to detect a compound depressed fracture with an associated dural tear is likely to result in meningitis or cerebral abscess.

Investigation

Double density appearance on *skull X-ray* suggests depression but tangential views may be required to establish the diagnosis. Impairment of conscious level or the presence of focal signs indicate the need for a *CT scan* to exclude underlying extradural haematoma or severe cortical contusion.

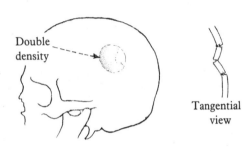

Management

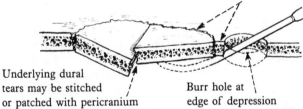

Bone edges nibbled away until fragments can be elevated and removed.

Underlying dural tears may be stitched or patched with pericranium

Burr hole at edge of depression

The aim of treatment is prevention of infection. The wound is debrided and the fragments elevated within 24 hours from injury. Bone fragments are either removed or replaced after washing with antiseptic. Antibiotics are not essential unless the wound is excessively dirty.

If the venous sinuses are involved in the depressed fracture, then operative risks from excessive bleeding may outweigh the risk of infection and antibiotic treatment alone is given.

Complications

Most patients make a rapid and full recovery, but a few develop complications:

Infection occurs when treatment is delayed, or debridement inadequate, and may cause meningitis or abscess formation. Infection seldom occurs after adequate wound toilet and is then usually superficial.

Epilepsy: Early epilepsy (in the first week) occurs in 10% of patients with depressed fracture. Late epilepsy develops in 15% over all, but is especially common when the dura is torn, when focal signs are present, when post-traumatic amnesia exceeds 24 hours or when early epilepsy has occurred (the risk ranges from 3–70%, depending on the number of the above factors involved). Elevation of the bone fragments does not alter the incidence of epilepsy.

Delayed Effects of Head Injury

EPILEPSY
Post-traumatic epilepsy
Post-traumatic epilepsy may be categorised into two types:

     early: occurring in the first week from injury.

Early Epilepsy   late: occurring after the first week from injury.

Early epilepsy occurs in 5% of patients admitted to hospital with non-missile (i.e. deceleration) injuries. It is particularly frequent in the first 24 hours after injury. Focal seizures are as common as generalised seizures. Status epilepticus occurs in 10%.

The risk of early epilepsy is high in – children.

          – patients with prolonged post-traumatic amnesia.

          – patients with an intracranial haematoma.

          – patients with a compound depressed fracture.

Late Epilepsy
Late epilepsy also occurs in about 5% of all patients admitted to hospital after head injury. It usually presents in the first year, but in some the first attack occurs as long as 10 years from the injury. Usually seizures are generalised, but temporal lobe epilepsy (complex partial seizures) occurs in 20%.

Late epilepsy is prevalent in patients with – early epilepsy.

          – intracranial haematoma.

          – compound depressed fracture.

Prophylactic anticonvulsants appear to be of little benefit in preventing the development of an epileptogenic focus.   Management is discussed on page 97.

CEREBROSPINAL FLUID (CSF) LEAK
After head injury a basal fracture may cause a fistulous communication between the CSF space and the paranasal sinuses or the middle ear. Profuse CSF leaks (rhinorrhoea or otorrhoea) are readily detectable, but brain may partially plug the defect and the leak may be minimal or absent. Failure to protect these patients with antibiotics may result in meningitis. When this is associated with anterior fossa fractures, it is usually pneumococcal; when associated with fractures through the petrous bone, a variety of organisms may be involved.

Clinical signs of a basal fracture have previously been described (page 209). The patient may comment on a 'salty taste' in his mouth. Anosmia suggests avulsion of the olfactory bulb from the cribriform plate.

Management

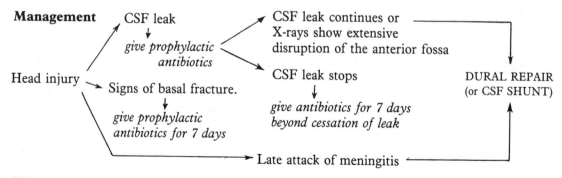

Delayed Effects of Head Injury

CSF leak *(continued)*

Pre-operative investigations

X-ray or *tomography* of the anterior fossa or petrous bone may help identify the fracture site.
CSF isotope infusion studies combined with pledget insertion into the nasal recesses may show the exact site of the leak, but results can be misleading.

A *high definition CT scan* combined with the introduction of *contrast into the basal cisterns* may also be of value.

Operation

As fractures of the anterior fossa often extend across the midline, a bifrontal exploration is required. The dural tear is repaired with fascia lata or lyophilised dural substitute. A CSF leak through the middle ear requires a subtemporal approach.

Failure to repair a CSF fistula may result from impaired CSF absorption with an intermittent or persistent elevation of ICP. In these patients a CSF shunt may be of benefit.

POST-CONCUSSIONAL SYMPTOMS

Even after relatively minor head injury, patients may have persistent symptoms of:

- headache, dizziness and increased irritability.
- difficulty in concentration and in coping with work.
- fatigue and depression.

This condition was once thought to be a purely psychological response, but it is now recognised that in an injury of sufficient severity to cause loss of consciousness or a period of post-traumatic amnesia some neuronal damage occurs; studies show a distinct delay in information processing in these patients, requiring several weeks to resolve. Vestibular 'concussion' (end-organ damage) may contribute to the symptomatology ('dizziness' and vertigo).

CUMULATIVE BRAIN DAMAGE

The effects of repeated neuronal damage is cumulative; when this exceeds the capacity for compensation, permanent evidence of brain damage ensues. The 'punch-drunk' state is well recognised in boxers but recent reports suggest that dementia may also occur from repeated head injury in jockeys.

Delayed Effects of Head Injury

CRANIAL NERVE DAMAGE

Cranial nerve damage occurs in about $\frac{1}{3}$ of patients with severe head injury. Although treatment is seldom required, these lesions may contribute towards the patient's residual disability.

Nerve	Cause of damage	Clinical problem	Management	Prognosis
I	Usually associated with anterior fossa fracture and CSF rhinorrhoea.	Anosmia.	Nil	Recovery is usual in a few months.
II	Optic nerve usually damaged in the optic foramen. Chiasmal damage occasionally occurs. [N.B. Visual loss may also occur from damage to the globe, occipital cortex or optic radiations.]	Visual loss or field defect in one eye. Bitemporal hemianopia.	Nil. Local eye/orbital damage may need treatment.	Recovery seldom occurs.
III IV VI	III nerve damage usually results from tentorial herniation but can also occur in fractures involving the superior orbital fissure or cavernous sinus. IV nerve damage is uncommon. VI nerve damage is usually associated with fractures of the petrous or sphenoid bones.	Pupil inequality, ptosis and disturbance of ocular movements.	Nil [other than removing cause of tentorial herniation].	Recovery usually occurs.
V	Occasionally follows petrous or sphenoid fractures.	Facial analgesia/ anaesthesia.	Nil	Usually permanent
VII	Associated with petrous fracture.	Immediate or delayed facial palsy.	Otologists occasionally recommend decompression. Early steroid therapy may benefit.	Immediate lesions have a poor prognosis; delayed lesions usually recover.
VIII	Petrous fracture may damage: – nerve – cochlea – ossicles Haemotympanum may result.	Vertigo, 'dizziness', hearing loss, tinnitus	Ossicular damage may benefit from operation.	Vestibular symptoms usually improve after several weeks. Nerve deafness is usually permanent. Conductive deafness from haemotympanum should gradually improve.
IX,X XI,XII	Associated with very severe basal fractures or extracranial injury.	Patient seldom survives primary damage.		

Delayed Effects of Head Injury

OUTCOME AFTER SEVERE HEAD INJURY

Head injury remains a major cause of death, especially in the young. Of those patients who survive the initial impact and remain in coma for at least 6 hours, approximately 40% die within 6 months. The extent of recovery in the remainder depends on the severity of injury. Residual incapacitating problems include both mental (impaired intellect and memory and altered personality) and physical defects (hemiparesis and dysphasia). Most recovery occurs within the first 6 months after injury, but improvement may continue for years. *Physiotherapy* and *occupational therapy* play an important role not only in minimising contractures and improving limb power and function but also in stimulating patient motivation.

Outcome is best assessed in terms of *dependence*. Even after severe injury most survivors regain an independent existence and may return to their premorbid social and occupational activities. Inevitably, some remain severely disabled requiring long-term care, but fortunately few are left in a persistent vegetative state with no awareness or ability to communicate with their environment.

Prognostic features

The duration of coma relates closely to the severity of injury and to the final outcome but in the early stages after injury the clinician must rely on other features – age, eye opening, verbal and motor responses, pupil response and eye movements.

Chronic Subdural Haematoma

Subdivision of subdural haematomas into acute and subacute forms serves no practical purpose. Chronic subdural haematoma however is best considered as a separate entity, differing both in presentation and management.

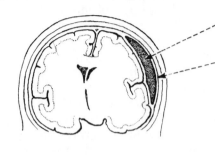

Chronic subdural haematoma – fluid may range from a faint yellow to a dark brown colour.

A membrane grows out from the dura to envelop the haematoma.

Chronic subdural haematomas occur predominantly in *infancy* and in the *elderly*. Trauma is the likely cause, although a history of this is not always obtained.

Predisposing factors:

- – Cerebral atrophy.
- – Low CSF pressure (after a shunt or fistula).
- – Alcoholism.
- – Coagulation disorder.

cause stretching of bridging veins.

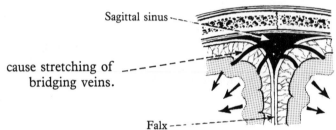

Breakdown of protein within the haematoma and a subsequent rise in osmotic pressure was originally believed to account for the gradual enlargement of the untreated subdural haematoma. Recent studies showing equality of osmotic pressures in blood and haematoma fluid cast doubt on this theory and recurrent bleeding into the cavity is now known to play an important role.

Clinical features tend to be non-specific.

- — Deterioration in conscious level, often with fluctuating course.
- — Dementia.
- — Symptoms and signs of raised ICP.
- — Focal signs occasionally occur, especially limb weakness. This may be ipsilateral to the side of the lesion i.e. a false localising sign (see page 211).

Chronic Subdural Haematoma

Diagnosis:

An *isotope brain scan* reliably detects chronic subdural haematomas, showing an area of increased uptake over the cortical surface.

Most patients with suspected chronic subdural haematoma are referred for a *CT scan*. Appearances depend on the time between injury and scan.

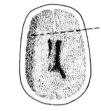

Injury >3 weeks old: low density seen over hemisphere convexity.

With injuries 1–3 weeks old, the subdural haematoma may be isodense with brain tissue.

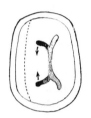

Extracerebral collection i.e. chronic subdural haematoma causes approximation of frontal and occipital horns.

If CT scan shows midline shift without any obvious extra- or intracerebral lesion, look at the shape of the ventricles.

Separation of the frontal and occipital horns suggests an intrinsic lesion e.g. encephalitis rather than a surface collection.

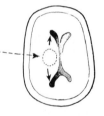

Management

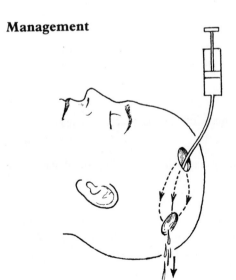

Adults

The haematoma is evacuated through two or three burr holes and the cavity is irrigated with saline. Drains may be left in the subdural space and nursing in the head down position may help prevent recollection.

Craniotomy with excision of the membrane is seldom required.

Infants

The haematoma is evacuated by repeated needle aspiration through the anterior fontanelle. Persistent subdural collections require a subdural peritoneal shunt. As in adults, craniotomy is seldom necessary.

Cerebrovascular Diseases

Vascular diseases of the nervous system are amongst the most frequent causes of admission to hospital. In a western population of 1 million, 2,500 'strokes' occur annually.

Better control of hypertension, reduced incidence of heart disease and a greater awareness of all risk factors have combined to reduce the frequency of 'stroke'. Despite this, 'stroke' still ranks third behind heart disease and cancer as a cause of death in affluent societies.

RISK FACTORS

Prevention of cerebrovascular disease is more likely to reduce death and disability than any medical or surgical advance in management. Prevention depends upon the identification of risk factors and their correction.

Hypertension

Hypertension is a major factor in the development of thrombotic cerebral infarction and intracranial haemorrhage.

There is no critical blood pressure level; the risk is related to the height of blood pressure and increases throughout the whole range from normal to hypertensive.

Systolic hypertension (frequent in the elderly) is also a significant factor and not as harmless as previously thought.

Cardiac disease

Cardiac enlargement, failure and arrhythmias as well as rheumatic heart disease, mitral valve prolapse and, rarely, cardiac myxoma are all associated with an increased risk of 'stroke'.

Diabetes

The risk of cerebral infarction is increased twofold in diabetes. More effective treatment of diabetes has not reduced the frequency of atherosclerotic sequelae.

Heredity

Close relatives are at only slightly greater risk than non-genetically related family members of a 'stroke' patient. Diabetes and hypertension show familial propensity thus clouding the significance of pure hereditary factors.

Blood lipids, Smoking, Diet/Obesity, Soft water

These factors are much less significant than in the genesis of coronary artery disease.

Race

Alterations in life style, diet and environment probably explain the geographical variations more than racial tendencies.

The STROKE PROFILE indicates the likelihood of 'stroke' occurring in an individual based on an analysis of the positive risk factors in that individual. E.g. a 60 year old man who is hypertensive, smokes, has elevated lipids, blood sugar and with cardiac enlargement on the ECG or chest X-ray, has a x10 greater risk than a 60 year old man with no such risk factors.

226

Cerebrovascular Disease – Mechanisms

'Stroke' is a generic term, lacking pathological meaning. Cerebrovascular diseases can be defined as those in which brain disease occurs secondary to a pathological disorder of blood vessels (usually arteries) or blood supply.

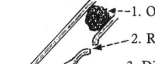

1. Occlusion by thrombus or embolus.

2. Rupture of vessel wall.

3. Disease of vessel wall.

4. Disturbance of normal properties of blood.

Whatever the mechanism, the resultant effect on the brain is either:
  ischaemia/infarction
  or haemorrhagic disruption.

Of all 'strokes':
  – 50% are THROMBOTIC in origin.
  – 30% are EMBOLIC in origin.
  – 15% are HAEMORRHAGIC in origin.

The less common causes e.g. arteritis (blood vessel wall disease) make up the remainder.

Rarely disease of the cerebral veins such as venous thrombosis causes cerebral infarction (venous infarction).

Cerebrovascular Disease – Natural History

Approximately $\frac{1}{3}$ of all 'strokes' are fatal. The age of the patient, the anatomical size of the lesion, the degree of deficit and the underlying cause all influence the outcome.

Immediate outcome

In cerebral haemorrhage, mortality approaches 70%.

Cerebral infarction fares better, with an immediate mortality of less than 25%, fatal lesions being large with associated cerebral oedema.

Embolic infarction carries a better outcome than thrombotic infarction.

Fatal cases of infarction die either at onset or else, more commonly, after the first week from cardiovascular or respiratory complications.

The level of consciousness on admission to hospital gives a good indication to immediate outcome. The deeper the conscious level the graver the prognosis.

Long term outcome

The prognosis following infarction due to thrombosis or embolisation from diseased neck vessels or heart is dependent on the progression of the underlying atherosclerotic disease. Recurrent cerebral infarction, symptoms of coronary artery disease and peripheral vascular disease may ensue.

The long term prognosis following survival from haemorrhage depends upon the cause and the treatment.

The outcome of infarction in young people with no identifiable explanation is variable with long term reinfarction rates between 20–40%.

Cerebrovascular Disease — Physiology

Standard techniques of cerebral blood flow (CBF) measurement provide information of both global and regional flow in patients with cerebral ischaemia or infarction. Recent availability of positron emission tomography (PET), recording oxygen and glucose metabolism as well as blood flow and blood volume, gives a more detailed and accurate understanding of pathophysiological changes after stroke.

Changes in cerebral infarction

NON-ISCHAEMIC HEMISPHERE

ISCHAEMIC HEMISPHERE

Mild reduction in global CBF – diaschisis – perhaps due to transneuronal depression of metabolism in the unaffected hemisphere.

Reduction in global CBF

In the infarcted area and its surroundings, more subtle changes in regional cerebral blood flow (r.CBF) are detected.

In the normal brain, cerebral blood flow to a particular part varies depending on the metabolic requirements, i.e. the supply of O_2 and glucose is 'coupled' to the tissue needs. After infarction, between areas of reduced flow and areas of luxury perfusion, lie areas of *relative luxury perfusion* where reduced flow exceeds the tissue requirements i.e. 'uncoupling' of flow and metabolism has occurred.

Areas of *reduced flow* are bordered by areas of increased flow – *luxury perfusion* – due to vasodilatation of arteriolar bed in response to lactic acidosis.

These changes in r.CBF are transient and revert to normal within days of the onset. The degree of disturbance of r.CBF correlates with outcome. Flow of <28 ml/min/100g result in the development of the morphological changes of infarction.

In patients with transient ischaemic attacks (TIA) a state of *misery perfusion* may exist in which flow is low relative to metabolism.

Clinical applications:

An appreciation of relationships between blood flow and metabolism explains why therapeutic procedures such as induced hypertension or carbon dioxide inhalation, designed to increase cerebral blood flow, do not necessarily improve outcome in 'stroke' patients.

Cerebrovascular Disease – Causes

OCCLUSION (Atheromatous/thrombotic)

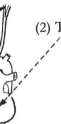

1. Large vessel occlusion or stenosis.

2. Branch vessel occlusion or stenosis.

3. Perforating vessel occlusion (lacunar infarction)

EMBOLISATION From:

(1) Atheromatous plaque in the internal carotid arteries or from the aortic arch.

(2) The heart
Rheumatic heart disease.
Ischaemic heart disease.
Bacterial endocarditis.
Atrial myxoma.
Prosthetic valves.
Prolapsing mitral valve.

(3) Miscellaneous
Fat emboli.
Air emboli.
Tumour emboli.

DISEASES of the VESSEL WALL

Arteritis
{
Rheumatoid vasculitis.
Systemic Lupus Erythematosus(SLE)
Polyarteritis nodosa.
Giant cell arteritis – Temporal arteritis,
Takayashu's disease.
}

Miscellaneous
{
Syphilitic vasculitis.
Fibromuscular hyperplasia.
Sarcoidosis.
Moya Moya disease.
}

Granulomatous vasculitis
{
Wegener's granulomatosis.
Granulomatous angiitis of the nervous system.
}

DISEASES of BLOOD

Coagulopathies.
Haemoglobinopathies.
Hyperviscosity syndromes.

Polycythaemia.
Idiopathic and thrombotic thrombocytopaenic purpura.
Thrombocythaemia.

VENOUS THROMBOSIS

Venous thrombosis within the nervous system may occur with infection and dehydration or in association with arterial occlusion when related to oestrogen excess e.g. the oral contraceptives or pregnancy.

HAEMORRHAGE

(1) Intracerebral haemorrhage (or intra-parenchymal haemorrhage) due to:
Hypertension. Aneurysm. Neoplasm. Trauma.
Arteriovenous malformation.
Anticoagulant therapy.   Septicaemia.
Disseminated intravascular coagulopathy.
Thrombotic thrombocytopaenic purpura.
Coagulation disorders e.g. haemophilia.

(2) Subarachnoid haemorrhage due to:
Aneurysm.
Arteriovenous malformation.
Trauma.
Tumour.
Anticoagulant therapy.
Coagulation disorders e.g.
haemophilia.

Occlusive and Stenotic Cerebrovascular Disease

PATHOLOGY

The normal vessel wall comprises:

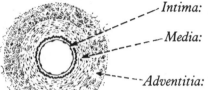

Intima: a single endothelial cell lining.

Media: fibroblasts and smooth muscle with collagen support and elastic tissue.

Adventitia: mainly composed of thick collagen fibres.

Within brain and spinal cord tissue the adventitia is usually very thin and the elastic lamina between media and adventitia less apparent.

The intima is an important barrier to leakage of blood and constituents into the vessel wall. In the development of the atherosclerotic plaque, damage to the endothelium of the intima is the primary event.

The Atherosclerotic plaque

Following intimal damage:

Intimal cells,
Smooth muscle cells laden with
cholesterol, lipids, phospholipids, } build up
Collagen and elastic fibres. subintimally.

Haemorrhage may occur within the plaque or the plaque may ulcerate into the lumen of the vessel forming an intraluminal mural thrombus. Either way, the lumen of the involved vessel is narrowed (stenosed) or blocked (occluded).

The plaque itself may give rise to emboli. Cholesterol is present partly in crystal form and fragments following plaque rupture may be sufficiently large to occlude the lumen of distal vessels. The cholesterol esters, lipids and phospholipids each play a role in the aggregation of such emboli.

The carotid bifurcation in the neck is a frequent site at which the atheromatous plaque causes stenosis or occlusion.

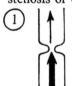 When stenosed by more than 80%, reduction of blood flow to brain occurs.

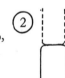 When occluded, the clinical outcome depends on speed of occlusion and the state of collateral circulation.

 When plaque has ulcerated – may result in cholesterol emboli or platelet emboli.

Platelet emboli arise from thrombus developed over the damaged endothelium. This thrombus is produced partly by platelets coming into contact with exposed collagen fibres. Platelets suppress the antiaggregatory agent PROSTACYCLIN and release the aggregating agent THROMBOXANE A2. Such a thrombus when formed may break off and pass distally to occlude a small vessel.

Occlusion of a vessel is also associated with proximal and distal thrombus formation.

Occlusive/Stenotic Cerebrovascular Disease

CLINICAL SYNDROMES

INTRODUCTION

Transient symptoms (transient ischaemic attacks, T.I.A.) precede infarction in 60–70% of patients. The investigation and treatment of these warning symptoms are dealt with on pages 244–249.

Thrombotic stroke develops over some hours, though with carotid occlusion may 'stutter' for some days. The stepwise progression is referred to as 'stroke in evolution'. Thrombotic infarction tends to occur during sleep, possibly due to the diurnal fluctuations in mean arterial blood pressure.

Headache is an occasional symptom of thrombotic infarction unless large vessels are involved → carotid occlusion — — — — vertebral occlusion — — —

Clinical examination should:
1. Document the neurological deficit.
2. Examine the vessels in the neck for presence or absence of pulsation and bruit.
3. Examine all other systems for evidence of coexisting peripheral vascular disease (PVD) or cardiac disease as well as stigmata of hypertension, diabetes etc.

Clinical Syndromes – Large Vessel Occlusion

OCCLUSION OF THE INTERNAL CAROTID ARTERY — may present in a 'stuttering' manner as the lumen progressively narrows.

The degree of deficit varies – occlusion may be asymptomatic and identified only at autopsy, or a catastrophic infarction may result.

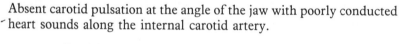

In the most extreme cases there may be:

Slow mentation → deterioration of conscious level.
Homonymous hemianopia of the contralateral side. —
Contralateral hemiplegia. —
Contralateral hemisensory disturbance.
Gaze palsy to the opposite side – eyes deviated to the side of the lesion.

A partial Horner's syndrome may be present on the side of the occlusion (involvement of sympathetic fibres on the internal carotid wall).

Occlusion of the dominant hemisphere side will result in a global aphasia.

Examination of the neck will reveal:

External carotid
Internal carotid
Bifurcation
Common carotid

Absent carotid pulsation at the angle of the jaw with poorly conducted heart sounds along the internal carotid artery.

Prodromal symptoms prior to occlusion may take the form of monocular blindness – AMAUROSIS FUGAX, and hemisensory and hemimotor disturbance of a transitory nature (see page 244).

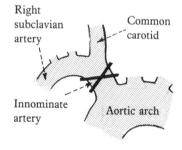

Right subclavian artery
Common carotid
Innominate artery
Aortic arch

The origins of the vessels from the aortic arch are such that an *innominate artery occlusion* will result not only in the clinical picture of carotid occlusion but will produce diminished blood flow and hence blood pressure in the right arm.

The outcome of carotid occlusion depends on the collateral blood supply.

The *anterior cerebral artery* may receive blood from:
1. The anterior communicating artery.
2. Anastomosis with meningeal branches of the external carotid.

The *middle cerebral artery* may receive blood from meningeal branches of the external carotid.

The intracranial portion of the *carotid artery* may receive blood from the external carotid circulation via retrograde flow in the ophthalmic artery.

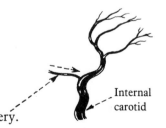

Internal carotid

Clinical Syndromes – Large Vessel Occlusion

ANTERIOR CEREBRAL ARTERY

Anatomy

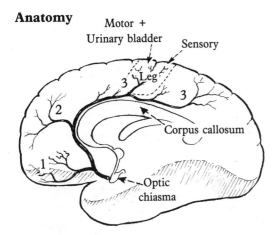

Medial surface of right cerebral hemisphere.

The anterior cerebral artery is a branch of the internal carotid and runs above the optic nerve to follow the curve of the corpus callosum. Soon after its origin the vessel is joined by the anterior communicating artery. Deep branches pass to the anterior part of the internal capsule and basal nuclei.

Cortical branches supply the medial surface of the hemisphere:

1. Orbital.
2. Frontal.
3. Parietal.

Clinical features

The anterior cerebral artery may be occluded by embolus or thrombus. The clinical picture depends on the site of occlusion (especially in relation to the anterior communicating artery) and the considerable anatomical variation – both anterior cerebral arteries may arise from one side by enlargement of the anterior communicating artery.

Occlusion proximal to the anterior communicating artery is normally well tolerated because of the cross flow.

Distal occlusion results in weakness and cortical sensory loss in the contralateral lower limb with associated incontinence. Occasionally a contralateral grasp reflex is present.

Proximal occlusion when both anterior cerebral vessels arise from the same side results in 'cerebral' paraplegia with lower limb weakness, sensory loss, incontinence and presence of grasp, snout and palmomental reflexes.

Bilateral frontal lobe infarction may result in *akinetic mutism* or deterioration in conscious level.

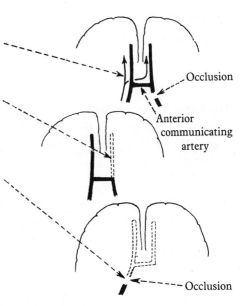

Clinical Syndromes – Large Vessel Occlusion

MIDDLE CEREBRAL ARTERY

Anatomy

Lateral surface of cerebral hemisphere.

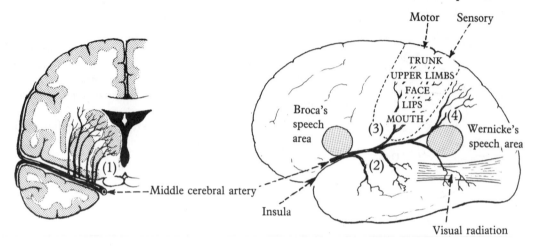

The middle cerebral artery is the largest branch of the internal carotid artery. It gives off (1) deep branches (perforating vessels – lenticulo-striate) which supply the internal capsule and basal nuclei. It then passes out to the lateral surface of the cerebral hemisphere at the insula of the lateral sulcus. Here, it gives off cortical branches (2) Temporal, (3) Frontal, (4) Parietal.

Clinical features

The middle cerebral artery may be occluded by embolus or thrombus. The clinical picture depends upon the site of occlusion and whether dominant or non-dominant hemisphere is affected.

Occlusion at the insula:

All cortical branches are involved —— Contralateral hemiplegia (leg relatively spared).
Contralateral hemianaesthesia and hemianopia.
Aphasia (dominant).
Neglect of contralateral limbs and
Dressing difficulty (non-dominant).

When cortical branches are affected individually, the clinical picture is less severe, e.g. involvement of parietal branches alone may produce Wernicke's dysphasia with no limb weakness or sensory loss.

The deep branches (perforating vessels) of the middle cerebral artery may be a source of haemorrhage or small infarcts (lacunes – see later).

234

Clinical Syndromes – Large Vessel Occlusion

VERTEBRAL ARTERY OCCLUSION

Anatomy   The Vertebral and Basilar arteries

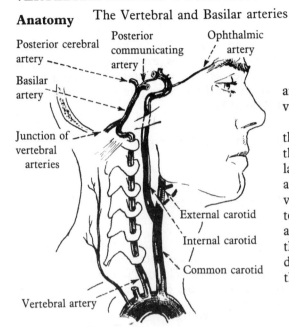

The vertebral artery arises from the subclavian artery on each side. Underdevelopment of one vessel occurs in 10%.

The vertebral artery runs from its origin through the foramen of the transverse processes of the lower five cervical vertebrae. It then passes laterally through the transverse process of the axis, then upwards to the atlas accompanied by a venous plexus and across the suboccipital triangle to the vertebral canal. After piercing the dura and arachnoid mater, it enters the cranial cavity through the foramen magnum. At the lower border of the pons, it unites with its fellow to form the basilar artery.

The vertebral artery and its branches supply the medulla and the inferior surface of the cerebellum before forming the basilar artery.

Clinical features

Occlusion of the vertebral artery, when low in the neck, is compensated by anastomotic channels.

When one vertebral artery is hypoplastic, occlusion of the other is equivalent to basilar artery occlusion.

Vertebral artery occlusion may be indistinguishable from the syndrome resulting from posterior inferior cerebellar artery occlusion (page 239).

The close relationship of the vertebral artery to the cervical spine is important. Damage at intervertebral foramina or the atlanto-axial joints following subluxation may result in intimal damage, thrombus formation and embolisation.

Vertebral artery compression during neck extension may cause symptoms of intermittent vertebrobasilar insufficiency.

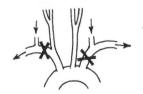

✗Stenosis of the proximal left or right subclavian artery may result in a retrograde flow down the vertebral artery when the arm is exercised. Symptoms of vertebrobasilar insufficiency arise – subclavian 'steal' syndrome. Surgical reconstruction or bypass of the subclavian artery may be indicated.

Clinical Syndromes – Large Vessel Occlusion

BASILAR ARTERY OCCLUSION

Anatomy

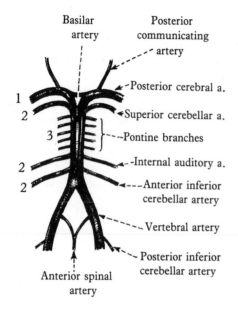

Basilar artery

Posterior communicating artery

- Posterior cerebral a.

1

2

3

- Superior cerebellar a.
- Pontine branches
- Internal auditory a.

2

2

- Anterior inferior cerebellar artery

- Vertebral artery

- Posterior inferior cerebellar artery

Anterior spinal artery

The basilar artery supplies the brain stem from medulla upwards and divides eventually into posterior cerebral arteries as well as posterior communicating arteries which run forward to join the anterior circulation (Circle of Willis).

Branches can be classified into:

1. Posterior cerebral arteries.
2. Long circumflex branches.
3. Paramedian branches.

Clinical features

Prodromal symptoms are common and may take the form of diplopia, visual field loss, intermittent memory disturbance and a whole constellation of other brain stem symptoms:
- vertigo.
- ataxia.
- paresis.
- paraesthesia.

The complete Basilar Syndrome following occlusion consists of:
Impairment of consciousness ⟶ coma.
Bilateral motor and sensory dysfunction, cerebellar signs and cranial nerve signs indicative of the level of occlusion.

The clinical picture is variable. Occasionally basilar thrombosis is an incidental finding at autopsy.

Bilateral lesions: Occlusion of the upper part of the basilar artery may result in cortical blindness often with denial of visual loss.

Involvement of the undersurface of both temporal lobes may produce severe amnesia.

Clinical Syndromes – Large Vessel Occlusion

POSTERIOR CEREBRAL ARTERY

Anatomy

Undersurface of left cerebral hemisphere.   Medial surface of right hemisphere.

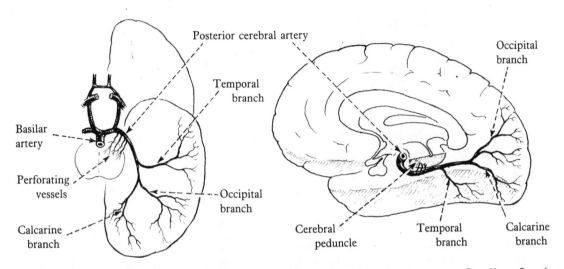

The posterior cerebral arteries are the terminal branches of the basilar artery. Small perforating branches supply midbrain structures, choroid plexus and posterior thalamus. Cortical branches supply the undersurface of the temporal lobe – temporal branch; and occipital and visual cortex – occipital and calcarine branches.

Clinical features

Proximal occlusion by thrombus or embolism will involve perforating branches and structures supplied –

Midbrain syndrome — III nerve palsy with contralateral hemiplegia — WEBER'S SYNDROME.

Thalamic syndromes — chorea or hemiballismus with hemisensory disturbance.

Occlusion of cortical vessels will produce a different picture with visual field loss (homonymous hemianopia) and sparing of macular vision (the posterior tip of the occipital lobe i.e. the macular area, is also supplied by the middle cerebral artery).

Posterior cortical infarction in the dominant hemisphere may produce problems in naming colours and objects.

Clinical Syndromes – Branch Occlusion

BASILAR ARTERY – LONG CIRCUMFLEX BRANCH OCCLUSION
Anatomy

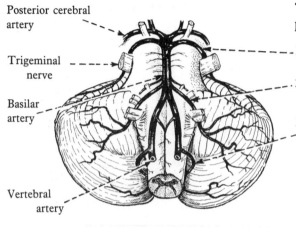

Posterior cerebral artery

Trigeminal nerve

Basilar artery

Vertebral artery

The cerebellum is supplied by three paired blood vessels:

1. Superior cerebellar artery ⎫ arise
2. Anterior inferior cerebellar artery ⎬ from basilar artery
3. Posterior inferior cerebellar artery (PICA) which arises from the vertebral artery.

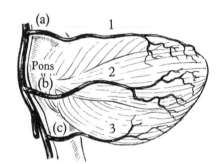

(a)

1

Pons

(b)

2

(c)

3

It can be seen that a vascular lesion in the territory of these vessels will produce not only cerebellar but also brain stem symptoms and signs localising to:

(a) superior pontine,
(b) inferior pontine and
(c) medullary levels.

Clinical features

Superior Cerebellar Artery Syndrome results in:

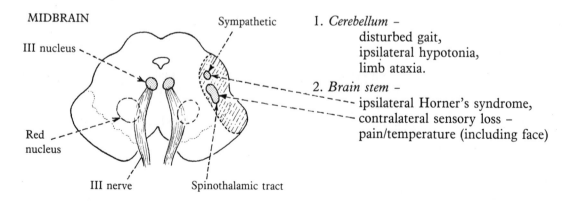

MIDBRAIN

III nucleus

Red nucleus

III nerve

Sympathetic

Spinothalamic tract

1. *Cerebellum* –
   disturbed gait,
   ipsilateral hypotonia,
   limb ataxia.
2. *Brain stem* –
   ipsilateral Horner's syndrome,
   contralateral sensory loss –
   pain/temperature (including face)

Clinical Syndromes – Branch Occlusion

Anterior Inferior Cerebellar Artery Syndrome results in:

PONS

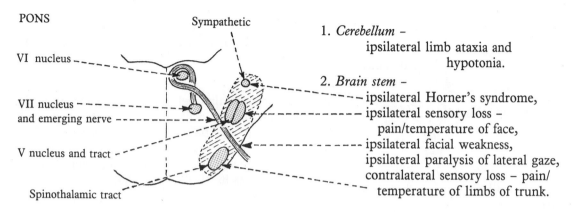

Sympathetic

VI nucleus

VII nucleus and emerging nerve

V nucleus and tract

Spinothalamic tract

1. *Cerebellum –*
   ipsilateral limb ataxia and
   hypotonia.
2. *Brain stem –*
   ipsilateral Horner's syndrome,
   ipsilateral sensory loss –
   pain/temperature of face,
   ipsilateral facial weakness,
   ipsilateral paralysis of lateral gaze,
   contralateral sensory loss – pain/
   temperature of limbs of trunk.

Posterior Inferior Cerebellar Artery Syndrome (lateral medullary syndrome) results in:

MEDULLA

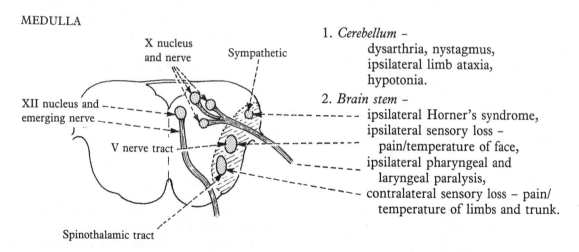

X nucleus and nerve

Sympathetic

XII nucleus and emerging nerve

V nerve tract

Spinothalamic tract

1. *Cerebellum –*
   dysarthria, nystagmus,
   ipsilateral limb ataxia,
   hypotonia.
2. *Brain stem –*
   ipsilateral Horner's syndrome,
   ipsilateral sensory loss –
   pain/temperature of face,
   ipsilateral pharyngeal and
   laryngeal paralysis,
   contralateral sensory loss – pain/
   temperature of limbs and trunk.

Clinical Syndromes – Branch Occlusion

BASILAR ARTERY – PARAMEDIAN BRANCH OCCLUSION

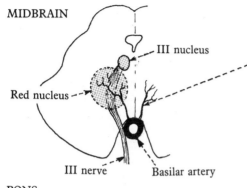

MIDBRAIN

III nucleus

Red nucleus

III nerve   Basilar artery

Paramedian branch occlusion is produced by occlusion of the penetrating mid-line branches of the basilar artery.

At the midbrain level damage to the nucleus or the fasciculus of the oculomotor nerve (III) will result in a complete or partial III nerve palsy; damage to the red nucleus (outflow from opposite cerebellar hemisphere) will also produce contralateral tremor – referred to as BENEDIKT's SYNDROME.

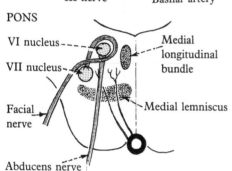

PONS

VI nucleus

VII nucleus

Medial longitudinal bundle

Facial nerve

Medial lemniscus

Abducens nerve

At the pontine level an abducens nerve (VI) palsy will occur with ipsilateral facial (VII) weakness and contralateral sensory loss – light touch, proprioception (medial lemniscus damage) when the lesion is more basal.

Abducens and facial palsy may be accompanied by contralateral hemiplegia – MILLARD – GUBLER SYNDROME.

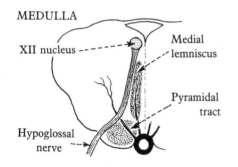

MEDULLA

XII nucleus

Medial lemniscus

Pyramidal tract

Hypoglossal nerve

At the medullary level, bilateral damage is usually sustained. A unilateral lesion is uncommon but, when present, will produce ipsilateral tongue weakness, contralateral sensory loss – light touch, proprioception (medial lemniscus damage) and contralateral hemiplegia (pyramidal tract damage).

Bilateral damage will produce the 'LOCKED-IN' or DE-EFFERENTATION SYNDROME.

The patient is awake and alert but is quadraplegic. Cranial nerve damage may result in extensive cranial nerve weakness with sparing of only the more laterally placed nuclei – the patient is literally 'locked in'. Sensory impairment due to medial lemniscus involvement and damage to the decussating fibres from the spinal tract of the trigeminal nerve is inevitable.

Clinical Syndromes – Perforating Vessel Occlusion

LACUNAR INFARCTION

Lacunes are small fluid filled cavities 0.5–1.5 cm in diameter. They are found in basal ganglia, internal capsule and pons. Lacunes are believed to represent small infarctions produced by occlusion of the small penetrating branches of the major intracranial arteries.

There are 2 possible causative mechanisms:

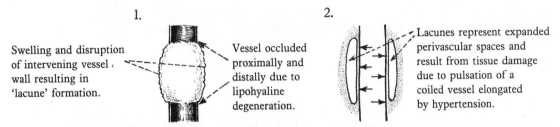

1.

Swelling and disruption of intervening vessel wall resulting in 'lacune' formation.

Vessel occluded proximally and distally due to lipohyaline degeneration.

2.

Lacunes represent expanded perivascular spaces and result from tissue damage due to pulsation of a coiled vessel elongated by hypertension.

Lacunes are found in hypertensive patients. Their formation is often unassociated with symptoms. However, certain clinical states are recognised:

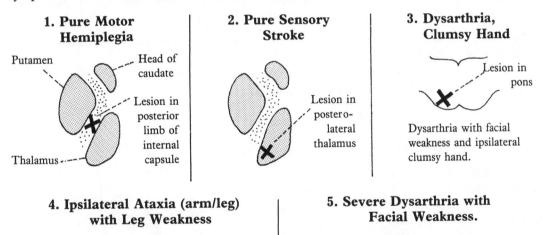

1. Pure Motor Hemiplegia

Putamen

Head of caudate

Lesion in posterior limb of internal capsule

Thalamus

2. Pure Sensory Stroke

Lesion in postero-lateral thalamus

3. Dysarthria, Clumsy Hand

Lesion in pons

Dysarthria with facial weakness and ipsilateral clumsy hand.

4. Ipsilateral Ataxia (arm/leg) with Leg Weakness

Lesion in pons

5. Severe Dysarthria with Facial Weakness.

Lesion in anterior limb of internal capsule

6. Multiple Lacunar Infarction 'État lacunaire'

The patient acquires a shuffling gait – 'marche à petits pas' – with features of pseudobulbar palsy and dementia.

The control of hypertension following initial lacunar infarction is essential to prevent future episodes.

Embolisation

Unlike thrombotic infarction, embolic infarction is very sudden in onset. The clinical picture depends upon the vessel involved. Anterior, middle or posterior cerebral artery branch occlusion is often presumed embolic in origin as thrombotic occlusion beyond the first main intracranial branches is unusual.

The diagnosis of embolic infarction depends upon:

1. The identification of an embolic source e.g. cardiac disease, carotid disease.
2. The clinical picture of sudden onset, with depression of consciousness if major vessel occlusion occurs.

Focal seizures are frequent at the onset and may persist for some time after the acute ischaemic episode.

EMBOLI originating from the INTERNAL CAROTID ARTERY and AORTA

Emboli from these sites are the commonest of non-cardiac origin. One third of all cerebral emboli arise from ulcerative plaques in the carotid arteries (see page 230). Emboli commonly produce *transient ischaemic attacks (T.I.A.)* as well as *infarction.*

Symptoms are referrable to the eye (retinal artery) and to the anterior and middle cerebral arteries, and take the form of:

Visual loss – with resolution *amaurosis fugax.*
Hemisensory and hemimotor disturbance.
Disturbance of higher function e.g. dysphasia.
Incidence of focal or generalised seizures is high.

When emboli arise from aorta (atheromatous plaque or aortic aneurysm) both hemispheres may be involved and renal (haematuria) and systemic cutaneous manifestations of embolisation may be apparent.

Embolisation

EMBOLI of CARDIAC ORIGIN

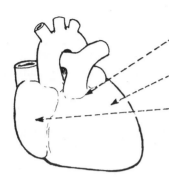

The heart represents a major source of cerebral emboli.

Valvular heart disease – rheumatic heart disease with mitral stenosis and atrial fibrillation.

Ischaemic heart disease – myocardial infarction with mural thrombus formation.

Arrhythmias – especially when of sinoatrial origin.

Bacterial endocarditis may give rise to septic cerebral embolisation with ischaemia → infection → abscess formation.
Neurological signs will occur in 30% of all cases of bacterial endocarditis, *S. aureus* and *streptococci* beng the offending organisms in the majority.

Non-bacterial endocarditis. Carcinomatous involvement of the heart may result in cerebral embolism.

Atrial myxoma is a rare cause of recurrent cerebral embolisation. Bihemisphere episodes with a persistently elevated ESR should arouse suspicion which may be confirmed by cardiac ultrasound.

Mitral valve prolapse is a cause of embolisation, again confirmed by cardiac ultrasound.

Patent foramen ovale may result in paradoxical embolisation; suspect in patient with deep venous thrombosis who develops cerebral infarction.

EMBOLI from OTHER SOURCES

Fat emboli: Following fracture, especially of long bones and pelvis, fat appears in the blood stream and may pass into the cerebral circulation, usually 3–6 days after trauma. Emboli are usually multiple and signs are diffuse.

Air emboli follow injury to neck/chest or follow surgery. Rarely air emboli complicate therapeutic abortion. Again the picture is diffuse neurologically. Onset is acute; if the patient survives the first 30 minutes, prognosis is excellent.
Nitrogen embolisation or decompression sickness (the 'Bends') produces a similar picture. If the patient survives, neurological disability may be profound.

Tumour emboli result in metastatic lesions; the onset is usually slow and progressive. Acute stroke-like presentation may occur, followed weeks or months later by the mass effects.

> Lung
> Melanoma
> Testicular tumours
> Lymphoblastic leukaemia } – Commonly metastasise to brain.
> Prostate
> Breast
> Renal

The clinical features of embolic vascular occlusion have already been discussed under Clinical Syndromes.

Transient Ischaemic Attacks (T.I.A's)

Transient ischaemic attacks are episodes of focal neurological symptoms of less than 24 hours duration occurring as a result of cerebrovascular disease. (Symptoms usually settle well within the 24 hour period.) Most episodes last for minutes rather than hours.

Exclude other causes of transient neurological symptoms – migraine, focal epilepsy, multiple sclerosis, entrapment neuropathy (e.g. carpal tunnel syndrome) – by careful history taking and examination. Also consider non-neurological causes of transient symptoms – anxiety, hyperventilation, hypoglycaemia and cardiac arrhythmia.

The pathogenesis of transient ischaemic attacks.

A reduction of cerebral blood flow below 20–30 ml 100g/min. renders patients neurologically unstable. The development of infarction is a consequence of the *degree* of reduced flow and the *duration* of such a reduction. If flow is restored to an area of brain within the critical period, ischaemic symptoms will reverse themselves. T.I.A's may be due to:

1. Reduced flow through a vessel.

A fall in perfusion pressure.
e.g. cardiac dysrhythmia
associated with localised
stenotic cerebrovascular
disease

– the *haemodynamic* explanation.

2. Blockage of the passage of flow by embolism.

arising from plaques in
aortic arch/extracranial
vessels or from the
heart.

– the *embolic* explanation.

Both mechanisms are important. Emboli are more widely accepted as the cause of T.I.A's in view of their occasional dramatic appearance in the retinal vessels in Amaurosis Fugax.

The symptomatology of T.I.A's

T.I.A's may be *posterior*.....

Vertebrobasilar territory
Loss of consciousness
Bilateral limb motor/sensory
           dysfunction.
Binocular blindness.

Vertigo, tinnitus, ⎤ not singly but in
diplopia, dysarthria ⎦ combination with each other.

.....or *anterior*

Carotid territory
  Hemiparesis,
  hemisensory disturbance,
  dysphasia,
  monocular blindness
    (Amaurosis Fugax).

Many transient ischaemic attacks are difficult to fit convincingly into either anterior or posterior circulation e.g. dysarthria with hemiparesis.

The natural history of T.I.A's.

Following a T.I.A., between 5–10% of patients will develop infarction in each year of follow-up, irrespective of the territory involved. The risk of infarction is probably at its greatest in the first 3–6 months after the initial T.I.A. Not all patients who develop cerebral infarction have had a warning T.I.A.

Stenotic/Occlusive Cerebrovascular Disease – Investigations

1. Confirm the diagnosis   – infarction ——— embolic
                                – haemorrhage ⟍ thrombotic

Computerised Tomography (CT scan)

Ideally, all patients should have a CT scan, but this is rarely possible in view of the frequency of stroke.

In practice, a CT scan is performed if:
  - there is doubt about the diagnosis.
  - symptoms progress.   ⎫ ? tumour ± haemorrhage
  - conscious level is depressed.   ⎬
  - neck stiffness is present.   ⎭   ? cerebral haemorrhage (see page 258).

or prior to any invasive investigation.

Infarction is evident as a low density lesion which conforms to a vascular territory i.e. usually wedge shaped. It is not immediately visible on CT but in most patients becomes apparent in 4–7 days.

CT scan also identifies:
  - the site and size of the infarct, providing a prognostic guide.
  - the presence of haemorrhagic infarction where bleeding occurs into the infarcted area.
  - intracerebral haemorrhage or tumour.

2. Demonstrate the site of the primary lesion.

(a) Non-invasive investigation

Non-invasive investigation of the extracranial vessels is preferable in the first instance and will, if normal, minimise the need for invasive tests.

Doppler ultrasonic imaging:

A transducer attached to a position detecting arm is passed backwards and forwards over the neck vessels, mapping out an image related to the moving column of red cells within the vessel.

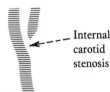

Internal carotid stenosis

Real time (B mode) ultrasound imaging:

This produces an image of vessels in longitudinal or transverse section.

Digital subtraction angiography:

This recent advance is described on page 44 and, with further development, is likely to become the non-invasive investigation of choice. At present, large volumes of contrast media are required for visualisation of the intracranial vessels making it unlikely to supercede conventional angiography.

(b) Invasive investigation

Often *cerebral angiography* is required as the definitive investigation, when the patient management is likely to be influenced by the result. There is no place for angiography in recent complete stroke due to either thrombosis or infarction until at least 1–2 weeks have elapsed. In the elderly or poor risk patients, negative non-invasive investigations may be considered sufficient, although with modern techniques the risks of angiography are small.

Stenotic / Occlusive Disease – Investigations

Indications for angiography:
- a recovered stroke patient at further risk.
- following transient ischaemic attacks.

Angiography identifies the site
and nature of the disease in intra-
and extracranial vessels, and indicates
the degree of collateral circulation.

 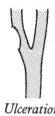 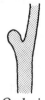

e.g.   *Stenosis*   *Ulceration*   *Occlusion*

Suspected carotid disease (bruit, clinical picture): demonstrate both carotids, intracranial vessels, the aortic arch and origins of the vertebrals. Approximately ⅓ of patients with carotid territory attacks will have angiographic abnormality.

Suspected vertebrobasilar disease (clinical picture): note the intracranial vessels and the course of the vertebral artery through the cervical foramina where osteophytic encroachment may occur. Note that proximal subclavian occlusion may result in retrograde flow down the vertebral arteries into the subclavian arteries, and cause T.I.A's aggravated by arm exercise – *subclavian steal* (page 235).

3. Identify factors which may influence treatment and outcome.

General investigations identify conditions which may predispose towards premature cerebrovascular disease. These are essential in all patients.

Chest X-ray — cardiac enlargement – hypertension/valvular heart disease

ECG — ventricular enlargement and/or
arrhythmias – hypertension/embolic disease.
recent myocardial infarct – embolic disease.
sino-atrial conduction defect – embolic disease/output failure.

Blood glucose — diabetes mellitus.
Serum lipids and cholesterol — hyperlipidaemia.
ESR — vasculitis.
Urine analysis — polyarteritis, thrombocytopenia.
Full blood count — polycythaemia, thrombocytopenia.

} See inflammatory vasculitis and blood diseases (page 250).

VDRL–TPHA — neurosyphilis
Note drug history — oral contraceptives, amphetamines, opiates.
Cervical spine X-ray — atlanto-axial subluxation.

Following the interpretation of these preliminary investigations, more detailed studies may be required e.g.

- echo cardiography
- cardiac catheterisation } cardiac embolic source.
- blood cultures ———— subacute bacterial endocarditis.
- sickle cell screen
- plasma electrophoresis } haematological disorder.

Cerebral Infarction – Management

The ACUTE STROKE

Clinical history, examination and investigation will separate thrombotic, embolic infarction and haemorrhage. Once the nature of the 'stroke' has been confidently defined, treatment should be instigated.

Treatment aims:
- Prevent progression of present event.
- Prevent immediate complication.
- Prevent the development of subsequent events.
- To rehabilitate the patient.

General measures

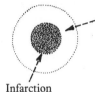

Infarction

Around the edge of an infarct, ischaemic tissue is at risk but is potentially recoverable. This compromised but viable tissue must be protected by ensuring a good supply of glucose and oxygen. Factors which might adversely affect this must be maintained – hydration, oxygenation, blood pressure. To this end, treat chest infections and cardiac failure/dysrhythmias.

Specific measures

Treatment of oedema

The degree of concomitant oedema relates to the magnitude of infarction. Oedema develops early and may cause ventricular displacement and transtentorial herniation with secondary brain stem damage. Controversy exists as to whether oedema is vasogenic or cytotoxic (as associated with metabolic encephalopathies) or a mixture of the two. Its effective treatment should lower morbidity and mortality but steroids and hyperosmolar agents (e.g. Mannitol) have been used with little effect on outcome. The poor response probably reflects the 'mixed' nature of the oedema.

Anticoagulant therapy

The use of anticoagulants to minimise the extent or reduce the risk of further infarction should in most cases be discouraged. Bleeding can occur into an infarct (haemorrhagic infarction) and anticoagulants may precipitate this. There are however exceptions to this rule:

1. In patients with a known cardiac source of emboli, the risk of recurrent embolic infarction is high and anticoagulant therapy should be commenced once CT scan and lumbar puncture have ruled out haemorrhagic infarction. In chronic valvular disease, treatment is long term; following myocardial infarction (with mural thrombus) – 6 months. With mitral valve prolapse, antiplatelet drugs will suffice.

2. Anticoagulants are also of value in the management of 'stroke in evolution'. The neurological deficit fluctuates but gradually worsens over some hours. The gradual progression is considered due to increasing thrombus formation with progressive 'silting' of collateral vessels and anticoagulant therapy should be commenced immediately after a CT scan.

Cerebral Infarction – Management

Specific measures *(continued)*

Blood viscosity

Cerebral blood flow will increase following haemodilution. Venesection, by lowering viscosity, would increase blood flow to the 'at risk' area. The value of venesection in improving morbidity and mortality is as yet unproven, although this should be considered in the polycythaemic stroke patient.

Inhibition of cerebral metabolism

Reduction in the brain's metabolic demands should theoretically protect further the 'at risk' area. The value of barbiturates, hypothermia and Naloxone to this end remains to be proven.

Prevention of further stroke

The recognition of risk factors and their correction to minimise the risk of further events forms a necessary and important step in long term treatment.

- Control hypertension.
- Emphasise the need to stop cigarette smoking.
- Correct lipid abnormality.
- Stop thrombogenic drugs e.g. oral contraceptives.
- Remove or treat embolic source.
- Treat inflammatory vascular or blood diseases.

Transient Ischaemic Attacks – Management

The aim of treatment is to prevent subsequent cerebral infarction:
    Establish diagnosis and exclude other pathologies causing transient neurological symptoms
        e.g. migraine.
    Establish which vessel is involved ⎯ Carotid territory.
                                         ⎯ Vertebrobasilar artery.
    Exclude predisposing condition.
    Examine patient thoroughly for evidence of extracranial vascular disease:
        Palpate carotids, upper limb pulses.   Auscultate the neck for bruits.
        Check blood pressure in both arms.   Examine heart.
    The rôle of the various available treatments still remains unclear.

Medical treatment:

General ⎯⎯ Reduce risk factors as described above.

Specific
Anticoagulation:
    There is no evidence that anticoagulated T.I.A. patients do more favourably than control groups, though studies are small and not all double blind; their rôle therefore remains unproven.

Antiplatelet agents:
    Canadian cooperative study is the most complete to date. Aspirin significantly reduced the risk of stroke in men but not in women, though this may be explained by smaller numbers of women in the study; it therefore has a rôle. Aspirin appears beneficial but the optimal dose is unclear (i.e. 300–1200 mg/day).

Surgical treatment:

The purpose of investigation is to define a surgically amenable lesion. However, the rôle of surgery is unclear. Generally, stenotic lesions are treated by carotid endarterectomy to restore normal perfusion pressure. The advantage of operative removal of an ulcerative lesion compared to antiplatelet drugs to minimise the risk of emboli has yet to be determined. The decision to operate may be influenced by the experience of the operator, the general condition of the patient and the quality of anaesthetic and post-operative care. Most surgery is confined to the carotid territory though osteophytic vertebral artery compression, subclavian steal syndrome and vertebral artery origin stenosis are all amenable to bypass techniques.

Superficial temporal to middle cerebral artery anastomosis (Anterior circulation).
The development of microsurgical bypass anastomosis has led to the rerouting of blood into an area of compromised circulation e.g. where T.I.A's occur distal to occlusion with an inadequate collateral supply.
Possible indications:
            – high cervical carotid stenosis (direct approach impossible).
            – carotid occlusion.   – middle cerebral artery stenosis or occlusion.
It appears that this technique does not influence the subsequent development of a completed stroke.

Occipital to posterior inferior cerebellar artery anastomosis is occasionally performed for posterior circulation ischaemia, but benefits remain undetermined.

Diseases of the Vessel Wall

INFLAMMATORY VASCULAR DISEASES (VASCULITIDES)

General principles

Involvement of cerebral vessels may present as an acute or subacute 'stroke-like' syndrome.

NECROTISING VASCULITIS

Systemic lupus erythematosus,   Takayashu's aortitis,
Polyarteritis nodosa,   Granulomatous vasculitis,
Hypersensitivity angiitis,   Granulomatous angiitis of CNS;
Giant cell arteritis,

    all can result in 'stroke' (infarction or haemorrhage)

Infections, toxins, chemicals may also produce vessel inflammation.

Mechanism

An immune basis for these disorders is likely.

In *Systemic Lupus Erythematosus:*

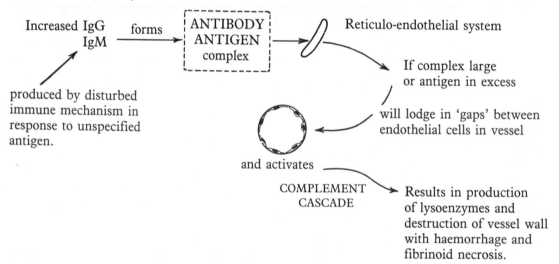

Increased IgG IgM — forms → ANTIBODY ANTIGEN complex → Reticulo-endothelial system

produced by disturbed immune mechanism in response to unspecified antigen.

If complex large or antigen in excess

will lodge in 'gaps' between endothelial cells in vessel

and activates

COMPLEMENT CASCADE

Results in production of lysoenzymes and destruction of vessel wall with haemorrhage and fibrinoid necrosis.

This is termed IMMUNE COMPLEX VASCULITIS.

Indirect immunofluorescent microscopy on biopsy material will demonstrate the presence of immune complexes.

In giant cell arteritis and granulomatous vasculitis, cellular immune mechanisms are probably to blame and vessels are directly attacked.

Diseases of the Vessel Wall

Vasculitis *(continued)*

CLINICAL PRESENTATIONS, DIAGNOSIS, MANAGEMENT

Systemic Lupus Erythematosus

In 75% of cases, neurological involvement precedes systemic manifestations.

- Personality change
- Seizures
- STROKE-LIKE SYNDROME
- Cranial or peripheral nerve involvement
- SPINAL STROKE
- Involuntary movements

Investigations

Blood

Elevated ESR.
Antinuclear antibodies – ANA (antiDNA).
Elevated immunoglobulins.
Depressed serum compliment levels.

Other

EEG – diffuse disturbance.
CT scan – multiple small contrast enhancing areas.
CSF – protein elevated (Ig), mononuclear cells,
          ANA, depressed compliment levels.
Angiography – vessels have beaded appearance.
Skin/lymph node or renal biopsy.

Treatment:

Steroids, immunosuppressive therapy.

Polyarteritis Nodosa

Nervous system involvement may occur in addition to systemic features.

- STROKE-LIKE SYNDROME – Microinfarction;
                                          Aneurysm formation with subarachnoid haemorrhage.
- SPINAL STROKE
- Peripheral nerve involvement.
- 'Cogan's' syndrome $\left\{ \begin{array}{l} \text{Interstitial keratitis} \\ \text{Deafness} \\ \text{Vertigo} \end{array} \right\}$ Progressing to $\longrightarrow$ Seizures/Stroke/Coma

Investigations

Blood

Elevated ESR.
Anaemia.
Leukopenia.
Eosinophilia.
Positive R.A. latex test.

Other

Biopsy – Skin/renal.
Microscopy — necrotic vessel,
          — lumen diminished,
          — leucocytes and eosinphils in
                    necrotic media and adventitia.
Positive indirect immunofluorescent microscopy.

Treatment

Steroids, immunosuppressive therapy.

Diseases of the Vessel Wall

Vasculitis *(continued)*

Hypersensitivity angiitis: caused by immune complex deposition in vascular basement membrane.   Neurological involvement in 30% of all cases.

Systemic symptoms

Fever   Followed by system involvement
Rash   ⟶   e.g. Cardiopulmonary.
Arthralgia   Gastro-intestinal.
                    Nervous system – neuropathy, STROKE-LIKE SYNDROME.

Causation	Investigation	
	Blood	*Other*
Bacterial or viral infection ⟶	Elevated ESR. ⟶	Biopsy – Skin.
Underlying neoplasia	Anaemia.	Small arteries/veins
	Leukopenia.	affected by fibrinoid necrosis
		with marked inflammatory cell
		infiltration.

Treatment

Remove or treat cause, and early high dose steroids ⟶ rapid improvement.

Giant Cell Arteritis (syn: Temporal arteritis)
Presents in patients 50 years +.

Systemic symptoms

Weight loss/lassitude invariable.
Polymyalgia Rheumatica may co-exist.
Headache.
Visual disturbance – short ciliary artery – blindness with a normal fundus.
Dementia.   vasa nervorum – ophthalmoplegia (N. III, IV, VI).
STROKE-LIKE SYNDROME – usually the superficial temporal branches of the external carotid are involved but the basilar artery and posterior cerebral artery involvement will result in stroke-like syndromes in these territories.

Fibrinoid necrosis in the media surrounded by macrophages.

Investigation

Blood	*Other*
⟶ Elevated ESR.	⟶ Temporal artery biopsy
Anaemia.	(Rarely) external carotid angiogram
Leukocytosis.	– beaded appearance.

Treatment

Steroids: Prednisolone 80–100 mg daily. Reduce to alternate day maintenance dose.
       Continue for 6–12 months.
Spontaneous recovery may occur at 6–12 months.

Diseases of the Vessel Wall

Vasculitis *(continued)*

Takayashu's disease

Aortic arch syndrome. Presents in young adults or children. It is an arteritis affecting major branches – round cell infiltration. When healing takes place, fibrosis narrows the vessels further.

Transient ischaemia.

Strokes.

Coronary artery involvement; cardiac symptoms.

Diagnosis is suspected by absence of pulses in limbs and neck. Confirmed by angiography and treated by surgical reconstruction.

Granulomatous vasculitis

Wegener's granulomatosis – twice as common in males aged 20–50 years.

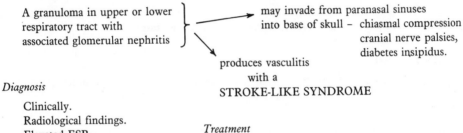

A granuloma in upper or lower respiratory tract with associated glomerular nephritis → may invade from paranasal sinuses into base of skull – chiasmal compression cranial nerve palsies, diabetes insipidus.

produces vasculitis with a STROKE-LIKE SYNDROME

Diagnosis

Clinically.

Radiological findings.

Elevated ESR.

Elevated IgA.

Elevated IgE.

Treatment

Responds to immunosuppressive therapy.

Granulomatous angiitis of the nervous system

Only central nervous system is involved.

Fever/headache/STROKE-LIKE SYNDROME.

Diagnosis

Difficult.

Laboratory findings unhelpful.

Meningeal biopsy diagnostic.

Treatment

Steroids are life-saving.

Diseases of the Blood

Disorders of the blood may manifest themselves as 'stroke-like' syndromes. Examination of the peripheral blood film is an important investigation in cerebrovascular disease. Where indicated, more extensive haematological investigation is necessary.

Disseminated Intravascular Coagulation (DIC)

A consequence of:

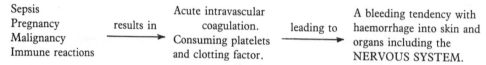

Sepsis
Pregnancy   results in → Acute intravascular coagulation. Consuming platelets and clotting factor.   leading to → A bleeding tendency with haemorrhage into skin and organs including the NERVOUS SYSTEM.
Malignancy
Immune reactions

Neurological involvement – a diffuse fluctuating encephalopathy, subarachnoid or subdural haemorrhage.

Diagnosis confirmed by – low platelet count – prolonged prothrombin time and reduced fibrinogen levels.

Treatment
Heparin. Fresh frozen plasma/vitamin K. Treatment of underlying cause.

HAEMOGLOBINOPATHIES

These are genetically determined disorders in which abnormal haemoglobin is present in red blood cells.

Sickle cell disease

The patient is of small stature, usually with chronic leg ulcers, cardiomegaly and hepatosplenomegaly. When arterial oxygen saturation is reduced, 'sickling' will occur, manifested clinically by abdominal pain/bone pain.

Neurological involvement – hemiparesis, optic atrophy, subarachnoid haemorrhage.

Diagnosis is confirmed in vitro by the 'sickling' of cells when O_2 tension is reduced and by haemoglobin electrophoresis.

Treatment
Analgesics for pain.
O_2 therapy or hyperbaric O_2.

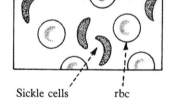

Sickle cells   rbc

Diseases of the Blood

Polycythaemia

Both polycythaemia rubra vera (primary) and secondary polycythaemia may result in *neurological* involvement – increased viscosity results in reduced cerebral blood flow and an increased tendency towards thrombosis.

Headaches, visual blurring and vertigo are common neurological symptoms.
Transient ischaemic attacks and thrombotic cerebral infarction occur.

Diagnosis

Hb and PCV are elevated.
Primary polycythaemia is confirmed by increased red cell count, white blood count and platelets.
Secondary polycythaemia – respiratory, renal or congenital heart disease are causal.

Treatment

Venesection with replacement of volume with low molecular weight dextran.
Antimitotic drugs may also be used.

Hypergammaglobulinaemia

An increase in serum gamma globulin may arise as a primary event or secondary to leukaemia, myeloma, amyloid. *Neurological* involvement develops in 20% of cases – due to increased viscosity.

Clinical features are similar to those of polycythaemia – peripheral nervous system involvement may also occur.

Diagnosis is confirmed by protein electrophoresis.

Treatment – underlying cause – plasmaphoresis.

Thrombotic Thrombocytopenic Purpura (syn: Moschkowitz's syndrome)

This is a fibrinoid degeneration of the subintimal structures of small blood vessels. Lesions occur in all organs including the brain.

Clinical features – Fever with purpura and multiorgan involvement and neurological features of diffuse encephalopathy or massive intracranial haemorrhage.

Haemolytic anaemia, haematuria and thrombocytopenia are the main laboratory features.

Treatment

Heparin, steroids and platelet inhibitors may be of value.

Thrombocytosis

This is an elevation in platelet count above 800,000 per mm^3 It may be part of a myeloproliferative disorder or 'reactive' to chronic infection. Patients present with recurrent thrombotic episodes.

Treatment

Plasmaphoresis and antimitotic drugs may be necessary.

Cerebrovascular Disease – Venous Thrombosis

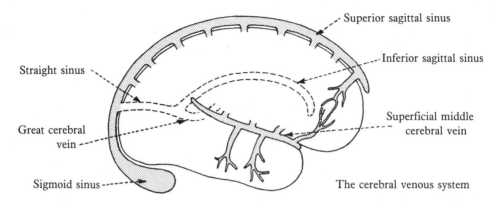

The venous sinuses play an important rôle in CSF absorption with arachnoid villi penetrating in particular the sagittal sinus.

Cerebral venous thrombosis may occur in pregnancy, with sepsis (sigmoid sinus thrombosis following mastoiditis), polycythaemia or sickle cell disease.

Infection with dehydration is a common causation in children.

Clinical features:

Headache with seizures at onset, progressing to coma in extreme cases. Bilateral signs are usually found because of the midline 'draining' nature of the sinuses.

CAVERNOUS SINUS THROMBOSIS

This commonly results from infection on the face spreading through the angular vein into the cavernous sinus.

Sphenoid, frontal and ethmoid sinuses may also act as infective sources.

Clinical features:

The clinical picture is characteristic with fevers, rigors, headache and involvement of III, IV, VI cranial nerves as well as the ophthalmic division of V.

Blockage of venous drainage results in oedema of the periorbital structures and forehead.

Retinal oedema and papilloedema will occur with loss of vision.

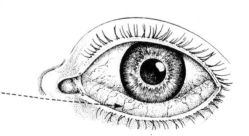

Treatment:

Adequate and appropriate antibiotics, with surgical drainage of sinuses if this is the source of infection.

Cerebrovascular Disease – Unusual Forms

ABNORMALITIES OF EXTRACRANIAL VESSELS
Fibromuscular dysplasia

The vessel has an appearance like a 'string of beads'; intracranial as well as extracranial vessels may also be involved. The patient presents with infarction as a result of thrombotic occlusion. There is a strong association with berry aneurysm.

Dilated and narrowed segments of vessel. Produced by fibrosis of the lamina media.

Internal carotid artery 'kinking'

A loop of redundant internal carotid artery – may be congenital or acquired as a consequence of atheromatous degenerative vascular disease.

The natural history of 'kinking' is unclear. The vessel may momentarily block during lateral head movement or damage to the endothelial lining might result in it becoming an embolic source. Treatment is usually conservative unless head turning clearly provokes symptoms, in which case reconstruction may be considered.

Cervical rib

Pressure from a cervical rib can result in aneurysmal formation in the subclavian artery with endothelial damage, thrombus formation and embolisation down the arm or retrograde thrombus spread and embolisation to the vertebral and common carotid arteries.

Veretebral artery

Common carotid artery

Cervical rib

Subclavian artery

The consequences of brachial plexus compression and its management are discussed on pages 430–433.

Trauma to carotid and vertebral vessels

A direct blow to the neck or a sustained tight grip around the neck may result in thrombotic occlusion.

A history of a hyperextension neck injury or an attempted 'throttling' with bruising of the neck is suggestive.

The vertebral arteries are particularly susceptible to trauma in view of their close relationship to the cervical spine at intervertebral foramina, atlanto-axial joint and the occipito-atlantal joint.

Angiography will confirm, and exploration and/or anticoagulant therapy may halt thrombus formation.

Inflammatory vessel occlusion

Infection in structures close to the carotid artery can result in inflammatory change in the vessel wall and secondary thrombosis. In children, infection in the retropharyngeal fossa (tonsillar infection) may cause cerebral infarction. Meningitis (especially pneumococcal) may result in secondary arteritis and occlusion of intracerebral vessels as they cross the subarachnoid space.

The Oral Contraceptive

Oral contraceptives increase the risk of stroke in young women. The risk is nine times that of age matched controls.

Pathology: Intimal hyperplasia is associated with thrombotic occlusion of large vessels. The risk of thromboembolism appears related to the oestrogen content of the 'pill' and its effect on platelet aggregation, antithrombin III and fibrinolysins.

257

Cerebrovascular Disease — Intracerebral Haemorrhage

By definition, 'intracerebral haemorrhage' occurs within the brain substance, but rupture through to the cortical surface may produce associated 'subarachnoid' bleeding. When the haemorrhage occurs deep in the hemisphere, rupture into the ventricular system is common.

Intraventricular haemorrhage

Intracerebral haematoma

Subarachnoid haemorrhage

Causes:

Aneurysm.
Arteriovenous malformation.
Trauma
Hypertension.

Blood dyscrasias.
Anticoagulant therapy.
Idiopathic.

In autopsy series, hypertension accounts for 40–50% of patients dying from non-traumatic haematomas. Aneurysms and arteriovenous malformations make up about 30%. In hypertensive patients, hyalinisation within the walls of small cerebral vessels results in the formation of *'microaneurysms'*. These are small outpouchings or local ectatic dilatations less than 1 mm in size, as initially described by Charcot and Bouchard. They tend to arise on intraparenchymal perforating vessels; rupture therefore occurs within the brain substance. In normotensive patients without any evident underlying pathology the cause remains unknown, but *cryptic arteriovenous malformations* are suspect especially in younger patients (i.e. less than 40 years) and when the haematoma is 'lobar' (i.e. frontal, temporal, parieto-occipital). In these patients, the haematoma may temporarily or permanently obliterate the lesion. Reinvestigation following haematoma resolution occasionally reveals previously undetected malformations.

Pathological effects:

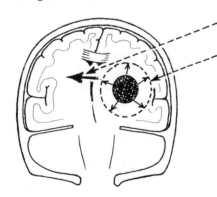

Space-occupying effect – brain shift.

48 hours after the bleed, the haematoma directly affects the adjacent brain substance producing a layer of necrosis surrounded by perivascular bleeding.

Oedema is seldom a prominent feature.

Haematoma resolution occurs in 4–8 weeks, leaving a cystic cavity.

Intracerebral Haemorrhage

Sites:

Frontal
Basal ganglia/thalamus
15%
37%
15%
21%
Parieto-occipital
Temporal
8%
Cerebellar
4%
Pontine

In hypertensive patients, up to 70% occur in the basal ganglia/thalamic region.

Clinical effects:

SUPRATENTORIAL HAEMATOMA

Mass effect: Sudden onset of headache followed by either a rapid loss of consciousness or a gradual deterioration in conscious level over 24–48 hours.

Focal signs: Hemiparesis, hemisensory loss and homonymous hemianopia are common. The patient may be aware of limb weakness developing prior to losing consciousness.
A III nerve palsy indicates transtentorial herniation.

CEREBELLAR HAEMATOMA — Sudden onset of headache with subsequent effects developing either acutely or subacutely –
Cerebellar and brainstem signs e.g. ataxia, dysarthria, nystagmus, vertigo and vomiting.
CSF obstruction ⟶ hydrocephalus with symptoms and signs of ↑ICP.

PONTINE HAEMATOMA — Sudden loss of consciousness.
Quadraplegia.
Respiratory irregularities ⟶ slowed respiration.
Pinpoint pupils, ↑temperature.
Skewed/dysconjugate eye movements.
Death usually follows.

Investigations:

A CT SCAN determines the exact site and size of the haematoma and excludes other pathologies.

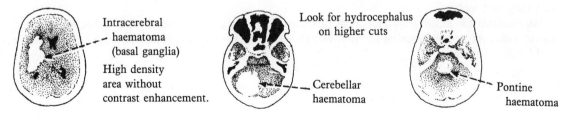

Intracerebral haematoma (basal ganglia)
High density area without contrast enhancement.

Look for hydrocephalus on higher cuts

Cerebellar haematoma

Pontine haematoma

ANGIOGRAPHY detects an underlying arteriovenous malformation (AVM) or aneurysm and is necessary before any operative intervention.

In patients with 'negative' angiography, managed conservatively, a late CT scan with contrast (double-dose) following haematoma reabsorption may demonstrate a small enhancing AVM.

Intracerebral Haemorrhage

Management:

Supratentorial haematoma:

Results of operative evacuation of intracerebral haematomas (through a craniotomy flap) are disappointing; a controlled study of conservative versus operative treatment by McKissock et al. in 1961 showed no difference in outcome. In general, haematoma evacuation is only indicated in patients who deteriorate or fail to improve as a result of the 'mass' effect; operation will not benefit moribund patients i.e. patients extending to painful stimuli with no pupil reaction.

Prognosis:

Poor prognostic features
– large, deep lesions (basal ganglia/thalamic).
  depth of conscious level (flexion or extension to painful stimuli).

Good prognostic factors
– small superficial lesions (i.e. frontal, temporal or parieto-occipital).
– conscious patients or patients localising to painful stimuli.

The overall mortality ranges from 50–65% (90% if the patient is in coma).

Cerebellar haematoma:

Small haematomas causing minimal effects may be managed conservatively. Otherwise, urgent evacuation through a suboccipital craniectomy is required. Relief of brainstem compression may be life saving and operative morbidity is low.

The overall mortality is approximately 30%.

Pontine haemorrhage:

Most patients with pontine haemorrhage die. A conservative approach is usually adopted although some advocate operative exploration.

INTRAVENTRICULAR HAEMORRHAGE

Haemorrhage into the ventricles causes a sudden loss of consciousness. With a large bleed, death may follow due to the pressure transmission throughout the ventricular system. Blood in the ventricles does not in itself cause brain damage and, following clot resolution, complete recovery may occur.

No treatment is required; attempts at flushing out the ventricles usually fail. If the blood 'cast' causes obstructive hydrocephalus, then ventricular drainage (although hampered by the presence of blood) is indicated.

Subarachnoid Haemorrhage (SAH)

Intracranial vessels lie in the *subarachnoid* space and give off small perforating branches to the brain tissue. Bleeding from these vessels or from an associated aneurysm occurs primarily into this space. Some intracranial aneurysms are imbedded within the brain tissue and their rupture causes intracerebral bleeding with or without subarachnoid haemorrhage.

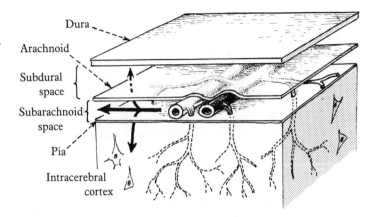

Occasionally the arachnoid layer gives way and a subdural haematoma results.

Incidence:

Subarachnoid haemorrhage occurs in approximately 10–15 per 100,000 per year.

Cause:

Cerebral aneurysms are the most frequent cause of subarachnoid haemorrhage, with arteriovenous malformations accounting for 6%.

In many patients detailed investigation fails to reveal a source of the haemorrhage. Some appear related to hypertension. Cryptic arteriovenous malformations or small thrombosed aneurysms may contribute to the remainder.

Causes of SAH	
Aneurysm	51%
A-V malformations	6%
Hypertension	15%
Tumours	
Bleeding diathesis	6%
Anticoagulants	
Idiopathic	22%

Symptoms and Signs:

The severity of the symptoms is related to the severity of the bleed.

Severe *headache* of instantaneous onset (often described as a 'blow to the head') may drop the patient to his knees. A transient or prolonged *loss of consciousness* or *epileptic seizure* may immediately follow. Nausea and *vomiting* commonly occur.

Rarely, the headache is mild and may represent a 'warning leak' of blood before a major bleed.

Subarachnoid Haemorrhage

Symptoms and Signs *(continued)*

Neck stiffness is present on passive neck flexion.

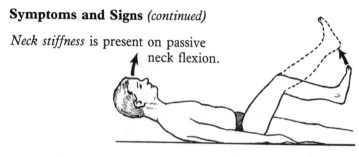

Kernig's sign:
stretching nerve roots by extending the knee causes pain.

Coma or *depression of conscious level* may result from the direct effect of the subarachnoid haemorrhage or from the mass effect of an associated intracerebral haematoma.

Focal damage from a haematoma will produce *focal signs* e.g. limb weakness, dysphasia. The presence of a III nerve palsy indicates either transtentorial herniation or direct nerve or oculomotor nucleus damage from a posterior communicating artery or basilar artery aneurysm.

Epilepsy frequently occurs and may mask other features.

Fundus examination may reveal *papilloedema* or a *subhyaloid haemorrhage* caused by the sudden rise in intracranial pressure.

A *'reactive hypertension'* commonly develops i.e. a rise in BP in patients with no evidence of pre-existing hypertension, and takes several days to return to normal levels.

Pyrexia is also a common finding; if severe and fluctuating, it may reflect ischaemic hypothalamic damage.

Investigative approach

Lumbar puncture establishes the diagnosis of subarachnoid haemorrhage, but in patients with a mass lesion, lumbar puncture could precipitate transtentorial herniation.

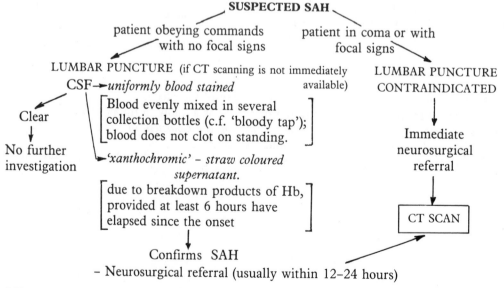

Subarachnoid Haemorrhage

Age limit for neurosurgical referral: Since mortality and morbidity increase with age, the traditional limit for aneurysm surgery is 65 years. With modern anaesthetic and operative techniques, however, this no longer applies. Some surgeons even consider patients over the age of 70 for further investigation with a view to direct or indirect operation (see below), provided their clinical state is satisfactory.

CT scan

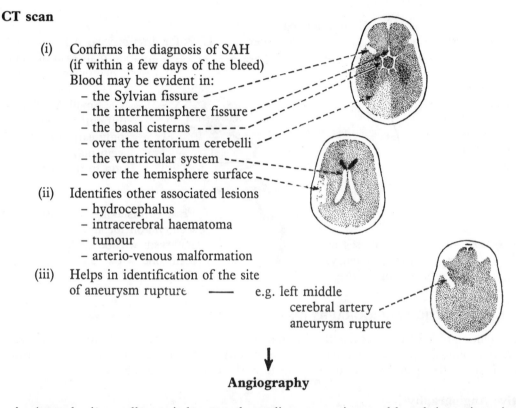

(i)   Confirms the diagnosis of SAH
      (if within a few days of the bleed)
      Blood may be evident in:
      – the Sylvian fissure
      – the interhemisphere fissure
      – the basal cisterns
      – over the tentorium cerebelli
      – the ventricular system
      – over the hemisphere surface

(ii) Identifies other associated lesions
      – hydrocephalus
      – intracerebral haematoma
      – tumour
      – arterio-venous malformation

(iii) Helps in identification of the site
      of aneurysm rupture ——— e.g. left middle
                                cerebral artery
                                aneurysm rupture

Angiography

Angiography is usually carried out at the earliest convenience, although in patients in poor clinical condition, the clinician may prefer to delay investigation until improvement has occurred. If a patient deteriorates from the mass effect of an intracranial haematoma, then emergency angiography is required prior to any decompressive operation.

Subarachnoid Haemorrhage

Angiography *(continued)*

Four vessel angiography is usually performed in all patients although in older patients vertebral angiography may be omitted in view of the greater operative risks for posterior circulation aneurysms.

Antero-posterior, lateral and *oblique* views are required.

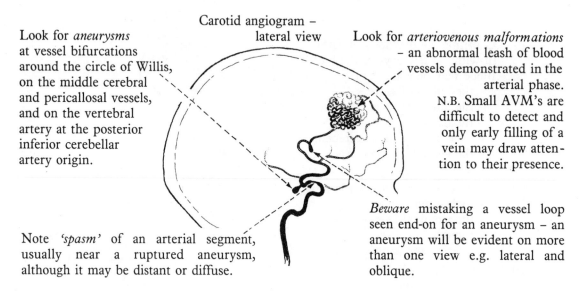

Carotid angiogram –
lateral view

Look for *aneurysms* at vessel bifurcations around the circle of Willis, on the middle cerebral and pericallosal vessels, and on the vertebral artery at the posterior inferior cerebellar artery origin.

Look for *arteriovenous malformations* – an abnormal leash of blood vessels demonstrated in the arterial phase. N.B. Small AVM's are difficult to detect and only early filling of a vein may draw attention to their presence.

Note *'spasm'* of an arterial segment, usually near a ruptured aneurysm, although it may be distant or diffuse.

Beware mistaking a vessel loop seen end-on for an aneurysm – an aneurysm will be evident on more than one view e.g. lateral and oblique.

DIGITAL SUBTRACTION ANGIOGRAPHY (DSA):

The resolution of DSA is as yet insufficient to detect small aneurysms. In the future, however, intra-arterial contrast injection DSA may replace standard angiographic techniques in permitting the use of far smaller quantities of contrast medium, thereby reducing the risks.

Negative Angiography

Angiography fails to reveal a source of the subarachnoid haemorrhage in approximately 20% of cases. In the presence of arterial spasm, reduction in flow may prevent the demonstration of an aneurysm and repeat angiography may be required at a later date.

Prognosis: In patients with negative angiography the outlook is excellent and the risk of rebleeding extremely small.

N.B. Rupture of a spinal angioma also results in SAH – if the patient's pain begins in the back before spreading to the head, or if any features of cord compression are apparent, then myelography should be the preliminary investigation (see page 408).

Cerebral Aneurysms

Incidence

At autopsy intracranial aneurysms are found in approximately 1 per cent of the British population.

Aneurysm rupture occurs in 6–12 per 100,000 per year.

Female : Male = 3 : 2
but this ratio varies with age $\Longleftarrow$ < 40 years, males > females.
$\Longrightarrow$ > 40 years, females ≫ males.

Age: — rupture is most common between 40 and 60 years but can occur in any age group, even in children.

Morphology

Intracranial aneurysms are usually *saccular*, – – – – – – – – – – – – occurring at vessel bifurcations.

Size varies from a few millimetres to several centimetres.
Those over 2.5 cm are termed 'giant' aneurysms.

Fusiform dilatation and ectasia of the carotid and the basilar artery may follow atherosclerotic damage. These aneurysms seldom rupture.
Mycotic aneurysms, secondary to vessel wall infection are now rare.

Aneurysm rupture: usually occurs at the fundus of the aneurysm and the risk appears related to size; rupture seldom occurs until the aneurysm is over 6 mm in diameter. In some, rupture occurs during exertion, straining or coitus, but in many there is no associated relationship. Giant aneurysms surprisingly are less likely to rupture, probably due to multiple layers of thrombus reinforcing the inner wall.

Sites of saccular aneurysm:

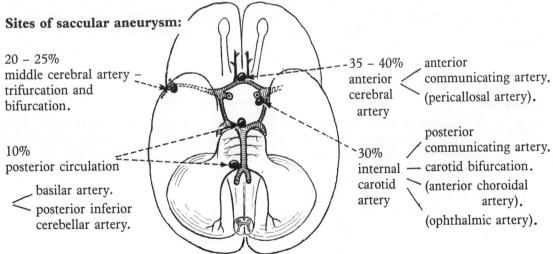

20 – 25%
middle cerebral artery – trifurcation and bifurcation.

10%
posterior circulation

< basilar artery.
< posterior inferior cerebellar artery.

35 – 40% anterior cerebral artery < anterior communicating artery. (pericallosal artery).

30% internal carotid artery

posterior communicating artery.
— carotid bifurcation.
< (anterior choroidal artery).
(ophthalmic artery).

Multiple aneurysms: in approximately 30% of patients with aneurysmal SAH, more than one aneurysm is demonstrated on angiography.

Cerebral Aneurysms

Pathogenesis: The exact cause of aneurysm formation remains unknown.

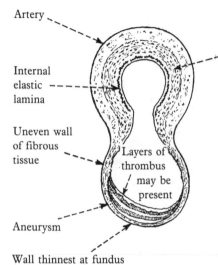

Artery

Internal elastic lamina

Uneven wall of fibrous tissue

Layers of thrombus may be present

Aneurysm

Wall thinnest at fundus

Aneurysms were once thought to be 'congenital' due to the finding of *developmental defects in the tunica media*. These defects occur at the apex of vessel bifurcation as do aneurysms, but they are also found in many extracranial vessels as well as intracranial vessels; saccular aneurysms in contrast are seldom found outwith the skull. Tunica media defects are often evident in children, yet aneurysms are rare in this age group. It now appears that *defects of the internal elastic lamina* are more important in aneurysm formation and these are probably caused by arteriosclerotic damage.

Hypertension may play a rôle; more than half the patients with ruptured aneurysm have pre-existing evidence of raised blood pressure. (Aneurysm formation is common in patients with hypertension from coarctation of the aorta.)

Clinical presentation:

1. Rupture (90%).

The features of SAH have already been described in detail (page 261); they include sudden onset of headache, vomiting, neck stiffness, loss of consciousness, focal signs and epilepsy.

Since the severity of the haemorrhage relates to the patient's clinical state and this in turn relates to outcome, much emphasis has been placed on categorising patients into 5 level grading systems e.g. 'Hunt and Hess', 'Nishioka'. Recently a new scale has been formed and approved by the World Federation of Neurosurgeons, incorporating the Glasgow Coma Scale (page 30):

Grade	Glasgow Coma Scale	
I	15	Neurologically intact (except for cranial nerve palsy).
II	15	Neurologically intact (except for cranial nerve palsy) with neck stiffness, headache or both.
III	13–14	(a) without focal neurological deficit. (b) with focal neurological deficit.
IV	8–12	With or without focal neurological deficit.
V	3–7	Unresponsive coma with or without abnormal posturing.

Glasgow Coma Score

eye opening	1–4	e.g.	no eye opening (1)
verbal response	1–5		no verbal response (1)
motor response	1–6		flexing to pain (3)
	3–15		= 5

This grading scale correlates well with final outcome and provides a prognostic index for the clinician. In addition, it enables matching of patient groups before comparing the effects of different management techniques.

Cerebral Aneurysm

Clinical presentation *(continued)*

2. Compression from aneurysm sac (7%)

A large *internal carotid artery aneurysm (or anterior communicating artery aneurysm)* may compress –

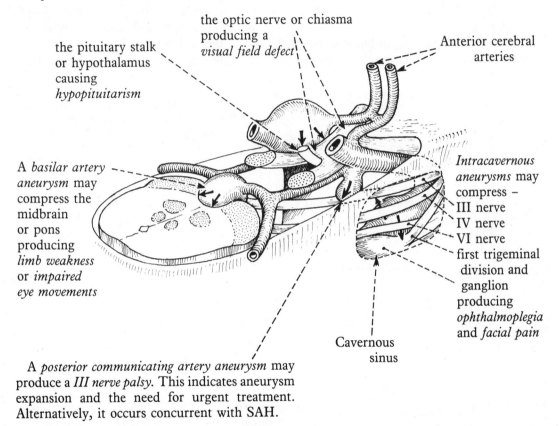

the pituitary stalk or hypothalamus causing *hypopituitarism*

the optic nerve or chiasma producing a *visual field defect*

Anterior cerebral arteries

A *basilar artery aneurysm* may compress the midbrain or pons producing *limb weakness* or *impaired eye movements*

Intracavernous aneurysms may compress –
III nerve
IV nerve
VI nerve
first trigeminal division and ganglion producing *ophthalmoplegia* and *facial pain*

Cavernous sinus

A *posterior communicating artery aneurysm* may produce a *III nerve palsy*. This indicates aneurysm expansion and the need for urgent treatment. Alternatively, it occurs concurrent with SAH.

3. Incidental finding (3%)

Angiography performed for reasons other than SAH, e.g. investigation of ischaemic or neoplastic disease, occasionally reveals previously undetected aneurysms.

Cerebral Aneurysm

Natural History of Ruptured Aneurysm

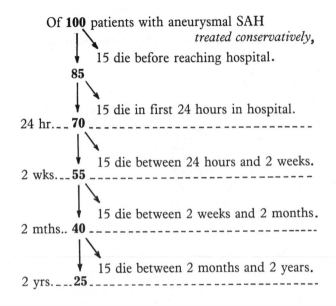

Of **100** patients with aneurysmal SAH *treated conservatively,*

15 die before reaching hospital.

85

15 die in first 24 hours in hospital.

24 hr. _ _ **70** _

15 die between 24 hours and 2 weeks.

2 wks. _ _ **55** _

15 die between 2 weeks and 2 months.

2 mths.. **40** _

15 die between 2 months and 2 years.

2 yrs. _ _ _ **25** _

SAH from ruptured aneurysm carries a high initial mortality which gradually declines with time. Of those who survive the initial bleed, rebleeding and cerebral infarction (see below) are the major causes of death.

These figures are based on studies of conservative treatment carried out in the 'sixties, at a time when the risks of operation were greater and benefits uncertain.

Complications of Aneurysmal SAH

INTRACRANIAL
– Rebleeding
– Cerebral ischaemia/infarction.
– Hydrocephalus.
– 'Expanding' haematoma.
– Epilepsy.

EXTRACRANIAL
– Myocardial infarction.
– Cardiac arrhythmias.
– Pulmonary oedema.
– Gastric haemorrhage (stress ulcer).

Cerebral Aneurysms — Complications

REBLEEDING

Rebleeding is a major problem following aneurysmal SAH. In the first 28 days (in untreated patients), approximately 30% of patients will rebleed; of these 70% die. In the following few months the risk gradually falls off but it never drops below 3.5% per year.

The chance of rebleeding after SAH   (A) in the first 6 months.

                                               (B) *per year,* in the subsequent decade.

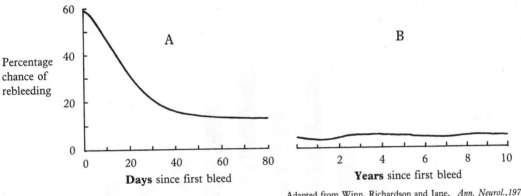

Adapted from Winn, Richardson and Jane,   *Ann. Neurol.,1977.*

Thus, even if patients survive the 'high risk' period in the first 6 months, there is a considerable chance of rebleeding and death in the subsequent ten years.

The clinical picture of rebleeding is that of SAH, but usually the effects are more severe than the initial bleed. Most patients lose consciousness; the risk of death from a rebleed is more than twice that from the initial bleed.

Investigation

All patients deteriorating suddenly require a CT scan. This helps in establishing the diagnosis of rebleeding and excludes a remediable cause of the deterioration e.g. acute hydrocephalus.

Cerebral Aneurysms — Complications

CEREBRAL ISCHAEMIA/INFARCTION

Following subarachnoid haemorrhage patients are at risk of developing cerebral ischaemia or infarction and this is an important contributory factor to mortality and morbidity. Approximately 25% of patients develop clinical evidence of ischaemia/infarction; of these 50% die as a result ; permanent neurological deficit persists in 50% of survivors. Cerebral ischaemia/infarction most frequently develops from the 4th to the 10th day from the onset – hence the term 'delayed cerebral ischaemia', but it can occur at any time from within 24 hours to several weeks, either before or after operation.

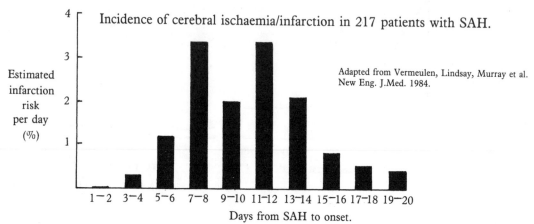

Incidence of cerebral ischaemia/infarction in 217 patients with SAH.

Adapted from Vermeulen, Lindsay, Murray et al. New Eng. J.Med. 1984.

Aetiology of Cerebral ischaemia/infarction

Arterial constriction ('vasospasm') was once thought to be the major factor responsible for delayed cerebral ischaemia; this may be so, but it is now recognised that other factors are likely to play an important rôle.

Vasospasm: Arterial narrowing on angiography occurs in up to 60% and is either focal (usually near the aneurysm) or diffuse. The development of vasospasm shows a similar delay to that of clinical ischaemia.

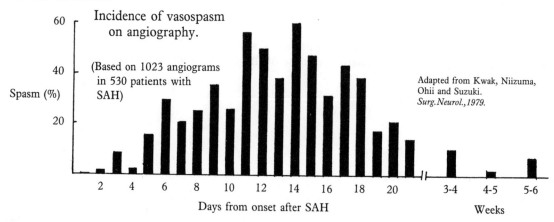

Incidence of vasospasm on angiography.

(Based on 1023 angiograms in 530 patients with SAH)

Adapted from Kwak, Niizuma, Ohii and Suzuki. *Surg.Neurol.,1979.*

Cerebral Aneurysms — Complications

Vasospasm (continued)

The exact cause of vasospasm remains unknown. Many substances, either released from the vessel wall or arising from the breakdown of blood clot, cause vasoconstriction e.g. serotonin, prostaglandin, oxyhaemoglobin; it is unlikely that any one factor is solely responsible. The greater the amount of blood in the basal cisterns (as shown on the CT scan), the higher the incidence of vasospasm and associated ischaemic deficits.

Reduced cerebral perfusion pressure:

Following SAH, intracerebral haematoma or hydrocephalus may cause a rise in intracranial pressure (ICP). Since cerebral perfusion pressure = Mean BP − ICP, a subsequent reduction in cerebral perfusion may occur.

Increased blood viscosity:

In a proportion of patients, the plasma volume falls in the first week after SAH. These patients are particularly at risk of developing cerebral ischaemic deficits probably as a result of increased blood viscosity.

Clinical effects of Cerebral ischaemia/infarction

This depends on the site and the extent of the ischaemic damage. After SAH, the anterior (carotid) circulation is most commonly involved.

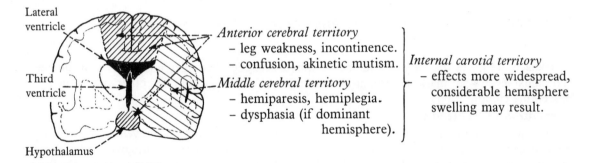

Lateral ventricle

Third ventricle

Hypothalamus

Anterior cerebral territory
 – leg weakness, incontinence.
 – confusion, akinetic mutism.
Middle cerebral territory
 – hemiparesis, hemiplegia.
 – dysphasia (if dominant
           hemisphere).

Internal carotid territory
 – effects more widespread, considerable hemisphere swelling may result.

HYDROCEPHALUS

Following SAH, cerebrospinal fluid drainage may be impaired by:

 – blood clot within the basal cisterns ⎱ 'communicating' hydrocephalus
 – obstruction of the arachnoid villi ⎰ (see page 359).
 – blood clot within the ventricular system – 'obstructive' hydrocephalus.

Hydrocephalus occurs in about 20% of patients, usually in the second week after the ictus; occasionally this is a late complication. In only $\frac{1}{3}$ are symptoms of headache, impaired conscious level, dementia, incontinence or gait ataxia severe enough to warrant treatment.

Cerebral Aneurysms — Complications

'EXPANDING' INTRACEREBRAL HAEMATOMA

Brain swelling around an intracerebral haematoma may aggravate the mass effect of the haematoma; this may cause a progressive deterioration in conscious level or progression of focal signs.

EPILEPSY

Epilepsy may occur at any stage after SAH, especially if a haematoma has caused cortical damage.

Seizures may be generalised or partial (focal).

EXTRACRANIAL COMPLICATIONS

MYOCARDIAL INFARCTION / CARDIAC ARRHYTHMIAS: electrocardiographic and pathological changes in the myocardium are occasionally evident after SAH, and ventricular fibrillation has been recorded. These problems are likely to occur secondarily to catecholamine release following ischaemic damage to the hypothalamus.

PULMONARY OEDEMA: this occasionally occurs after SAH, probably as a result of massive sympathetic discharge; note the 'pink, frothy' sputum and typical auscultatory and chest X-ray findings.

GASTRIC HAEMORRHAGE: bleeding from gastric erosions occasionally occurs after SAH but rarely threatens life.

Cerebral Aneurysms — Management following SAH

Headache requires *analgesia* - codeine or dihydrocodeine. Stronger analgesics may depress conscious level and mask neurological deterioration. Management is otherwise aimed at preventing complications –

Prevention of Rebleeding

OPERATION: Clipping of the aneurysm neck is the only certain way of preventing rebleeding, but this technique is not always possible and other methods are sometimes employed. The timing of operation is a controversial topic. The earlier the operation – the fewer patients die from rebleeding, but the greater is the operative morbidity and mortality.

BED REST: Usually enforced after SAH, although there is no evidence that this reduces the rebleed risk. If conservative treatment is planned, most restrict bed rest to 2–3 weeks.

ANTIFIBRINOLYTIC AGENTS: tranexamic acid, epsilon aminocaproic acid.

These agents have been used for many years with the aim of preventing rebleeding by delaying clot dissolution around the aneurysm fundus. A recent large multicentre trial showed that tranexamic acid does reduce bleeding (by more than 50%) but at the expense of increasing the incidence of cerebral ischaemia. The overall results showed no improvement in mortality or morbidity.

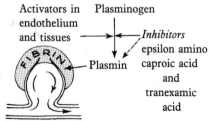

Fibrinolytic Mechanism

Activators in endothelium and tissues → Plasminogen ← *Inhibitors* epsilon amino caproic acid and tranexamic acid

Plasmin

Cerebral Aneurysms — Management following SAH

OPERATIVE METHODS

Direct clipping of the aneurysm neck is the optimal method of treatment and prevents further rupture; aneurysm clips rarely slip after application. The operating microscope and improved anaesthetic techniques have considerably lowered mortality and morbidity. Careful dissection of arachnoid tissue around the neck of the aneurysm enables accurate positioning of the clip.
The use of hypotension during dissection and clipping may also aid handling and reduce tension within the aneurysm sac.

Wrapping: If the width of the aneurysm neck or its involvement with adjacent vessels prevents clipping then muslin gauze may be wrapped around the fundus. This may provide some protection but the long term benefits are uncertain.

Some surgeons cover the aneurysm fundus with a solidifying acrylic agent, but this is a difficult technique which has not gained widespread popularity.

Trapping: Clipping of proximal and distal vessels is the only possible treatment for some aneurysms e.g. 'giant' and intracavernous aneurysms. This prevents rebleeding but carries a high risk of producing an ischaemic deficit. A bypass procedure – superficial temporal to middle cerebral anastomosis, prior to trapping – may help minimise the risk of this complication.

Induced thrombosis: Several methods have been employed to induce thrombosis within the aneurysm sac. These include insertion of yards of fine wire into the exposed sac and stereotactic insertion of an electrode. Even external electromagnetic induction has been used. These methods, however, are not without risk; thrombus formation may be short lived and rebleeding may occur.

Cerebral Aneurysms — Management following SAH

Operative Methods (continued)

Proximal occlusion

– *anterior cerebral artery occlusion:* if difficulty is encountered in directly clipping anterior communicating artery aneurysms, some advocate occlusion of the anterior cerebral artery, proximal to the aneurysm. Provided this vessel is not the sole supplier of both distal anterior cerebral arteries, the risk of ischaemia is small. The reduction in intraarterial pressure reduces the risk of rebleeding, but not on a permanent basis.

– *common carotid ligation:* this technique is used for aneurysms arising directly from the carotid artery where clipping has failed or was not attempted e.g. an intracavernous aneurysm or 'giant' ophthalmic artery aneurysm. Most patients tolerate common carotid occlusion; collateral circulation through the circle of Willis and perhaps from reverse flow in the external carotid artery usually provides sufficient hemispheric flow to prevent ischaemic complications.

Ligation of the common carotid artery (rather than the internal carotid artery) permits retrograde flow in the external carotid artery from anastomosis with vessels on the opposite side and may help prevent ischaemic complications.

Efforts are made to predict patients who will not tolerate common carotid occlusion.
– Compression of the carotid artery during angiography demonstrates the extent of cross circulation from the other side.
– Cerebral blood flow studies performed preoperatively (Xenon inhalation) and peroperatively (intraarterial Xenon) before and during temporary occlusion are of value in identifying those patients with an inadequate collateral circulation. Pressure from the internal carotid artery stump provides additional information.
– Alternatively, the common carotid artery is temporarily occluded under local anaesthetic for a 30 minute period; if no neurological deficit develops, the vessel is permanently ligated.

These methods are not infallible and late ischaemic deficits occasionally occur.

Carotid ligation prevents the patient from rebleeding in the 'high risk' period. Beyond the first 6 months, the rebleed risk reverts to that of an untreated aneurysm i.e. 3.5% per year.

274

Cerebral Aneurysms — Management following SAH

TIMING OF OPERATION

Pioneers of aneurysm surgery found that operation within a day or two of the haemorrhage carried an unacceptably high risk. Operative mortality rates dramatically fell when operation was delayed for several weeks. The longer the delay, the better the results; but the longer the delay, the greater the possibility of death from rebleeding. The clinical condition or 'grade' of the patient also played a major part; the worse the grade the worse the outcome. As a result, surgeons adopted an optimal delay period of *6–14 days from the haemorrhage, the exact time depending on the patient's clinical condition.*

Improved operative and anaesthetic techniques in recent years again led surgeons to attempt operation within 48 hours of the haemorrhage. Although operative mortality is higher than for those patients undergoing delayed operation, the reduced mortality from rebleeding may offset this. Clarification of the optimal time for aneurysm surgery requires further study, but *initial results suggest that, for patients in good clinical condition (grade I), operation within 2–3 days prevents a proportion from rebleeding, yet adds little additional risk.*

OPERATIVE MORTALITY (i.e. mortality rate in patients undergoing operation) ranges from 5–50% depending on the patient's clinical condition and the timing of operation. *Management mortality* figures are of more value when comparing results of different management regimes.

Operative Mortality (at 3 months)			**Management Mortality** (at 3 months)		
Patients undergoing operation No. = 187			Patients admitted to the neurological/neurosurgical unit within 3 days from the haemorrhage. No. = 479		
	No.	Mortality		No.	Mortality
Preoperative Grade (Hunt and Hess) 1	82	5%	Grade on admission (Hunt and Hess) 1	79	22%
2	55	24%	2	180	32%
3	46	20%	3	132	31%
4	4	50%	4	82	63%
5	-	-	5	6	100%

Adapted from Vermeulen, Lindsay, Murray et al.
New Eng. J. Med (1984)

275

Cerebral Aneurysms — Management following SAH

Prevention of Cerebral Ischaemia/Infarction

Despite considerable clinical and experimental research, cerebral ischaemia remains a major problem following SAH. Recent advances may prove beneficial –

Avoidance of antihypertensive therapy: antihypertensive therapy is widely used after SAH to reduce 'reactive' hypertension and to theoretically minimise the risk of rebleeding. In the normal subject a drop in BP results in cerebral vasodilatation to maintain cerebral blood flow (autoregulation, page 74). After SAH, autoregulation is often impaired; a drop in BP causes a reduction in cerebral blood flow with a subsequent risk of cerebral ischaemia. Accumulated evidence shows that patients with SAH on antihypertensive therapy have a significantly higher risk of cerebral infarction.

Hypertensive therapy and plasma volume expansion: since autoregulation commonly fails after SAH, artificial means of blood pressure elevation (peripheral vasoconstriction – metaraminol or dopamine infusion combined with plasma volume expansion) increase cerebral blood flow. In 1972, Kosnik and Hunt demonstrated that ischaemic neurological deficits developing after aneurysm operations could be reversed by inducing hypertension. Often a critical level of blood pressure was evident.

Early recognition and treatment of a developing neurological deficit may prevent progression from ischaemia to infarction. Delayed treatment may merely aggravate vasogenic oedema in an ischaemic area. This technique of induced hypertension is now widely applied – with good results, although it is possible that patients who benefit would have recovered spontaneously with time.

Antispasmodic agents: despite numerous trials in the last 10–20 years, antispasmodic drugs remain a dismal failure in the prophylaxis of 'vasospasm' and cerebral ischaemia. Recent interest centres around the calcium antagonist NIMODIPINE. One multicentre study demonstrated a promising reduction of severe ischaemic deficits in patients on nimodipine. Whether this is due to an antispasmodic effect remains unknown; further confirmation is required.

Steroids/Rheomacrodex/Mannitol: many clinicians use steroids or a combination of rheomacrodex and mannitol infusion either prophylactically or following the development of a neurological deficit, but since there are no adequate trials of their use in SAH, benefits remain unknown.

Cerebral Aneurysms — Management following SAH

Hydrocephalus

Hydrocephalus causing acute deterioration in conscious level requires urgent CSF drainage with a ventricular catheter (in 'communicating' hydrocephalus lumbar puncture may provide temporary benefit).

Gradual deterioration or failure to improve in the presence of enlarged ventricles indicates the need for permanent CSF drainage with either a ventriculo-peritoneal or ventriculo-atrial shunt.

Expanding Intracerebral Haematoma

Intracerebral haematomas from ruptured aneurysms do not require specific treatment unless 'mass' effect causes a deterioration of conscious level. This necessitates urgent angiography followed by evacuation of the haematoma and clipping of the aneurysm; under these circumstances, operative mortality is high.

OUTCOME AFTER SUBARACHNOID HAEMORRHAGE

Of patients surviving the initial bleed and admitted within 3 days to the neurosurgical unit, approximately one third die within the following 3 months. Almost half make a good recovery and regain former employment, although in a proportion, minor personality change and intellectual deficit persist.

Factors providing a prognostic guide are: age, loss of consciousness at the ictus, clinical condition on admission and the presence of pre-existing hypertension or arterial disease.

Comparing different operative or management policies: Comparison of different treatments for ruptured aneurysms is difficult, unless conducted under the confines of a randomised controlled trial. 'Operative mortality' provides little information unless patient groups are carefully matched for age, clinical condition and timing of operation. 'Management mortality' (e.g. outcome of all admitted patients up to 3 months from the ictus) is of more practical value, but even then, admission policies require careful scrutiny.

Cerebral Aneurysms — Management following SAH

ANEURYSMS CAUSING COMPRESSIVE SYMPTOMS AND SIGNS

Aneurysms may present as a result of compression of adjacent neurological structures. A III nerve palsy from a posterior communicating aneurysm often precedes rupture by a few days or weeks and indicates the need for urgent operative treatment.

A giant aneurysm (over 25 mm in diameter) causing compressive problems, seldom ruptures but the symptoms and signs are unlikely to resolve unless spontaneous thrombosis occurs.

Direct clipping and aspiration or excision of the sac provides the best treatment. In some patients the size of the aneurysm neck prevents clipping and either common carotid ligation (if a carotid aneurysm) or 'trapping' provide alternative methods. Prior to 'trapping, superficial temporal middle cerebral anastomosis may help prevent ischaemic complications.

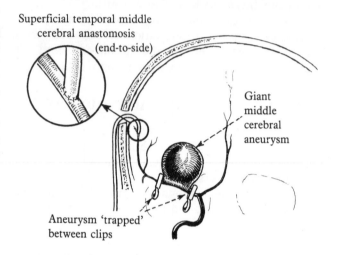

Superficial temporal middle cerebral anastomosis (end-to-side)

Giant middle cerebral aneurysm

Aneurysm 'trapped' between clips

INCIDENTAL ANEURYSMS

Opinions vary as to whether incidental aneurysms (i.e. aneurysms not causing symptoms or signs) require operation. Recent studies suggest that the risk of bleeding from a previously unruptured aneurysm is approximately 1% per year, with aneurysms over 10 mm in diameter carrying the highest risk.

Operative mortality of aneurysm clipping in the absence of SAH lies well below 5%. Thus, younger patients (e.g. under 45 years) with an otherwise normal life expectancy may well benefit from operation.

When angiography after SAH reveals multiple aneurysms the neurosurgeon must decide whether to operate on the intact as well as the ruptured aneurysm. If accessible through the one craniotomy flap, many clip unruptured aneurysms at the initial operation, although delayed clipping at a second operation several weeks later minimises the risk of ischaemic complications.

Arterio-Venous Malformations

Arterio-venous malformations (AVM's) are developmental anomalies of the intracranial vasculature; they are not neoplastic despite their tendency to expand with time and the descriptive term 'angioma' occasionally applied.

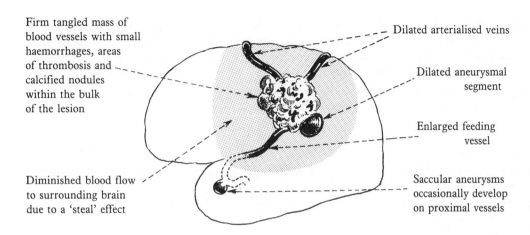

Firm tangled mass of blood vessels with small haemorrhages, areas of thrombosis and calcified nodules within the bulk of the lesion

Dilated arterialised veins

Dilated aneurysmal segment

Enlarged feeding vessel

Diminished blood flow to surrounding brain due to a 'steal' effect

Saccular aneurysms occasionally develop on proximal vessels

Dilated arteries feed directly into a tangled mass of blood vessels of varying calibre; they by-pass the capillary network and shunt oxygenated blood directly into the venous system. As a result of raised intraluminal pressure, veins may adopt an 'aneurysmal' appearance. Arterio-venous malformations may occur at any site but are commonest in the middle cerebral artery territory.

Occasionally, different forms of vascular malformation exist:

Capillary telangiectasis: an area of dilated capillaries, like a small petechial patch on the brain surface – especially in the pons. These lesions are often only revealed at autopsy.

Cavernous malformation/angioma: plum coloured sponge-like mass composed of a collection of blood filled spaces, but without enlargement of feeding or draining vessels.

Clinical presentation:

HAEMORRHAGE: About 40–60 per cent of patients with an AVM present with haemorrhage – often with an intracerebral or intraventricular component. In comparison with saccular aneurysms, AVM's tend to bleed in younger patients i.e. 20–40 years, and are less likely to have a fatal outcome. In addition, vasospasm and delayed ischaemic complications rarely develop. Small AVM's are at greater risk of bleeding than larger lesions.

Risk of initial and recurrent bleeding: the risk of haemorrhage over a 5 year period in patients with a previously unruptured AVM is approximately 15 per cent (i.e. 2–3 per cent per year); however this risk increases to 50 per cent for lesions under 3 cm in size.

After a haemorrhage, the chance of a further bleed is slightly increased in the first year but beyond that the risk reverts to that of an unruptured AVM.

Mortality from haemorrhage: in contrast to the high mortality following aneurysm rupture, haemorrhage from an AVM carries the relatively low mortality rate of approximately 10 per cent.

Arterio-Venous Malformations

Clinical presentation (continued)

EPILEPSY: Generalised or partial seizures commonly occur in patients with arterio-venous malformation either before or after haemorrhage, especially if the lesion involves the cortical surface.

NEUROLOGICAL DEFICIT: Large AVM's, especially those involving the basal ganglia, may present with a slowly progressive dementia, hemiparesis or visual field defect, probably as a result of a 'steal' effect. The infrequent brain stem AVM may also produce a motor or sensory deficit, with or without cranial nerve involvement.

HEADACHE: Attacks of well localised headache – unilateral and throbbing – occur in a proportion of patients subsequently shown to have an AVM.

CRANIAL BRUIT: Auscultation, especially over the eyeball, occasionally reveals a bruit.

Investigations:

CT scan: Most AVM's are evident on CT scan unless masked by the presence of an intracranial haematoma.

A double dose of intra-venous contrast may aid visualisation, especially with small 'cryptic' lesions.

Before i.v. contrast

Area of mixed density with high density patches (calcification) = AVM.

High density area = intracerebral haematoma

After i.v. contrast

Lesion irregularly enhanced

Streaks of enhancement represent dilated feeding and draining vessels.

ANGIOGRAPHY Four vessel angiography confirms the presence of an AVM and delineates the feeding and draining vessels. Occasionally small AVM's are difficult to detect and only early venous filling may draw attention to their presence.

N.B. If angiographic investigation of patients with intracranial haematoma is unexpectedly negative (e.g. in younger, normotensive patients with a lobar haematoma) repeat investigation with CT scan and double dose of contrast following haematoma resolution is advisable.

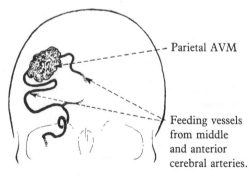

Parietal AVM

Feeding vessels from middle and anterior cerebral arteries.

Arterio-Venous Malformations

Management:

Various methods of treating arteriovenous malformations are available, but all risk further damage. The urgency of the patient's clinical condition and the risks of treatment must be weighed against the risk of a conservative approach.

Indications for intervention:

- 'expanding' haematoma associated with the AVM.
- risk of haemorrhage, especially in younger patients with many years 'at risk'.
- progressive neurological deficit.

N.B. Operative removal appears to have little effect on the control of epilepsy; epilepsy is therefore not a reason for intervention.

Methods of treatment:

Operation: *Excision* – complete excision of the AVM (confirmed by per- or post-operative angiography) is the most effective method of treatment, but some deeply situated lesions in the basal ganglia or brain stem are inoperable in view of the risk of neurological deficit.

Occlusion of feeding vessels – widely used in the past, this method is no longer acceptable since repeat investigation inevitably shows persistent filling of the AVM from dilated collateral vessels.

Embolisation: Skilled catheterisation techniques permit selective embolisation of feeding vessels with sponge, muscle, beads, pieces of lyophilised dura or detachable balloons. Long term benefits of this technique still require assessment; it is not without risk and recurrence rates may be high.

Radiotherapy: In the past, standard radiotherapy was employed in many patients with inoperable AVM's; although some workers claimed limited success, this approach has not been generally adopted. Recent developments include the use of a *focussed proton beam* (only available in centres with a cyclotron) and *focussed beams of irradiation from multiple sources sited on a stereotactic frame* (only available in a few centres). Preliminary results with these treatments look promising, especially for small lesions. The advantage of both techniques is the minimal damage to surrounding tissue; the disadvantage is a delay of up to two years before complete tissue destruction occurs. Despite this, these methods may prove ideal for some deeply situated lesions.

Arterio-Venous Malformations

ANEURYSM OF THE VEIN OF GALEN

This is a type of arterio-venous malformation in which arteries feed directly into the great vein of Galen causing massive aneurysmal dilatation. Patients present either in the neonatal period with severe high output cardiac failure due to the associated arterio-venous shunt, in infancy with cranial enlargement due to an obstructive hydrocephalus, or in childhood with subarachnoid haemorrhage. A cranial bruit is always evident. Cardiac failure usually develops in the neonatal period and is invariably fatal. In the other groups operation is feasible; ventricular drainage combined with clipping of feeding vessels from the carotid and basilar circulation may cure, but mortality and morbidity are high.

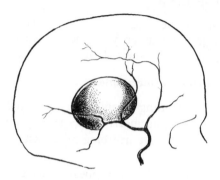

Presentation rarely occurs in later years when operative results are more favourable.

STURGE-WEBER SYNDROME

Angiomatosis affecting the facial skin, eyes and leptomeninges produces the characteristic features of the Sturge-Weber syndrome – a capillary naevus over the forehead and eye, epilepsy and intracranial calcification. See page 543.

Arterio-Venous Malformations

CAROTID-CAVERNOUS FISTULA

A fistulous communication between the internal carotid artery and the cavernous sinus may follow skull base trauma either immediately or after a delay of several days or weeks. Less often carotid-cavernous fistulae occur spontaneously when a saccular aneurysm ruptures.

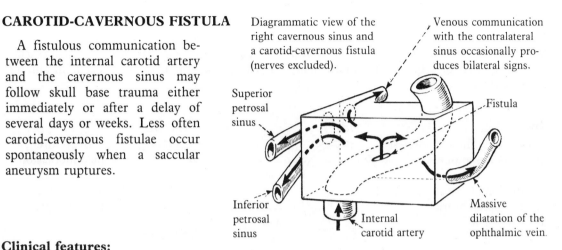

Diagrammatic view of the right cavernous sinus and a carotid-cavernous fistula (nerves excluded).

Venous communication with the contralateral sinus occasionally produces bilateral signs.

Superior petrosal sinus

Fistula

Inferior petrosal sinus

Internal carotid artery

Massive dilatation of the ophthalmic vein.

Clinical features:

Symptoms develop *suddenly* (cf. cavernous sinus thrombosis) – the patient becomes aware of a 'noise' inside his head. Pain may follow. Examination reveals definitive signs:

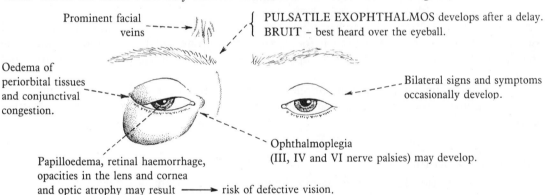

Prominent facial veins

PULSATILE EXOPHTHALMOS develops after a delay.
BRUIT – best heard over the eyeball.

Oedema of periorbital tissues and conjunctival congestion.

Bilateral signs and symptoms occasionally develop.

Ophthalmoplegia (III, IV and VI nerve palsies) may develop.

Papilloedema, retinal haemorrhage, opacities in the lens and cornea and optic atrophy may result ⟶ risk of defective vision.

Methods of fistula repair:

Trapping: ligation of the supraclinoid carotid and ophthalmic arteries intracranially, followed by ligation of the internal carotid artery in the neck.

Direct operative repair: repair of the fistula within the cavernous sinus with the aid of cardiopulmonary bypass.

Embolisation: – with muscle emboli or plastic beads introduced into the internal carotid artery.
– with detachable balloon catheterisation.

The multiplicity of methods of fistula repair reflect the difficulties and limitations of each technique. None are without risk. The recently developed method – detachable balloon catheterisation – in expert hands may prove to be the most satisfactory.

N.B. In a proportion of patients in whom treatment failed or was postponed, symptoms and signs resolve, presumably due to spontaneous thrombosis.

Intracranial Tumours

Incidence:

Primary brain tumours occur in approximately 6 persons per 100,000 per year. Fewer patients with metastatic tumours reach a neurosurgical centre, although the actual incidence must equal, if not exceed that of primary tumours. About 1 in 12 primary brain tumours occur in children under 15 years.

Site:

In adults, the commonest tumours are gliomas, metastases and meningiomas; most lie in the supratentorial compartment.

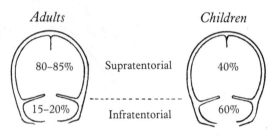

Adults — 80–85% Supratentorial, 15–20% Infratentorial

Children — 40% Supratentorial, 60% Infratentorial

In children, medulloblastomas and cerebellar astrocytomas predominate.

Pathology:

Intracranial tumours are often described as 'benign' or 'malignant', but these terms cannot be directly compared with their extracranial counterparts:

A *benign* intracranial tumour may have devastating effects if allowed to expand within the rigid confines of the skull cavity. A benign astrocytoma may infiltrate widely throughout brain tissue preventing complete removal, or may occupy a critical neurological site preventing even partial removal.

A *malignant* intracranial tumour implies rapid growth, poor differentiation, increased cellularity, mitosis, necrosis and vascular proliferation, but metastases to extracranial sites rarely occur.

Pathological Classification:

In 1979, the World Health Organisation drew up an internationally agreed classification of intracranial tumours based on the tissue of origin. This system avoids the term 'glioma' – previously encompassing astrocytoma, oligodendroglioma, ependymoma and glioblastoma multiforme. Since the cell origin of the highly malignant glioblastoma is unrecognisable, this is classified along with tumours of embryonic origin.

Intracranial Tumours — Pathological Classification

NEUROEPITHELIAL

┌ Astrocytes → **ASTROCYTOMA:** The most common primary brain tumour. Histological features permit separation into four grades depending on the degree of malignancy. Grading is of limited accuracy and only reflects the features of the biopsy specimen and not necessarily those of the whole tumour. The most malignant type – anaplastic astrocytoma (grade IV) – occurs most frequently and widely infiltrates surrounding tissue. The less common low grade astrocytomas include the pilocytic (juvenile) type and fibrillary, protoplasmic and gemistocytic types.

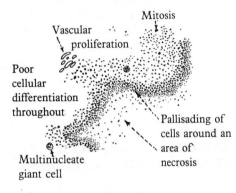

Composite diagram showing the characteristic features of a malignant astrocytoma.

Mitosis

Vascular proliferation

Poor cellular differentiation throughout

Pallisading of cells around an area of necrosis

Multinucleate giant cell

├ Oligodendrocytes → **OLIGODENDROGLIOMA:** Usually a slowly growing, sharply defined tumour. Variants include an anaplastic (malignant) form and a 'mixed' astrocytoma oligodendroglioma.

├ Ependymal cells and choroid plexus

→ **EPENDYMOMA:** Occurs anywhere throughout the ventricular system or spinal canal, but is particularly common in the 4th ventricle and cauda equina. It infiltrates surrounding tissue and may spread throughout the CSF pathways. Variants include an anaplastic type and a subependymoma arising from subependymal astrocytes.

→ **CHOROID PLEXUS PAPILLOMA:** Rare tumours and an uncommon cause of hydrocephalus due to excessive CSF production. They are usually benign but occasionally occur in a malignant form.

├ Neurones → **GANGLIOGLIOMA/GANGLIOCYTOMA/NEUROBLASTOMA:** Rare tumours containing ganglion cells and abnormal neurones. Occur in varying degrees of malignancy.

├ Pineal cells → **PINEOCYTOMA/PINEOBLASTOMA:** Extremely rare tumours. The latter are less well differentiated and show more malignant behaviour.

└ Poorly differentiated and embryonic cells

→ **GLIOBLASTOMA MULTIFORME:** A highly malignant tumour with no cell differentiation, preventing identification of its tissue origins.

→ **MEDULLOBLASTOMA:** A malignant tumour of childhood arising from the cerebellar vermis. Small closely packed cells are often arranged in rosettes surrounding abortive axons. - - - - - - - - May seed through the CSF pathways.

Intracranial Tumours — Pathological Classification

MENINGES → MENINGIOMA: Arise from the arachnoid granulations, usually closely related to the venous sinuses but also found over the hemispheric convexity.

The tumours compress rather than invade adjacent brain. They also occur in the spine and orbit. Most are benign (despite their tendency to invade adjacent bone) but some undergo sarcomatous change.

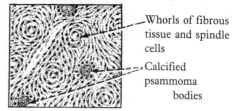

Whorls of fibrous tissue and spindle cells

Calcified psammoma bodies

Histological types – syncytial, transitional, fibroblastic and angioblastic.

↳ MENINGEAL SARCOMA and primary MENINGEAL MELANOMA: Exceedingly rare tumours.

NERVE SHEATH CELLS Intracranial tumours of the nerve sheath cells usually involve the acoustic nerve, rarely the trigeminal nerve.

→ NEURILEMMOMA (syn. schwannoma, neurinoma): - a non-invasive slowly growing tumour lying in close apposition to the nerve of origin.

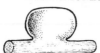

Different histological types exist:

Antoni type A – shoals and whorls of tightly packed cells in groups or pallisades.
Antoni type B – a meshwork of interlinked, loosely packed stellate cells.

↳ NEUROFIBROMA: – A diffuse tumour, expanding the whole nerve, through which the nerve fibres course. This tumour is associated with *Von Recklinghausen's syndrome* and has a greater tendency to undergo malignant change than the neurilemmoma.

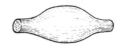

BLOOD VESSELS → HAEMANGIOBLASTOMA: Occurs within the cerebellar parenchyma or spinal cord.

In 1926, Lindau described a syndrome relating cerebellar and/or spinal haemangioblastomas with similar tumours in the retina (Von Hippel's disease) and cystic lesions in the pancreas and kidney.

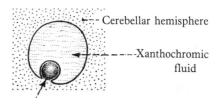

Cerebellar hemisphere

Xanthochromic fluid

Reddish brown tumour nodule lying in the wall of the cyst. Histology shows a mass of blood vessels separated by clear, foamy vacuolated cells.

Intracranial Tumours — Pathological Classification

GERM CELLS

- GERMINOMA: Primitive spheroidal cell tumour comparable to seminoma of the testis.
- TERATOMA: A tumour containing a mixture of well differentiated tissues – dermis, muscle, bone.

} Uncommon tumours of the pineal region (not arising from pineal cells)

TUMOURS OF MAL-DEVELOP-MENTAL ORIGIN

- CRANIOPHARYNGIOMA: Arises from cell rests of buccal epithelium and lies in close relation to the pituitary stalk. Usually a nodular tumour with cystic areas containing greenish fluid and cholesteatomatous material.
- EPIDERMOID/DERMOID CYSTS: Rare cystic tumours arising from cell rests predetermined to form epidermis or dermis.
- COLLOID CYST: A cystic tumour arising from an embryological remnant in the roof of the 3rd ventricle.

ANTERIOR PITUITARY GLAND

- PITUITARY ADENOMA: Benign tumour, usually secreting excessive quantities of prolactin, growth hormone or adrenocorticotrophic hormone.
- ADENOCARCINOMA: Malignant tumour occasionally arises in the pituitary.

LOCAL EXTENSION FROM ADJACENT TUMOURS

- CHORDOMA: Rare tumour arising from cell rests of the notochord. May occur anywhere from the sphenoid to the coccyx – but commonest in the basi-occipital and the sacrococcygeal region, invading and destroying bone at these sites.
- GLOMUS JUGULARE TUMOUR (syn. chemodectoma):   Vascular tumour arising from 'glomus jugulare' tissue lying either in the bulb of the internal jugular vein or in the mucosa of the middle ear. The tumour invades the petrous bone and may extend into the posterior fossa or neck.
- Other local tumours include CHONDROMA, CHONDROSARCOMA and CYLINDROMA.

PRIMARY MALIGNANT LYMPHOMA   (syn. microgliomatosis):   Forms around parenchymal blood vessels. May be solitary or multifocal. A proportion of patients have evidence of extracranial involvement; in those the primary site (i.e. intra- or extracranial) remains unknown.

METASTATIC TUMOURS: May arise from any primary site but most commonly spread from the bronchus or breast.

Intracranial Tumours — Classification according to Site

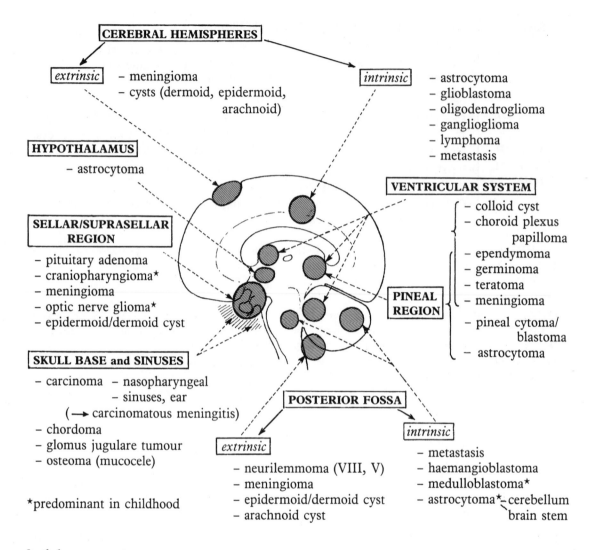

CEREBRAL HEMISPHERES

extrinsic
- meningioma
- cysts (dermoid, epidermoid, arachnoid)

intrinsic
- astrocytoma
- glioblastoma
- oligodendroglioma
- ganglioglioma
- lymphoma
- metastasis

HYPOTHALAMUS
- astrocytoma

SELLAR/SUPRASELLAR REGION
- pituitary adenoma
- craniopharyngioma★
- meningioma
- optic nerve glioma★
- epidermoid/dermoid cyst

VENTRICULAR SYSTEM
- colloid cyst
- choroid plexus papilloma
- ependymoma
- germinoma
- teratoma
- meningioma
- pineal cytoma/blastoma
- astrocytoma

PINEAL REGION

SKULL BASE and SINUSES
- carcinoma – nasopharyngeal
  – sinuses, ear
  (→ carcinomatous meningitis)
- chordoma
- glomus jugulare tumour
- osteoma (mucocele)

POSTERIOR FOSSA

extrinsic
- neurilemmoma (VIII, V)
- meningioma
- epidermoid/dermoid cyst
- arachnoid cyst

intrinsic
- metastasis
- haemangioblastoma
- medulloblastoma★
- astrocytoma★–cerebellum
  brain stem

★predominant in childhood

Aetiology:

The cause of most intracranial tumours remains unknown, but in some, predisposing factors are recognised:

Cranial irradiation: long term follow-up after whole head irradiation (e.g. for tinea capitis) shows an increased incidence of both benign and malignant tumours – astrocytoma, meningioma.

Immunosuppressive therapy: leads to an increased incidence of lymphoma and lymphoreticular tumours.

Neurofibromatosis: linked to an increased incidence of optic nerve glioma and meningioma (page 541).

Tuberose sclerosis: related to the formation of subependymal astrocytomas.

Intracranial Tumours — Incidence

The table below details the incidence of intracranial tumours examined by the Neuropathology Department, Institute of Neurological Sciences, Glasgow (population 2.7 millions) over a 5 year period.

SUPRATENTORIAL	Adults		Children (<15 years)	
Anaplastic astrocytoma (including glioblastoma multiforme)	347	(40%)	5	(7%)
Meningioma	134	(15%)	—	
Metastasis	105	(12%)	—	
Astrocytoma	73	(8%)	5	(7%)
Pituitary adenoma	31	(4%)	—	
Craniopharyngioma	13	(1%)	9	(13%)
Oligodendroglioma	9	(1%)	1	(1%)
Colloid cyst	4	(<1%)	—	
Lymphoma	2	(<1%)	—	
Others	11	(1%)	6	(9%)
INFRATENTORIAL				
Neurilemmoma	50	(6%)	—	
Metastasis	39	(4%)	—	
Haemangioblastoma	17	(2%)	—	
Astrocytoma	12	(1%)	19	(27%)
Meningioma	12	(1%)	—	
Medulloblastoma	6	(<1%)	17	(24%)
Dermoid/epidermoid	3	(<1%)	1	(1%)
Ependymoma			4	(6%)
Others	8	(1%)	3	(4%)
Total	876		70	

(Adapted from Adams, Graham and Doyle, Brain Biopsy, 1982.)

Intracranial Tumours – Clinical Features

Symptoms tend to develop insidiously, gradually progressing over a few weeks or years, depending on the degree of malignancy (cf. acute onset of a cerebrovascular accident followed by a gradual improvement if the patient survives). Occasionally tumours present acutely due to haemorrhage or the development of hydrocephalus.

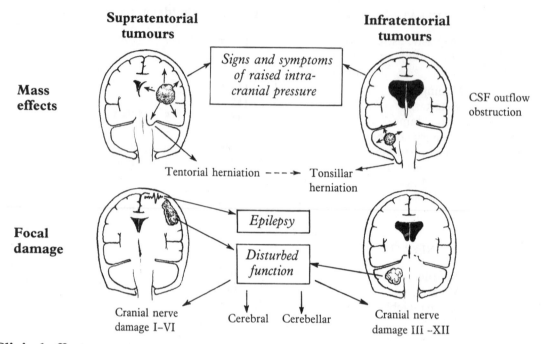

Supratentorial tumours

Infratentorial tumours

Mass effects

Signs and symptoms of raised intra-cranial pressure

CSF outflow obstruction

Tentorial herniation ---→ Tonsillar herniation

Focal damage

Epilepsy

Disturbed function

Cranial nerve damage I–VI

Cerebral   Cerebellar

Cranial nerve damage III –XII

Clinical effects:

- **RAISED INTRACRANIAL PRESSURE** – headache, vomiting, papilloedema ⎱ see pages
- **BRAIN SHIFT** – deterioration of conscious level, pupillary dilatation ⎰ 76–78

EPILEPSY (see page 87)

– generalised ⎫
– partial (focal) ⎪ occur in 30% of
– partial ⎬ patients with brain tumours
  progressing to ⎪
  generalised ⎭

Partial seizures help localise the tumour site.

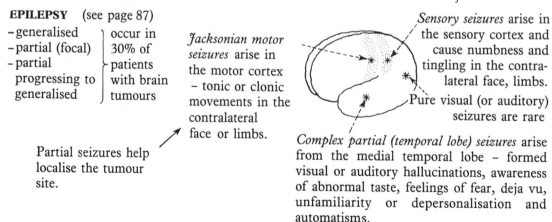

Jacksonian motor seizures arise in the motor cortex – tonic or clonic movements in the contralateral face or limbs.

Sensory seizures arise in the sensory cortex and cause numbness and tingling in the contra-lateral face, limbs.

Pure visual (or auditory) seizures are rare

Complex partial (temporal lobe) seizures arise from the medial temporal lobe – formed visual or auditory hallucinations, awareness of abnormal taste, feelings of fear, deja vu, unfamiliarity or depersonalisation and automatisms.

290

Intracranial Tumours – Clinical Features

DISTURBED FUNCTION

Supratentorial – See higher cortical dysfunction, pages 104–112.

FRONTAL LOBE

Contralateral face,
  arm or leg weakness.
Expressive dysphasia
  (dominant hemisphere).
Personality change
  – antisocial behaviour
  – loss of inhibitions
  – loss of initiative
  – intellectual impairment
  → profound dementia
    especially if the corpus
    callosum is involved.

N.B. Involvement of the fronto-
  ponto-cerebellar pathway may
  mimic cerebellar disease.

OCCIPITAL LOBE

Visual field defect
  – homonymous hemianopia.

CORPUS CALLOSUM – dysconnection
syndromes
Apraxia.
Word blindness.

PARIETAL LOBE

Disturbed Sensation
  – localisation of touch
  – two point discrimination
  – passive movement
  – astereognosis
  – sensory inattention.
Visual field defect
  – lower homonymous
      quadrantanopia.
Receptive dysphasia ⎤
Right/left confusion ⎟ Dominant
Finger agnosia   ⎬ hemisphere.
Acalculia   ⎟
Agraphia   ⎦

Apraxia ⎤ Non-dominant
Agnosia ⎦   hemisphere.

TEMPORAL LOBE

Receptive dysphasia (dominant hemisphere).
Visual field defect
  – upper homonymous quadrantanopia.

Supratentorial tumours may directly damage
the I and II cranial nerves. Cavernous sinus
compression or invasion may involve the III–VI
cranial nerves.

HYPOTHALAMUS/PITUITARY

Endocrine dysfunction.

Infratentorial

MIDBRAIN/BRAIN STEM

Cranial nerve lesions III–XII.
Long tract signs
  – motor and sensory.
Deterioration of conscious level.
Tremor (red nucleus).
Impaired eye movements.
Pupillary abnormalities.
Vomiting, hiccough (medulla).

CEREBELLUM – see cerebellar
  dysfunction, pages 167–170.
Ataxic gait.
Intention tremor.
Incoordination.
Dysarthria.
Nystagmus.

N.B. Intrinsic brain stem tumours in contrast to extrinsic tumours are more likely to produce long
  tract (motor and sensory) signs early in the
  course of the disease.

Intracranial Tumours — Investigation

Chest X-ray: ⎫
ESR: ⎭ The high incidence of metastatic tumour makes these tests mandatory in patients with suspected intracranial tumour.

Skull X-ray Note:

Calcification
  – oligodendroglioma.
  – meningioma (look for hyperostosis of adjacent bone)
  – craniopharyngioma.

Osteolytic lesion
  – primary or secondary bone tumour.
  – dermoid/epidermoid.
  – chordoma.
  – nasopharyngeal carcinoma.
  – myeloma.
  – reticulosis.

Signs of raised intracranial pressure
-- Suture diastasis (in infants).
-- 'Beaten brass' appearance – of limited value since it may occur normally in children and in some adults.
- *erosion of the posterior clinoids* (may also occur from local pressure e.g. craniopharyngioma.

Lateral view

Towne's view

Pineal shift (ensure 'shift' is not due to film rotation).

CT scanning: Note:
  Site:
    e.g. frontal, occipital
    – *extrinsic:* outwith brain substance
        e.g. meningioma.
    – *intrinsic:* within brain substance
        e.g. astrocytoma.
  Mass effect
    – midline shift.
    – ventricular compression.
    – hydrocephalus (secondary to 3rd ventricular or posterior fossa lesion).

Effect on adjacent bone i.e. meningioma → hyperostosis.

Single or multiple lesions i.e. if multiple → metastasis.

Effect of contrast enhancement. e.g. none – low grade astrocytoma. irregular – malignant astrocytoma. homogeneous – meningioma.

High definition scans (i.e. narrow slice width) – useful in the detection of pituitary, orbital and posterior fossa tumours.

Coronal and sagittal reconstruction ⎫
Direct coronal scanning ⎭ – useful in demonstrating the vertical extent and relationships of tumours – especially when intraventricular or arising from the pituitary fossa or skull base.

Intracranial Tumours — Investigation

Angiography: although angiography may reveal a tumour 'blush' or vessel displacement, it is only occasionally required to supplement CT scanning. In some patients, it provides useful preoperative information e.g. identifies feeding vessels to a vascular tumour or tumour involvement and constriction of major vessels.

Nuclear magnetic resonance scanning: this may well become a valuable investigation in the diagnosis of intracranial tumours – especially around the skull base, but possible advantages over CT scanning await further evaluation.

Isotope scanning: useful in the detection of intracranial pathology if CT scanning is unavailable – but will not distinguish the nature of the lesion.

CSF examination: lumbar puncture is contraindicated if the clinician suspects intracranial tumour. If CSF is obtained by another source e.g. ventricular drainage or during shunt insertion, then cytological examination may reveal tumour cells.

Tumour markers: as yet attempts to find a substance in blood or CSF which reflects growth of a specific tumour have been limited – only the link between elevated alpha fetoprotein and human chorionic gonadotrophins with germinomas of the third ventricle aids diagnosis. The development of monoclonal antibodies, with further improvements in their specificity may provide a useful approach to tumour localisation and identification in the future.

CAUSES of INTRACRANIAL MASS LESIONS (other than tumour)

VASCULAR – haematoma.
– giant aneurysm.
– arteriovenous malformation.
– infarct with oedema.
– venous thrombosis.

INFECTION – abscess.
– tuberculoma.
– sarcoidosis.
– encephalitis.

TRAUMA – haematoma.
– contusion

CYSTS – arachnoid.
– parasitic (hydatid).

Intracranial Tumours – Management

Steroid therapy

Steroids dramatically reduce oedema surrounding intracranial tumours, but appear unlikely to directly affect tumour growth.

A loading dose of 12 mg i.v. dexamethasone followed by 4 mg q.i.d. often reverses progressive clinical deterioration within a few hours. After several days treatment, gradual dose reduction minimises the risk of unwanted side effects.

Sellar/parasellar tumours occasionally present with steroid insufficiency. In these patients, steroid cover is an essential prerequisite of any anaesthetic or operative procedure.

Operative management:

Most patients with intracranial tumours require one or more of the following approaches:

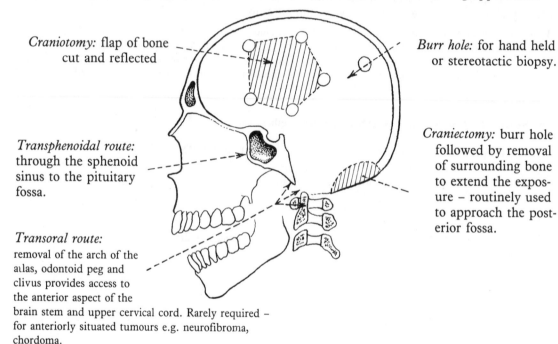

Craniotomy: flap of bone cut and reflected

Burr hole: for hand held or stereotactic biopsy.

Transphenoidal route: through the sphenoid sinus to the pituitary fossa.

Craniectomy: burr hole followed by removal of surrounding bone to extend the exposure – routinely used to approach the posterior fossa.

Transoral route: removal of the arch of the atlas, odontoid peg and clivus provides access to the anterior aspect of the brain stem and upper cervical cord. Rarely required – for anteriorly situated tumours e.g. neurofibroma, chordoma.

The subsequent procedure – *biopsy, partial tumour removal/internal decompression* or *complete removal* – depends on the nature of the tumour and its site. The infiltrative nature of primary malignant tumours prevents complete removal and often operation is restricted to biopsy or tumour decompression. Prospects of complete removal improve with benign tumours such as meningioma or craniopharyngioma; if any tumour tissue is overlooked, or if fragments remain attached to deep structures, then recurrence may result.

Intracranial Tumours – Management

Radiotherapy:

Present day treatment of intracranial tumours with radiotherapy utilises one of the following:
- *megavoltage X-rays.*
- γ rays from *cobalt 60.*
- electron beam from a *linear accelerator.*
- *accelerated particles from a cyclotron* e.g. neutrons, nuclei of helium, protons.

Alternatively the tumour is treated from within (brachytherapy) by the implantation of a radioactive seed e.g. yttrium[90]

In contrast to older methods of 'deep X-ray therapy', these modern techniques produce greater tissue penetration and avoid radiation damage to the skin surface.

The effect of radiotherapy depends on the total dose – usually up to 6,000 rads, and the treatment duration. This must be balanced against the risk to adjacent normal structures. In general, the more rapidly the tumour cells divide, the greater the sensitivity. Radiotherapy is of particular value in the management of malignant tumours – malignant astrocytoma, metastasis, medulloblastoma and germinoma, but also plays an important part in the management of some benign tumours – pituitary adenoma, craniopharyngioma. Since some tumours seed throughout the CSF pathways e.g. medulloblastoma, *whole neural axis irradiation* minimises the risk of a distant recurrence.

Complications of radiotherapy: following treatment, deterioration in a patient's condition may occur for a variety of reasons:

during treatment – increased oedema – reversible.
after weeks, months – demyelination.
6 months–10 years – *radionecrosis* – irreversible.
(usually 1–2 years)

Similar complications may involve the spinal cord after irradiation of spinal tumours.

Hypoxic cell sensitisers: during radiotherapy, part of the destructive process involves conversion of oxygen to hydroxyl ions. The presence of hypoxic areas within the tumour substance increases radioresistance. Recent use of hypoxic cell sensitisers e.g. misonidazole, aims to increase sensitivity within these regions. Benefits of these drugs await evaluation.

Intracranial Tumours – Management

Chemotherapy:

Chemotherapeutic agents have been used for many years in the management of malignant brain tumours, but benefits remain uncertain.

Drugs most commonly employed include BCNU, CCNU, methyl CCNU, procarbazine, vincristine and methotrexate.

The ideal chemotherapeutic drug selectively kills tumour cells; but tumour cell response relates directly to the dose. Inevitably, high drug dosage causes *bone marrow toxicity*. In practice, failure to produce signs of marrow depression (e.g. leucopenia) indicates an inadequate dose.

Side effects preclude the use of chemotherapy in benign or 'low grade' tumours. In patients with malignant tumours, some studies demonstrate that individual or combined therapy produces some tumour remission, but randomised controlled trials show disappointing results. In malignant astrocytoma however, BCNU may produce a modest benefit. In medulloblastoma combined therapy including CCNU and vincristine may delay recurrence.

In vitro chemosensitivity: the vast array of available drugs and the infinite permutations of combined therapy create difficulties in drug selection. One approach, currently under study, utilises cultured tumour cells from biopsy material. In vitro analysis of growth inhibition or the rate of cell death following application of a specific drug, points to the tumour 'sensitivity' of the drug under test. Future refinements of this technique may lead to the wider use of chemotherapy in brain tumour management.

Future Prospects: The recently acquired technique of monoclonal antibody production raises new possibilities in the management of malignant brain tumours, although problems of delivery and localisation still require development. Monoclonal antibodies may serve as carriers, taking cytotoxic drugs, toxins or radionuclides directly to the tumour site.

Prognosis of Intracranial Tumours:

Patient prognosis depends on the specific tumour type; this is described for individual tumours in subsequent pages.

Tumours of the Cerebral Hemispheres – Intrinsic

Intrinsic tumours arise within the brain substance.

ASTROCYTOMA (and glioblastoma multiforme)
Astrocytomas may occur in any age group, but are commonest between 40 and 60 years.
Male : female = 2 : 1.

Primary sites: Found in equal incidence throughout the frontal, temporal, parietal and thalamic regions, but less often in the occipital lobe. Microscopic classification defines 4 grades (Kernohan I–IV), but this is of limited accuracy. A more practical description for the clinician divides tumours into either 'malignant' or 'low grade'.

'Malignant' astrocytoma/glioblastoma multiforme

Malignant astrocytoma (grade III/IV) and glioblastoma multiforme (grade IV) constitute over 40% of all primary intracranial tumours. Peak age incidence is 55 years. These tumours widely infiltrate adjacent brain; growth is rapid. At autopsy, microscopic examination usually reveals spread to multiple distant sites.

Malignant astrocytoma

Overlying gyri flattened and pale

At autopsy 75% show microscopic spread to the contralateral hemisphere. Some patients may present with a bilateral corpus callosal tumour or 'butterfly' astrocytoma

Necrotic areas may coalesce and form cystic cavities

'Low grade' astrocytoma

Low grade astrocytomas (grade I/II) make up 14% of all primary intracranial tumours and occur on average at an earlier age than their malignant counterparts (about 40 years).

Fibrillary astrocytoma

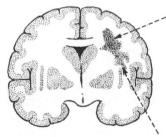

Firm, rubbery texture with or without cystic regions

Infiltrates surrounding brain with minimal mass effect and neuronal damage.

These tumours are diffuse and slowly growing, and composed of well differentiated astrocytic cells subdivided into fibrillary, protoplasmic or gemistocytic types. Although 'benign' they widely infiltrate surrounding brain and lack a definitive edge or capsule. A further 'low grade type – the pilocytic (or 'juvenile') astrocytoma occurs in the hypothalamic region as well as in the optic nerve (page 327) and cerebellum (page 310). Since partial resection may result in a cure, some believe pilocytic astrocytomas are 'hamartomas' rather than true tumours.

Tumours of the Cerebral Hemispheres — Intrinsic

ASTROCYTOMA

Clinical features:

Astrocytes may present with:
- epilepsy.
- signs and symptoms of focal brain damage – dysphasia, hemiparesis, personality change.
- signs and symptoms of raised intracranial pressure – headache, vomiting, depression of conscious level.

With the exception of epilepsy, symptoms usually develop gradually, progressing over several weeks, months or years, the rate depending on the degree of malignancy. Sudden deterioration suggests haemorrhage into a necrotic area. In a patient with long standing epilepsy, the rapid development of further symptoms may result from malignant change within a previously 'low grade' lesion.

Investigations:

Skull X-ray: of limited value; shift of a calcified pineal or erosion of the dorsum sella indicates the presence of an intracranial mass.

CT scan: appearances vary considerably; in general, malignant and low grade lesions show different characteristics –

Malignant astrocytoma/glioblastoma multiforme

The lesion,
site and
associated mass
effect
– ventricular compression
– midline shift
are clearly demonstrated.

Surrounding regions
of low density
indicate either
oedema or
infiltrative
     tumour.

Areas of mixed density, irregularly enhance with contrast. No plane exists between tumour and brain indicating infiltration.

Central, low density regions represent necrotic areas or cystic cavities; neither enhances with contrast.

Low grade astrocytoma

A low density region, usually un-enhancing with contrast suggests a low grade infiltrative lesion; detection is often difficult in early stages.
Calcification occasionally occurs.

Some low grade tumours secrete fluid which may encircle the lesion – 'benign cystic astrocytoma'.

Tumours of the Cerebral Hemispheres — Intrinsic

ASTROCYTOMA

Management:

Management varies for patients presenting with a mass lesion causing a rise in intracranial pressure or focal signs, and for those who present with epilepsy resulting from a small infiltrative tumour.

(a) In patients with raised intracranial pressure or focal signs

Steroid therapy: A loading dose of dexamethasone 12mg i.v. followed by 4mg q.i.d. reduces peritumour oedema and leads rapidly to an improvement in symptoms. After several days, a gradual reduction in dose avoids toxicity.

Confirmation of diagnosis: CT scan appearance alone is seldom sufficient to diagnose a malignant tumour with complete certainty. Lack of confirmation of the nature of the lesion may result in the incorrect treatment of a benign condition such as abscess, tuberculoma or sarcoidosis or omission of radiotherapy in a highly radiosensitive lesion such as lymphoma. *Thus tissue acquisition for histological examination is essential.* Identification of tumour type and grade by either a burr hole or open biopsy provides a prognostic guide and aids further management.

Burr hole biopsy: A brain cannula inserted into the abnormal region permits aspiration of a small quantity of tissue for immediate (smear and frozen section) and delayed (paraffin section) examination. Provided patients receive steroid cover the risks are small, but occasionally biopsy produces or increases a focal deficit or causes a fatal haemorrhage.

Controlled suction

Dandy brain cannula – on introduction, a change in consistency may be detected on encountering tumour tissue.

Aspiration of fluid from a cystic cavity may provide a temporary decompression.

For deep inaccessible lesions (e.g. hypothalamus), a *stereotactic method*, guided by CT scan (see page 370), permits accurate placement of a fine cannula at a predetermined site. Although minimising tissue damage the minute specimen size makes histological examination difficult.

N.B. The degree of malignancy may vary from region to region within the one lesion and this limits the accuracy of biopsy. If findings vary, then the region of greatest malignancy dictates the tumour grade.

Tumours of the Posterior Fossa — Intrinsic

ASTROCYTOMA
Management of patients with raised intracranial pressure or focal signs *(continued)*

Craniotomy – *open biopsy*
             – *internal tumour decompression*
             – *lobectomy*

A bone flap turned over the appropriate region allows direct inspection of the cortical surface.

The surgeon may insert a brain cannula into the abnormal area to obtain an 'open' biopsy, open into the tumour cavity and remove as much tissue as is feasible – internal decompression, or following histological confirmation perform a lobectomy (frontal, occipital or non-dominant temporal) in the hope that most tumour tissue is included.

Radiotherapy: Most active in rapidly growing malignant tumours – grade III and IV. Radiotherapy extends survival, but does not cure.

Chemotherapy: Various combinations of chemotherapeutic agents (e.g. BCNU, 5-fluorouracil, PCV) have been used in the management of malignant astrocytoma and glioblastoma multiforme. Although a proportion of tumours undoubtedly respond to chemotherapy, studies have as yet failed to demonstrate any significant prolongation of survival.

Treatment Selection and Prognosis

After establishing the diagnosis, further treatment depends on the degree of malignancy, the tumour site, the extent of any presenting neurological deficit and the patient's age. Quality of survival must be considered as well as duration.

Malignant astrocytoma/glioblastoma multiforme: Despite modern techniques, these common primary tumours still carry an extremely grave prognosis, irrespective of the selected treatment.

Although there are many protagonists for aggressive operative treatment, benefits remain unconvincing. Extensive tumour resection extends average survival by only one or two months; at one year, the percentage of patients surviving varies little, irrespective of whether burr hole biopsy or tumour resection was performed. Complete removal is impossible; even the formidable 'hemispherectomy' fails due to interhemispheric spread.

	Median survival (months)
Burr hole biopsy	3–4
Tumour resection	6
Burr hole biopsy + radiotherapy	6–8
Tumour resection + radiotherapy	9–10

Radiotherapy appears to have the greatest effect, extending the mean survival period by 3–4 months.

Management policies vary widely. In Britain, most neurosurgeons now adopt a relatively conservative policy, combining burr hole biopsy with radiotherapy. In general, *'partial'* or *'complete'* resection (with radiotherapy) is only considered in:

      – younger patients.
      – patients with 'accessible' lesions e.g. frontal pole.
      – patients with pressure symptoms, yet no disabling focal signs.

A *diagnostic burr hole biopsy* alone is appropriate in:

      – elderly patients.   – patients with marked disability (e.g. severe dysphasia).

Tumours of the Cerebral Hemispheres — Intrinsic

ASTROCYTOMA

Low grade astrocytoma: If biopsy reveals a low grade astrocytoma (grade I and II), then prognosis relatively improves but median survival is only 2 years for grade II and 4 years for grade I. In some instances, however, patients survive for more than 20 years. If the CT scan shows a well defined tumour mass, then operative decompression is worthwhile; in some, the diffuse infiltrative nature of the tumour limits resection. Many clinicians advise radiotherapy despite the expected limited sensitivity.

(b)   **Management in patients with epilepsy alone**

A small poorly defined region of low density on the CT scan, without contrast enhancement, suggests a low grade astrocytoma. In these patients, the clinician may defer biopsy until follow-up CT scans or the development of focal signs indicate progression.

OLIGODENDROGLIOMA

Oligodendrogliomas are far less common than astrocytomas. They occur in a slightly younger age group – 30–50 years, and usually involve the frontal lobes. Occasionally involvement of the ventricular wall results in CSF seeding. Radiological calcification occurs in 40%.

In contrast to astrocytomas, the tumour margin often appears well defined. The rate of growth of oligodendrogliomas and the degree of malignancy are variable. Many tumours exhibit a 'mixed' histological picture with areas of astrocytic change scattered between the oligodendroglia. In these, grading is judged by the astrocytic component. Malignant change may result in a histological pattern resembling glioblastoma multiforme.

Oligodendroglioma

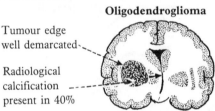

Tumour edge well demarcated

Radiological calcification present in 40%

Some tumours involve the ventricular wall – CSF seeding may occur.

Management: matches that of astrocytomas. Low grade lesions may benefit from 'complete' or 'partial' excision. In malignant tumours, radiotherapy may have the greatest effect.

Prognosis: depends on the tumour grade. Long term survival (over 20 years) is occasionally recorded, but in tumours showing malignant change, expected survival compares closely with the depressing figures for malignant astrocytoma.

HYPOTHALAMIC ASTROCYTOMA

Hypothalamic tumours usually occur in children; they are usually astrocytomas of the pilocytic (juvenile) type.

Clinical presentation takes different forms. Initially the child *fails to thrive* and becomes *emaciated*. Signs of *panhypopituitarism* may be evident. Eventually an anabolic phase results in *obesity* accompanied by *diabetes insipidus* and *delayed puberty.*

Upward tumour extension may obstruct the foramen of Munro and cause *hydrocephalus.*

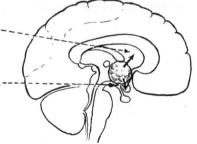

Involvement of the tuberal region may result in the rare presentation of *precocious puberty* with secondary sexual characteristics developing in children perhaps only a few years old.

Downward extension invades the optic chiasma and *impairs vision.*

Management: The site of the lesion prevents operative removal; a stereotactic biopsy may aid tumour identification. If hydrocephalus is present, a bilateral ventriculoperitoneal/atrial shunt relieves pressure symptoms. Radiotherapy is of doubtful value.

Tumours of the Cerebral Hemispheres — Intrinsic

METASTATIC TUMOURS

Any malignant tumour may metastasise to the brain. Malignant melanomas show the highest frequency (66% of patients); this contrasts with tumours of the cervix and uterus where <3% develop intracranial metastasis. The most commonly encountered metastatic intracranial tumours arise from the bronchus and the breast; of patients with carcinomas at these sites, 25% develop intracranial metastasis.

In up to 50% of patients, the tumours are multiple.

Spread: usually haematogenous. Occasionally a metastasis to the skull vault may result in a nodule or plaque forming over the dural surface.

Common primary sites
- bronchus
- breast
- kidney
- thyroid
- stomach
- prostate
- testis
- melanoma

Intracranial sites:

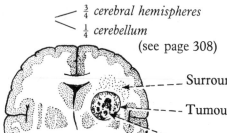

$\frac{3}{4}$ *cerebral hemispheres*
$\frac{1}{4}$ *cerebellum*
(see page 308)

Involvement of the ventricular wall or encroachment into the basal cisterns may result in tumour cells seeding through the CSF pathways.

Surrounding oedema is often marked.

Tumour margin – well defined.

Necrotic areas may break down to form cystic cavities containing a pus-like fluid.

Clinical features:

Patients with supratentorial metastatic tumours may present with epilepsy, or with signs and symptoms occurring from focal damage or raised intracranial pressure. Cerebellar metastases are discussed on page 308. Carcinomatous meningitis causes single or multiple cranial nerve palsies and may obstruct CSF drainage.

Investigations:

A CT scan shows single or multiple well demarcated lesions of variable size. Often an extensive low density area, representing oedema, surrounds the lesion.

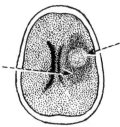

Metastatic lesions usually enhance with contrast. A ring-like appearance may resemble an abscess – but the wall is irregular and thickened.

The search for a primary lesion must include a thorough clinical examination and a chest X-ray. Other investigations including barium studies, abdominal CT scans, ultrasound and sputum and urine cytology have questionable value, unless clinically indicated.

302

Tumours of the Cerebral Hemispheres — Intrinsic

METASTATIC TUMOURS

Management and prognosis:

(a) Solitary lesions: If the tumour lies in an accessible site, complete excision followed by radiotherapy provides good results – survival usually depends on the extent of extracranial disease and its ability to respond to treatment rather than on intracranial recurrences.

In general, in patients with no other evidence of systemic cancer, the median survival period approaches 2 years after the intracranial operation. In patients with other evidence of systemic disease, results are less good with a median survival of 8 months.

(b) Multiple lesions: In these patients, operative removal is seldom practical or possible. Provided no doubt exists about the diagnosis (i.e. multiple abscesses or tuberculomata may resemble metastatic deposits) then whole brain irradiation is administered.

LYMPHOMA (syn. MICROGLIOMATOSIS)

Single or multifocal tumours occurring at any hemispheric site. Some are discreet lesions, others extensively invade surrounding brain. They are prone to develop in immunosuppressed patients. Histology shows sleeves of primitive reticulum cells around and extending outwards from the blood vessels.

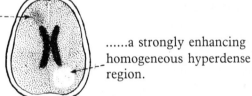

CT scan: shows either a poorly enhancing low density region or......

......a strongly enhancing homogeneous hyperdense region.

Multiplicity also suggests lymphoma.

Management: Biopsy confirms the nature of the lesion. Radiotherapy may produce dramatic results.

GANGLIOGLIOMA

This is a rare tumour occurring in the younger age group (<30 years), composed of abnormal neuronal growth mixed with a glial component. The proportion of each component varies from patient to patient. Growth is slow and malignant change uncommon; when this occurs it probably develops in the glial component.

Management follows that of low grade astrocytomas.

NEUROBLASTOMA

Rarely occurs intracranially in children <10 years. Highly cellular, malignant lesion composed of small round cells, some showing neuronal differentiation.

Tumours of the Cerebral Hemispheres – Extrinsic

Extrinsic tumours arise outwith the brain substance.

MENINGIOMA

Meningiomas constitute about one fifth of all primary intracranial tumours. They are slowly growing and arise from the arachnoid granulations. These lie in greatest concentration around the venous sinuses, but they also occur in relation to surface tributary veins. Meningiomas may therefore develop at any meningeal site. Occasionally they are multiple.

Meningiomas present primarily in the 40–60 age group and have a slight female preponderance. They are principally benign tumours although a malignant form exists.

Sites of intracranial meningioma

The remainder arise from the middle fossa, orbital roof and lateral ventricle.

Pathology:

Various histological types are described – syncytial, transitional, fibroblastic and angioblastic; different types may coexist within the same tumour. These distinctions serve little clinical value, although it is important to identify the haemangiopericytic variant of the angioblastic group as well as the malignant type, as these indicate the likelihood of rapid growth and a high rate of recurrence following removal.

Macroscopic appearance

The dural origin usually incorporates the main arterial supply.

The tumour surface, although often lobulated, is well demarcated from the surrounding brain and attached only by small bridging vessels.

Marked *oedema* often develops in the surrounding brain.

A reactive *hyperostosis* develops in adjacent bone, forming a swelling on the inner table. Hyperostosis affecting the outer table may produce a palpable lump. Tumour tissue may infiltrate adjacent bone.

Parasagittal tumours may invade and obstruct the sagittal sinus.

Tumour texture and vascularity varies considerably from patient to patient – some are firm and fibrous, others soft. *Calcified deposits* (psammoma bodies) are often found.

En-plaque meningioma: In some patients, rather than developing a spherical form, the meningioma spreads 'en-plaque' over the dural surface. This type often arises from the outer aspect of the sphenoid wing.

304

Tumours of the Cerebral Hemispheres — Extrinsic

MENINGIOMA Clinical features:

Approximately a quarter of patients with meningioma present with epilepsy – often with a focal component. In the remainder, the onset is insidious with pressure effects (headache, vomiting, papilloedema) often developing before focal neurological signs become evident.

Notable characteristic features occur, dependent on the tumour site – PARASAGITTAL/PARA-FALCINE tumours lying near the vertex affect the 'foot' and 'leg' area of the motor or sensory strip. *Partial seizures* or a *'pyramidal' weakness* may develop in the leg (i.e. primarily affecting foot dorsiflexion, then knee and hip flexion). Extension of the lesion through the falx can produce *bilateral leg weakness.* Posteriorly situated parasagittal tumours may present with a *homonymous hemianopia.* Tumours arising anteriorly may grow to extensive proportions before causing focal signs; eventually minor *impairment of memory, intellect* and *personality* may progress to a *profound dementia.*

INNER SPHENOIDAL WING tumours may compress the optic nerve and produce *visual impairment.* Examination may reveal a central *scotoma* or *field defect* and *optic atrophy.*

N.B. The FOSTER KENNEDY syndrome denotes a tumour causing optic atrophy in one fundus from direct pressure and papilloedema in the other due to increased intracranial pressure.

Involvement of the cavernous sinus or the superior orbital fissure may produce *ptosis* and *impaired eye movements* (III, IV and VI nerve palsies) or *facial pain and anaesthesia* (V_1 nerve damage) – see diagram on page 140. *Proptosis* occasionally results from venous obstruction or tumour extension into the orbit.

OLFACTORY GROOVE tumours destroy the olfactory bulb or tract causing unilateral followed by bilateral *anosmia.* Often this passes unnoticed by the patient; with tumour expansion, dementia may gradually ensue.

SUPRASELLAR tumours – see page 327.

Investigations:

SKULL X-RAY: note:

Associated signs of
long standing
increased ICP i.e.
posterior clinoid erosion.

----Bony hyperostosis – radiating spicules
occasionally seen ('sunray' effect).

15% show calcification.

Dilated middle meningeal groove.

CT SCAN

Before i.v. contrast   Meningioma – well circumscribed lesions
of a density usually greater than
or equal to brain with a surrounding
area of low attenuation (oedema).
Calcification may be evident.

The lesion abuts the dura overlying the hemispheric cavity,
the falx or the sagittal sinus
or arises from the skull base.

After i.v. contrast

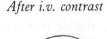

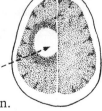

A dense, usually
homogeneous
enhancement
occurs after
contrast injection.

305

Tumours of the Posterior Fossa — Extrinsic

MENINGIOMA Investigations *(continued)*

ANGIOGRAPHY: characteristically shows a highly vascular lesion with a typical tumour 'blush'. It provides useful preoperative information – identifying the site of major feeding vessels e.g. inner sphenoid wing meningioma may encircle and ·constrict the internal carotid artery.

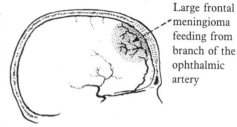

Large frontal meningioma feeding from branch of the ophthalmic artery

Selective catheterisation and embolisation of external carotid feeding vessels can reduce tumour vascularity and diminish operative risks from excessive haemorrhage.

Management:

Management aims at complete removal of both the tumour and its origin without damaging adjacent brain; but this depends on the tumour site and its nature. Even with 'convexity' tumours where complete excision of the dural origin is possible, overlooking a small piece of tumour imbedded in adjacent brain will result in recurrence. This is particularly likely with malignant meningiomas where the plane of cleavage is often obscured.

Parasagittal meningioma

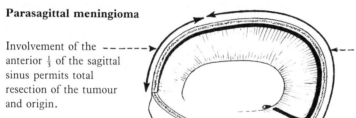

Involvement of the anterior $\frac{1}{3}$ of the sagittal sinus permits total resection of the tumour and origin.

Resection of the posterior $\frac{2}{3}$ of the sagittal sinus carries an unacceptably high risk of bilateral venous infarction; in this region tumours are dissected off the sinus and the origin diathermied.

Tumours arising from the skull base seldom permit excision of the origin. Occasionally the patient's age or the tumour site prevents operation or allows only a limited removal; in these patients radiotherapy is often administered but its value remains unknown. Radiotherapy should be administered in malignant tumours.

Operative results: With modern techniques, operative mortality has fallen to between 5–10% depending on the position and the size of the tumour.

Tumour recurrence: depends predominantly on the completeness of removal. Tumour type seems less important although a higher rate of recurrence has been reported in the haemangiopericytic variant of the angioblastic group as well as in tumours showing malignant features.

Meningiomas recur in up to $\frac{1}{3}$ of patients followed up for more than 10 years.

Tumours of the Cerebral Hemispheres — Extrinsic

ARACHNOID CYSTS

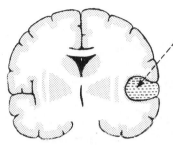

These cystic collections of CSF-like fluid lie in the Sylvian fissure, the chiasmatic cistern, the cisterna magna or over the hemisphere convexity. Some are related to a previous infective meningitis with subsequent adhesions but in most, the cause remains unknown. Those occurring in the Sylvian fissure may be associated with temporal lobe agenesis.

Occasionally arachnoid cysts present as an intracranial mass, but more often they are found by chance on CT scan.

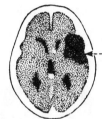

CT scan: shows a low density (CSF density well demarcated lesion, occasionally producing expansion of the overlying bone.

Treatment: only required if the mass effect becomes symptomatic – *marsupialisation* or *cystoperitoneal shunt*

EPIDERMOID/DERMOID CYSTS

These cysts, more commonly found in the posterior fossa (page 316), occasionally develop in the Sylvian or interhemispheric fissure. They may present with epilepsy, features of raised intracranial pressure or with focal neurological signs. Rupture into the subarachnoid space causes a chemical meningitis.

On CT scan, the extreme low attenuation of the cyst contents is characteristic. Symptoms may necessitate operative evacuation of the cyst contents. Removal of the cyst wall is often impossible and reaccumulation may occur.

Tumours of the Posterior Fossa — Intrinsic

CEREBELLAR METASTASIS

In adults, metastasis is the commonest tumour of the cerebellar hemisphere. Primary sites match those of supratentorial lesions (page 302).

Clinical features: may present acutely or progress over several months.

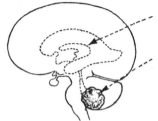

CSF obstruction   *hydrocephalus* – signs and symptoms of raised intracranial pressure.

Cerebellar signs – ataxia, nystagmus, dysarthria, incoordination.

Extension into the cerebello-pontine angle may damage cranial nerves V–XII – especially if a *carcinomatous plaque* develops.

Investigations:

CT scan shows a well defined solid or cystic lesion lying within the cerebellar hemisphere and enhancing irregularly with contrast.

Obstructive hydrocephalus often evident on higher scan cuts

4th ventricle displaced

Management:

Operative removal of a single metastasis through a suboccipital craniectomy is worthwhile provided the patient has a reasonable prognosis from the primary tumour. Risks are small – extensive cerebellar hemisphere resection (on one side) seldom produces any significant permanent deficit. A course of *radiotherapy* should follow operation. Persistence of obstructive hydrocephalus requires a ventriculo-peritoneal or atrial shunt.

HAEMANGIOBLASTOMA

This tumour of vascular origin occurs primarily in the middle aged; it is slightly more prevalent in males. In some patients, haemangioblastomas occur at other sites e.g. the spinal cord and retina and may be associated with other pathologies e.g. poly-cythaemia and cysts in the pancreas and kidneys – *Von Hippel Lindau disease* (page 543).

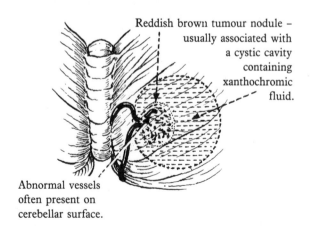

Reddish brown tumour nodule – usually associated with a cystic cavity containing xanthochromic fluid.

Abnormal vessels often present on cerebellar surface.

Tumours of the Posterior Fossa — Intrinsic

HAEMANGIOBLASTOMA *(continued)*

Clinical features:

Cerebellar signs and symptoms or the effects of CSF obstruction usually develop insidiously. Occasionally a subarachnoid haemorrhage occurs. In female patients, symptoms often appear during pregnancy.

Investigations:

CT scan shows a well defined low density cystic region in the cerebellum with a strongly enhancing nodule in the wall. Occasionally multiple lesions are evident.

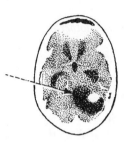

Management:

In most patients *operative removal* of the tumour nodule is straightforward, but recurrences (or further tumours at other sites e.g. spine) develop in 20%.

MEDULLOBLASTOMA

Medulloblastomas occur predominantly in childhood, with a peak age incidence of about 5 years. They arise in the cerebellar vermis and usually extend into the 4th ventricle. All are highly malignant and spread readily throughout the CSF pathways, often seeding to the lateral ventricles or the spinal theca.

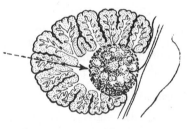

Clinical features:

Destruction of the cerebellar vermis causes truncal and gait ataxia often developing over a few weeks.

Alternatively, the patient presents with signs and symptoms of raised intracranial pressure due to blockage of CSF drainage. In the very young, failure to recognise these features has resulted in permanent visual loss from severe papilloedema.

Investigations:

CT scan shows an isodense midline lesion in the cerebellar vermis, compressing and displacing the 4th ventricle and enhancing strongly with contrast.

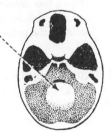

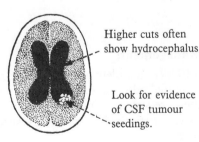

Higher cuts often show hydrocephalus

Look for evidence of CSF tumour seedings.

Tumours of the Posterior Fossa — Intrinsic

MEDULLOBLASTOMA *(continued)*

Management:

Operation: — the aim is to remove as much tumour as possible, yet producing minimal damage to surrounding tissue, in particular the floor of the 4th ventricle. Some patients require a CSF shunt, although this provides a further potential route for tumour seeding.

Radiotherapy: — medulloblastomas are radiosensitive. Whole neural axis irradiation attempts to cover any undetected CSF seeding.

Chemotherapy: — appears to provide effective supplementary treatment, but initial encouraging results await full evaluation.

Prognosis:

Studies in the last decade show a 5 year survival of approximately 40–50%. With present treatment methods, it is hoped this figure will extend to 60–70%.

CEREBELLAR ASTROCYTOMA

In contrast to astrocytomas of the cerebral hemispheres, cerebellar astrocytomas are usually low grade tumours of the fibrillary or pilocytic types. They are particularly common in children and carry an excellent prognosis. Occasionally a more diffuse or anaplastic type occurs with a less favourable outcome. They usually lie in the cerebellar hemisphere or vermis but occasionally extend through a peduncle into the brain stem. Many have cystic components.

Clinical features:

Cerebellar signs and symptoms tend to develop gradually over many months; if CSF obstruction occurs, the patient may present acutely with headache, papilloedema and deteriorating conscious level.

Investigations:

CT scan – density changes and the degree of contrast enhancement are variable.

Often a low density cystic area abuts or encircles the tumour mass

Displaced 4th ventricle

Management:

Ideally, complete *operative removal* is attempted provided the brain stem is not involved. With 'juvenile' pilocytic tumours, long term survival is likely. Even after partial removal 'cures' have been reported; although histologically similar to some supratentorial lesions, growth characteristics clearly differ. Persistent hydrocephalus may require a ventriculoperitoneal/atrial shunt.

Tumours of the Posterior Fossa — Intrinsic

BRAIN STEM ASTROCYTOMA

Rarely, astrocytomas arise within the brain stem. Most are of the fibrillary or pilocytic types and diffusely expand the pontine region. They develop mainly in children or young adults.

Clinical features:

Cranial nerve palsies and long tract signs gradually develop as the tumour progresses. Eventually conscious level is impaired.

Investigations:

CT scan shows:

– absence of the cisterns surrounding the brain stem.

– posterior displacement of the 4th ventricle.

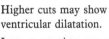

Higher cuts may show ventricular dilatation.

Low attenuation area often evident within the pons.

Management:

Operative expolration is rarel indicated. Usually radiotherapy is administered without histological confirmation of the diagnosis.

Prognosis:

Most patients die within a few years, although some may survive for up to 20 years with minimum disability.

Tumours of the Posterior Fossa — Extrinsic

ACOUSTIC NEURILEMMOMA / NEUROFIBROMA

Nerve sheath tumours are the commonest infratentorial tumours, constituting 6% of all primary intracranial tumours. They usually present in middle age (40–50 years) and occur more frequently in women.

They are benign, slowiy growing tumours which arise primarily from the vestibular portion of the VIII cranial nerve and lie in the cerebello-pontine angle – a wedge shaped area bounded by the petrous bone, the pons and the cerebellum. Rarely these tumours arise from the V cranial nerve.

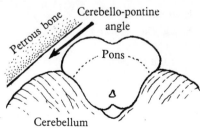

Tumours of the Posterior Fossa — Extrinsic

ACOUSTIC NEURILEMMOMA/NEUROFIBROMA *(continued)*

Pathology: Two types of nerve sheath tumour exist:

NEURILEMMOMA (syn. schwannoma, neurinoma) – arises from the Schwann cells but grows on the surface of the nerve trunk.

NEUROFIBROMA – also arises from Schwann cells but diffusely expands the nerve trunk, separating nerve fibres and fascicles.

Neurofibromas form part of *Von Recklinghausen's disease* and may be associated with other lesions e.g. meningioma, aqueduct stenosis, café au lait spots. Neurilemmomas are usually solitary lesions, but in Von Recklinghausen's disease multiple tumours may also occur. Malignant change occasionally develops, more commonly in neurofibromas.

Clinical features:

Patients with acoustic tumours often complain of *occipital pain* on the side of the tumour. In addition:

VIII nerve damage causes a *gradually progressive sensorineural deafness* noted over many months or years. *Vertigo* is rarely troublesome since slow tumour growth readily permits compensation. Similarly *tinnitus* is usually minimal.

V nerve damage causes *facial pain, numbness* and *paraesthesia. Depression of the corneal reflex* is an important early sign.

Compression of the aqueduct and the 4th ventricle may result in hydrocephalus with *symptoms and signs of raised intracranial pressure.*

N.B. Tentorium cerebelli and left cerebellar hemisphere removed.

Facial weakness is surprisingly *uncommon* despite marked VII nerve compression

IX, X and XI nerve damage seldom occurs but occasionally large tumours cause *swallowing difficulty, voice change* and *palatal weakness.*

Cerebellar and pontine damage – large tumours may compress the cerebellum causing *ataxia, ipsilateral incoordination* and *nystagmus.* Pontine damage may produce a *contralateral hemiparesis.*

312

Tumours of the Posterior Fossa — Extrinsic

ACOUSTIC NEURILEMMOMA/NEUROFIBROMA *(continued*

Investigations:

Neuro-otological tests (see page 58)

- audiometry
- tone decay
- loudness recruitment test
- speech discrimination
- brain stem auditory evoked potential

} help differentiate deafness due to:

conductive deficit

sensorineural — cochlear deficit

retrocochlear deficit (e.g. acoustic tumour)

- caloric testing – invariably shows absence or impairment of the response on the affected side.

Tomography of the internal auditory meatus (IAM) may show erosion and dilatation on the affected side.

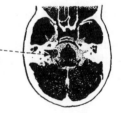

CT scan

Acoustic neurilemmoma

Look for dilatation of the IAM

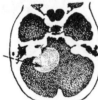

I.V. contrast is essential, since acoustic tumours are often iso-dense. After contrast the tumour, lying adjacent to the IAM enhances strongly. Low density cystic areas are occasionally seen. Patients with 4th ventricle compression may show associated dilatation of the 3rd and lateral ventricles.

Metrizemide CT scan – the introduction of contrast into the *basal cisterns* (by lumbar or cisternal puncture) helps outline small acoustic tumours projecting from the internal auditory meatus. Alternatively, *air* insufflation may be used.

[This CT scan technique replaces *myodil encephalography* – failure to run myodil into the internal auditory meatus, indirectly indicates the presence of an acoustic tumour.]

CSF examination often shows exceptionally high protein levels i.e. up to 10g/l. (Note lumbar puncture is contraindicated with large tumours.)

Tumours of the Posterior Fossa — Extrinsic

ACOUSTIC NEURILEMMOMA/NEUROFIBROMA — Management:

The treatment of acoustic tumours is operative removal. A conservative approach gains nothing; operative risks relate directly to tumour size – the larger the tumour, the higher the operative mortality and the smaller the chance of preserving VII nerve function.

Technique:

Middle fossa approach: temporal lobe retraction exposes the acoustic tumour and facial nerve from above. The tentorium cerebelli and the superior petrosal sinus are divided if necessary.

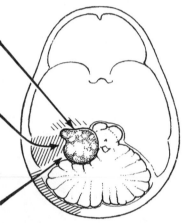

TRANSLABYRINTHINE APPROACH: approaching the tumour through the mastoid air cells and the labyrinth permits early identification of the facial nerve; tumour decompression and removal follows.

SUBOCCIPITAL APPROACH: the cerebello-pontine angle is approached from below by removing occipital bone and retracting the cerebellum.

Tumour debulking aids dissection of the tumour capsule from the surrounding structures, including the facial nerve. Drilling away the roof of the internal meatus exposes the tumour and facial nerve lying within the canal.

All methods have their advocates. Limited visualisation of the brain stem structures through a translabyrinthine approach makes this unsuitable for large tumours. Inevitably this approach damages hearing. With very small tumours (which usually arise from the vestibular portion of the nerve), careful removal via the suboccipital route may preserve cochlear nerve as well as facial nerve function.

Results:

The mortality rate relates to tumour size and approaches 20% for very large tumours. Death usually results from damage to important vascular structures (e.g. anterior inferior cerebellar artery) or from post-operative cerebellar swelling. The incidence of facial nerve preservation also depends on tumour size. In most patients with small tumours (e.g. under 2cm) facial nerve integrity is preserved compared to only 20% of patients with large tumours (e.g. over 4cm), although recovery may take many months. Incomplete eyelid closure may require *tarsorrhaphy* to prevent corneal ulceration. When facial nerve palsy persists, *hypoglossal-facial anastomosis* may alleviate the final cosmetic result.

Swallowing difficulty from X cranial nerve damage seldom persists; intravenous or cautious oral fluid administration during this period should prevent aspiration.

In 10–30% of patients, incomplete tumour removal results in a late recurrence and further operations are required. In the elderly, an intentional intracapsular subtotal removal may provide the safest approach.

Tumours of the Posterior Fossa — Extrinsic

TRIGEMINAL NEURILEMMOMA

Rarely neurilemmomas arise from the trigeminal ganglion or nerve root. These lie in the middle fossa or extend into the cerebello-pontine angle, compress surrounding structures – cavernous sinus, midbrain and the pons – and erode the apex of the petrous bone.

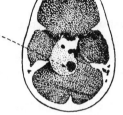

Clinical features are usually long standing – facial pain, paraesthesia and numbness. Compression of posterior fossa structures results in nystagmus, ataxia and hemiparesis.

Skull X-ray shows erosion of the petrous apex and CT scan demonstrates an enhancing lesion extending into the middle and/or posterior fossa.

Management: Operative removal, even if subtotal, should provide long lasting benefit. The tumour is approached through either the middle fossa or through a suboccipital craniectomy depending on the predominant site.

MENINGIOMA

Approximately 8% of all intracranial meningiomas arise in the posterior fossa.

Clinical features:

These depend on the exact tumour site. Those arising over the *cerebellar convexity* may not present until the mass obstructs CSF drainage. Meningiomas arising in the *cerebello-pontine angle* may involve any cranial nerve from V to XII. A *clivus* meningioma may present with bilateral VI nerve palsies before pontine pressure causes long tract signs.

Tumours growing at the *foramen magnum,* compressing the cervico-medullary junction, produce characteristic effects – pyramidal weakness initially affecting the ipsilateral arm, followed by the ipsilateral leg, spreading to the contralateral limbs with further tumour growth.

Investigations:

CT scan identifies the exact tumour site.

Most meningiomas enhance homogeneously with contrast.

Management:

As with supratentorial meningiomas, treatment aims at complete tumour removal. In the posterior fossa, cranial nerve involvement makes this difficult and tedious; exciaion of the tumour origin is seldom possible.

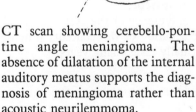

CT scan showing cerebello-pontine angle meningioma. The absence of dilatation of the internal auditory meatus supports the diagnosis of meningioma rather than acoustic neurilemmoma.

Tumours of the Posterior Fossa — Extrinsic

EPIDERMOID/DERMOID CYSTS

These cysts of embryological origin develop from cells predestined to become either epidermis or dermis. They most commonly arise in the cerebello-pontine angle but may also occur around the suprasellar cisterns, in the lateral ventricles and in the Sylvian fissures, often extending deeply into brain tissue.

Pathology: Depends on cell of origin:

Epidermoid (epidermis – a thin transparent cyst wall often adheres firmly to surrounding tissues; the contents – keratinised debris and cholesterol crystals produce a 'pearly' white appearance.

Dermoid (dermis) – as above, but thicker walled and, in addition, containing hair follicles and glandular tissue. Midline dermoid cysts lying in the posterior fossa often connect to the skin surface through a bony defect. This presents a potential route for infection.

Clinical features:

When lying in the cerebello-pontine angle, epidermoid/dermoid cysts often cause *trigeminal neuralgia* (see page 150). Neurological findings may range from a depressed corneal reflex to multiple cranial nerve palsies. Rupture and release of cholesterol into the subarachnoid space produces a severe and occasionally fatal *chemical meningitis*. The presence of a *suboccipital dimple* combined with an attack of infective meningitis should raise the possibility of a posterior fossa dermoid cyst with a cutaneous fistula.

Investigations:

CT scan shows a characteristic low density (often 'fat' density) - - - - - lesion, unchanged after contrast enhancement or showing only slight peripheral enhancement.   Calcification may be evident.

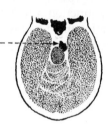

Treatment:

Adherence of the cyst wall to important structures invariably prevents complete removal but evacuation of the contents provides symptomatic relief. Recollection of the keratinised debris usually takes many years.

Sellar/Suprasellar Tumours — Pituitary Adenoma

Tumours of the pituitary gland constitute about 5% of intracranial tumours. They arise from the anterior portion of the gland and are usually benign.

Previous Classification:
   Previously based on the light microscopic appearance of the tumour cell type.

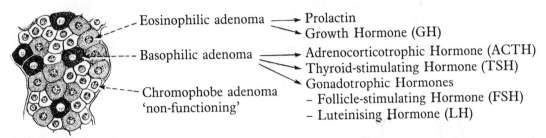

   Eosinophilic adenoma ——→ Prolactin
                            ↘ Growth Hormone (GH)

   Basophilic adenoma ——→ Adrenocorticotrophic Hormone (ACTH)
                        ——→ Thyroid-stimulating Hormone (TSH)
                        ↗ Gonadotrophic Hormones
                            – Follicle-stimulating Hormone (FSH)
                            – Luteinising Hormone (LH)

   Chromophobe adenoma
   'non-functioning'

PRESENT Classification

   Recent immuno-assay techniques permit a more practical classification based on the hormone type secreted. About half of the 'non-functioning' chromophobe adenomas secrete prolactin.

- **Prolactinoma.**
- **GH secreting tumour.**
- **ACTH secreting tumour.**
- **TSH secreting tumour** ⎫
- **FSH/LH secreting tumour** ⎭ rare.

Clinical Presentation:

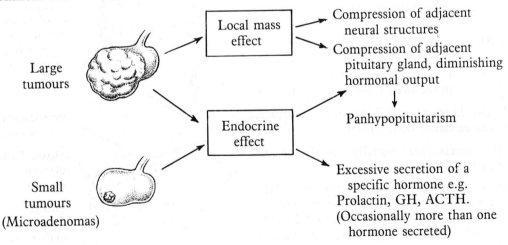

Large tumours →

Small tumours (Microadenomas) →

Local mass effect
→ Compression of adjacent neural structures
→ Compression of adjacent pituitary gland, diminishing hormonal output
   ↓
   Panhypopituitarism

Endocrine effect
→ Excessive secretion of a specific hormone e.g. Prolactin, GH, ACTH. (Occasionally more than one hormone secreted)

Sellar / Suprasellar Tumours — Pituitary Adenoma

LOCAL MASS EFFECT

Headache: occurs in most patients with enlargement of the pituitary fossa. It is not specific in site or nature.

Visual Field Defects

Pressure on the inferior aspect of the optic chiasma causes *superior temporal quadrantanopia* initially, with progression to bitemporal hemianopia.

Cavernous Sinus Compression

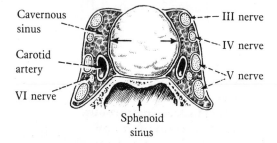

Cavernous sinus

Carotid artery

VI nerve

III nerve

IV nerve

V nerve

Sphenoid sinus

In some pituitary tumours, lateral expansion may compress nerves lying within the walls of the cavernous sinus. The III nerve is especially vulnerable.

ENDOCRINE EFFECT

1. HYPERSECRETION The clinical syndrome produced is dependent on the hormone secreted.

GROWTH HORMONE (GH) stimulates growth and plays a part in control of protein, fat and carbohydrate metabolism. Excess GH in the adult causes ACROMEGALY.

In childhood, prior to fusion of bone sutures, GH excess causes GIGANTISM.

GH levels are usually increased to >10ng/ml.

Hyperglycaemia normally suppresses GH secretion. GH samples are taken in conjunction with blood glucose during a glucose tolerance test. The lack of GH suppression after glucose administration confirms the presence of a tumour.

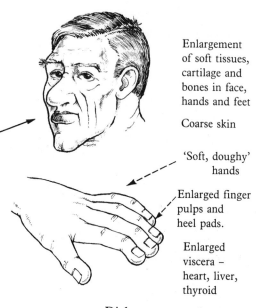

Enlargement of soft tissues, cartilage and bones in face, hands and feet

Coarse skin

'Soft, doughy' hands

Enlarged finger pulps and heel pads.

Enlarged viscera – heart, liver, thyroid

Diabetes occurs in 10%

Sellar / Suprasellar Tumours — Pituitary Adenoma

PROLACTIN

This hormone helps to promote lactation. The introduction of immuno-assay techniques has shown prolactinaemias to be the commonest type of pituitary tumour and aided early detection of prolactin microadenomas.

This tumour may present with

- INFERTILITY
- AMENORRHOEA
- GALACTORRHOEA

In males, the tumour may present with IMPOTENCE or remain undetected until local pressure effects occur.

In most centres, a serum prolactin of 360mU/l is considered abnormal, but before assuming the presence of a prolactin secreting tumour, other causes must be excluded.

Causes of Hyperprolactinaemia

1. Stress.
2. Pregnancy.
3. Drugs (especially dopamine antagonists).
4. Hypothyroidism
5. Renal disease.
6. Pituitary adenoma.
7. Hypothalamic lesion or
   pituitary stalk section.

Many drugs including chlorpromazine, methyl dopa and oestrogens elevate serum prolactin. Since thyrotrophic hormone (TRH) stimulates prolactin release, prolactin levels are high in hypothyroidism.

Prolactin differs from other anterior pituitary hormones in that it is under tonic inhibitory control from the hypothalamus. Hypothalamic lesions or pituitary stalk section lead to a deficiency of prolactin inhibitory factor (PIF) producing a rise in the serum prolactin.

The following tests suggest the presence of a prolactin secreting tumour, but these are of limited reliability:

1. Loss of the normal diurnal fluctuation in prolactin levels.
2. Loss or reduction in response to TRH injection (normal increases x 500).
3. Loss of response to metoclopramide (normal increases x 2000).

Sellar / Suprasellar Tumours — Pituitary Adenoma

ADRENOCORTICOTROPHIC HORMONE (ACTH)

ACTH stimulates secretion of cortisol and androgens. Hypersecretion causes adrenal hyperplasia which presents with the characteristic features of CUSHING's SYNDROME.

This syndrome may also be produced by an adrenal tumour or by ectopic secretion from a bronchial carcinoma, but steroid administration is the commonest cause.

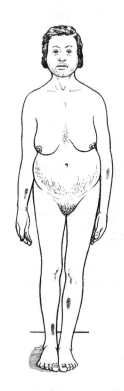

Features:

Moon face.
Buffalo-type obesity.
Purple striae over flanks and abdomen.
Bruising.
Muscle weakness and wasting.
Osteoporosis.
Latent diabetes mellitis.
Hypertension.
Acne.
Hirsutism and baldness.
Increased susceptibility to infection.

The diagnosis is established by the finding of elevated urine and plasma cortisol levels which are not suppressed by dexamethasone administration.

Bilateral adrenalectomy for Cushing's disease is sometimes followed by the development of Nelson's syndrome – high ACTH levels, pituitary enlargement and marked skin pigmentation.

TSH – stimulates thyroid hormone secretion.
FSH – controls growth of ovarian follicles/spermatogenesis.
LH – induces ovulation/testosterone secretion.

} Hypersecreting tumours very rare.

Sellar / Suprasellar Tumours — Pituitary Adenoma

2. HYPOSECRETION

Many pituitary tumours are diagnosed before panhypopituitarism develops, but large tumours may cause gradual impairment of pituitary hormone secretion. Growth hormone and the gonadotrophins are first affected, followed by TSH and ACTH. Panhypopituitarism only occurs when more than 80% of the anterior pituitary is destroyed.

Impaired secretion	ADULTS	CHILDREN
GH	—	pituitary dwarfism – diminished skeletal growth, retarded sexual development, hypoglycaemic episodes, normal intelligence.
Gonadotrophins –	amenorrhoea, sterility, loss of libido.	
ACTH ——	glucocorticoid and androgen deficiency, muscle weakness and fatigue.	
TSH ——	secondary hypothyroidism, low BMR, sensitivity to cold, physical and mental sluggishness, coarseness of hair.	
Prolactin* ——	failure of lactation.	

*Prolactin secretion is most resistant to pituitary damage. Deficiency is seldom evident, usually only presenting after post-partum haemorrhage (Sheehan's syndrome) as a failure of lactation associated with the other features of panhypopituitarism.

Pituitary hormone assay cannot distinguish low 'normal' levels from impaired secretion, *but low levels of pituitary hormone in the presence of low target gland hormones* confirm hyposecretion e.g. low TSH levels despite a low serum thyroxine.

The lack of response to tests designed to increase specific pituitary hormones provides additional confirmation of hypofunction:

1. GH ⎱ — *Insulin Tolerance Test:* Hypoglycaemia acting via the hypothalamic
    ACTH ⎰ pituitary axis should elevate GH and ACTH levels, the latter causing a significant rise in plasma cortisol.

2. Gonadotrophin — *Gonadotrophin Releasing Hormone (GnRH) injection* should produce a rapid rise in LH and a slower rise in FSH.

3. TSH ⎱ — *Thyrotrophin Releasing Hormone (TRH) injection* should increase
    Prolactin ⎰ plasma levels of both TSH and prolactin.

The above tests can be carried out simultaneously as the *Combined Pituitary Stimulation Test.* Insulin, GnRH and TRH are injected intravenously and all anterior pituitary hormones measured from repeated blood samples taken over a 2 hour period. Glucose levels are also checked to ensure adequacy of the hypoglycaemia.

PITUITARY APOPLEXY

This is an uncommon complication of pituitary tumours due to the occurrence of haemorrhage into the tumour substance. Severe headache of sudden onset, rapidly progressive visual failure and extraocular nerve palsies accompany acute pituitary insufficiency. Death may follow unless urgent treatment is instituted.

Sellar / Suprasellar Tumours — Pituitary Adenoma

NEURORADIOLOGICAL INVESTIGATION

Skull X-ray

Large tumours cause expansion or 'ballooning' of the pituitary fossa and may erode the floor

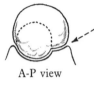

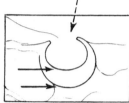

A-P view

Asymmetrical fossa expansion gives the appearance of a 'double floor' effect on the lateral view

Tomography is useful to delineate erosion of the fossa floor.

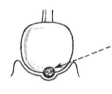

Microadenomas may produce a small erosive cup on the floor, best seen on an anterioposterior view.

CT scan

CT scan with contrast enhancement clearly demonstrates large tumours filling the pituitary fossa and expanding into the suprasellar compartment.

Suprasellar extension

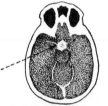

Axial view

High definition CT scanning provides most information:

Large tumours: Coronal and axial views of the pituitary region obtained either by reconstruction or direct scanning demonstrate the exact extent of the suprasellar extension.

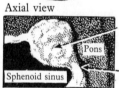

Large tumour with suprasellar extension

Pons

Sphenoid sinus

4th ventricle

Coronal view

Microadenomas: One or two millimetre slices may demonstrate a low density region within the gland tissue or may show deviation of the pituitary stalk from the midline. The incidence of false negatives, however, is high.

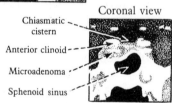

Chiasmatic cistern

Anterior clinoid

Microadenoma

Sphenoid sinus

Basal Cisternogram

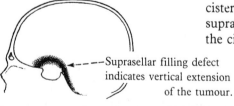

Suprasellar filling defect indicates vertical extension of the tumour.

If high definition scanning is not available, then a basal cisternogram will clearly demonstrate the extent of the suprasellar extension. Radiopaque contrast is injected into the cisterna magna and runs along the skull base.

Angiography may be required in the investigation of a pituitary lesion to exclude the presence of an aneurysm presenting as a suprasellar mass.

A **cavernous sinogram** may help by demonstrating the extent of cavernous sinus involvement.

322

Sellar / Suprasellar Tumours — Pituitary Adenoma

MANAGEMENT

Management of pituitary tumours depends on the mode of presentation. Those presenting as mass lesions require decompression and correction of endocrine abnormalities. With microadenomas, treatment of the hormonal disturbance is the main priority. Early treatment may prevent later development of mass lesions.

Methods include: Operative decompression,
Radiotherapy, Drugs.

OPERATIVE APPROACH
From BELOW:

1. Trans-sphenoidal

Through an incision in the upper gum the nasal mucosa is stripped from the septum and the pituitary fossa approached through the sphenoid sinus.

2. Trans-ethmoidal

An incision is made on the medial orbital wall and the pituitary fossa approached through the ethmoid and sphenoid sinuses.

With the trans-ethmoidal and trans sphenoidal routes the pituitary gland can be directly visualised and explored for micro-adenoma. Even large tumours with supra-sellar extensions may be removed from below, avoiding the need for craniotomy.

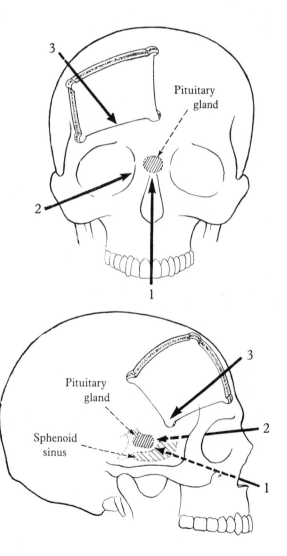

From ABOVE:

3. Trans-frontal

Through a craniotomy flap the frontal lobe is retracted to provide direct access to the pituitary tumour. This approach is usually reserved for tumours with large frontal or lateral extensions.

N.B.   All patients require steroid cover before any anaesthetic or operative procedure.

Sellar/Suprasellar Tumours — Pituitary Adenoma

MANAGEMENT

RADIOTHERAPY

Pituitary adenomas are radiosensitive and irradiation is most commonly employed externally. Occasionally radioactive seeds of yttrium or gold are implanted into the pituitary fossa either via a trans-sphenoidal approach or stereotactically through a frontal burr hole.

DRUGS

Bromocriptine is a dopamine agonist which lowers abnormal circulating hormone concentrations, especially prolactin. In high doses, it may also reduce growth hormone secretion.

Which Treatment?

Treatment choice depends on presenting features.

LARGE TUMOURS – Further expansion of a tumour already extending outside the pituitary fossa risks permanent visual damage. *Operative* removal provides rapid decompression and with the trans-sphenoidal or trans-ethmoidal approach, risks are minimal. With large tumours there is never certainty of complete removal and *radiotherapy* is a useful supplementary treatment. If radiotherapy is used primarily, there is a likelihood of tumour swelling; subsequent reduction in size and correction of hormone levels is usually considerably delayed. A few advocate initial treatment of prolactinomas with bromocriptine but only 60% decrease in size and occasionally tumour growth continues.

MICROADENOMAS – If the tumour is contained wholly within the pituitary fossa there is little immediate risk of visual damage and treatment is directed at reducing hormone levels. Trans-sphenoidal or trans-ethmoidal operation provides a rapid return to normal hormonal levels in 80–90%. Bromocriptine provides an alternative approach to the treatment of prolactin secreting microadenomas. With a resultant reduction in prolactin levels, pregnancy may follow and this occasionally induces rapid tumour expansion. There is also a theoretical but unsubstantiated risk of teratogenicity. Drugs are of less benefit in the control of GH and ACTH secreting tumours.

Sellar/Suprasellar Tumours

CRANIOPHARYNGIOMA

These cystic tumours constitute about 3% of all primary intracranial tumours. They present predominantly in children and in young adults but symptoms may develop at any age. Although benign, their proximity to crucial structures poses complex problems of management. Most craniopharyngiomas have solid components of squamous epithelium with calcified debris and one or more cystic regions containing greenish cholesteatomatous fluid. In some, the tumour is solid throughout. Although the tumour capsule appears well defined, histological examination reveals finger-like projections extending into adjacent tissue with marked surrounding gliosis.

Sites: Growth usually begins near the pituitary stalk, but may extend in many directions.

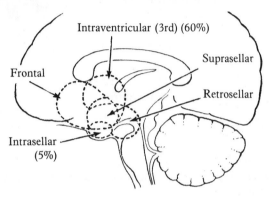

Clinical features: depend on the exact site and size of the tumour. Growth is slow and most signs and symptoms develop insidiously.

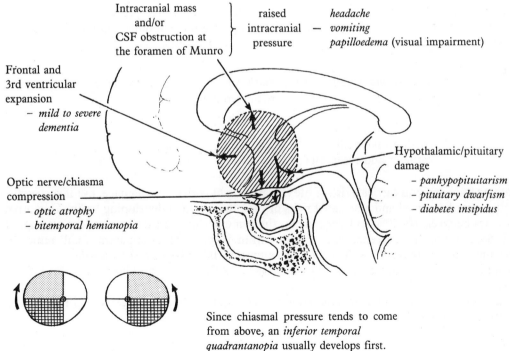

Intracranial mass and/or CSF obstruction at the foramen of Munro } raised intracranial pressure — *headache* *vomiting* *papilloedema* (visual impairment)

Frontal and 3rd ventricular expansion
- *mild to severe dementia*

Optic nerve/chiasma compression
- *optic atrophy*
- *bitemporal hemianopia*

Hypothalamic/pituitary damage
- *panhypopituitarism*
- *pituitary dwarfism*
- *diabetes insipidus*

Since chiasmal pressure tends to come from above, an *inferior temporal quadrantanopia* usually develops first.

325

Sellar/Suprasellar Tumours

CRANIOPHARYNGIOMA *(continued)*

Investigations:

Skull X-ray: shows calcification above or within the pituitary fossa in 80%.

CT scan: shows a lesion of mixed density containing solid and cystic components lying in the suprasellar region.

In children, CT scan invariably shows calcification

Coronal or sagittal reconstruction helps by demonstrating the exact relationships of the tumour to the 3rd ventricle.

The cyst capsule often enhances with contrast.

Pituitary function studies (page 321): often demonstrate the need for hormone replacement.

Management:

Several options exist; the more aggressive the treatment, the higher the risks, but the lower the recurrence rate.

All patients require steroid cover before any anaesthetic or operative procedure.

Operative removal usually involves a subfrontal or subtemporal craniotomy, although the trans-sphenoidal route may permit removal of purely intrasellar tumours.

Methods:

1. *Total tumour excision (+ radiotherapy if recurrence develops)*
2. *Subtotal tumour excision + radiotherapy*
3. *Cyst drainage +* ⎯⎯⎯ *radiotherapy*
   (with an indwelling   or
   catheter and reservoir)   implantation of yttrium^{90}

Attempted total excision carries a risk of life threatening hypothalamic damage, but if successful avoids the immediate need and associated risks of radiotherapy to a developing brain. Operative mortality lies between 10–30% and depends on the tumour site and the extent of the attempted removal. Some report a recurrence rate of 50% within 10 years of an apparent 'total' removal. This presumably results from residual tumour extensions lying beyond the capsule.

With subtotal removal the recurrence rate approaches 90%, but with radiotherapy this falls to 30–50%.

The decision to aim for total or subtotal removal requires careful judgement. Preoperative investigations help but the final decision often awaits direct exploration.

326

Sellar/Suprasellar Tumours

OPTIC NERVE (GLIOMA) ASTROCYTOMA

This rare tumour usually presents in children under 10 years. Up to one-third are associated with Von Recklinghausen's disease. Tumour growth expands the nerve in a fusiform manner. Some extend anteriorly into the orbit, others posteriorly to involve the optic chiasma. All are of the pilocytic type and growth is slow.

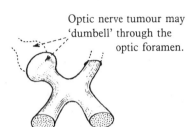

Optic nerve tumour may 'dumbell' through the optic foramen.

Clinical features:

Visual field scotomas gradually progress to *complete visual loss.*
Orbital extension causes *proptosis.*
In some patients posterior expansion beyond the chiasma causes *hypothalamic damage* and/or *hydrocephalus.*
X-rays of the orbital foramen show dilatation and *CT scans* demonstrate an enhancing mixed attenuation mass within the orbit or lying in the suprasellar region.

Management:

			Prognosis
Unilateral lesion	—	complete excision with orbital enucleation if necessary.	— Excellent
Lesion involving the optic chiasma	—	conservative approach (the value of radiotherapy is not known)	— Patients may retain vision for many years; survival is often long-term. Those with hypo-thalamic damage have a poor prognosis.

SUPRASELLAR MENINGIOMA

Meningiomas arising from the tuberculum sellae often present early as a result of chiasmal compression and visual field defects – usually with *bitemporal hemianopia.*

Straight X-rays may show *hyperostosis* of the tuberculum sellae or planum sphenoidale.

CT scan shows a rounded, often partly calcified suprasellar mass homogeneously enhancing with contrast.

Unfortunately the visual defect often persists after operation, but attempted removal is essential to prevent further progression.

Hyperostotic sphenoid

MENINGIOMA OF THE OPTIC NERVE SHEATH

Rarely, meningiomas arise from the optic nerve sheath, usually extending in dumbell fashion through the optic foramen. Some penetrate the orbital dura and invade the orbital contents. Total excision is impossible without sacrificing the adjacent optic nerve.

SUPRASELLAR EPIDERMOID/DERMOID (see page 316).

Note: large aneurysms or granulomas (TB, sarcoid) may simulate a sellar/suprasellar tumour on CT scan. If in doubt, perform angiography prior to operative exploration.

Pineal Region Tumours

Pineal region tumours are relatively uncommon. They consist of a variety of different pathological types and as a result of the direct anatomical relationship with the third ventricle include tumours arising at this site. Less than 20% actually originate from 'pineal' cells.

Pathological types:

TERATOMA: well differentiated tumour occurring predominantly in males, and formed from various cell types – muscle, bone, cartilage, dermis.

Tumour consistency depends on the predominant cell type. In most patients the tumour margin is well defined. Malignant, poorly differentiated forms occasionally occur.

GERMINOMA: a malignant tumour, resembling seminoma of the testis. The tumour adhees firmly to the surrounding tissues and cells readily spread to the floor or anterior wall of the third ventricle. Cells may also seed through the CSF pathways to the spinal cord or cauda equina.

PINEOCYTOMA: well differentiated, slowly growing tumour. ⎫ rare tumours of true
PINEOBLASTOMA: poorly differentiated, highly malignant tumour. ⎬ 'pineal' origin.

GLIAL CELL TUMOURS – ASTROCYTOMA – arising from cells within the pineal gland, or from adjacent brain.

MENINGIOMA ⎫
DERMOID ⎬ rarely occur in the pineal region.
EPIDERMOID ⎭

EPENDYMOMA – arising from cells lining the third ventricle.

Clinical features: develop due to:

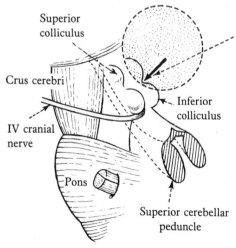

Superior colliculus
Crus cerebri
IV cranial nerve
Pons
Inferior colliculus
Superior cerebellar peduncle

LOCAL MASS EFFECT

Pressure on the tectal plate
– PARINAUD's *syndrome (impaired upward gaze, pupillary abnormalities)* (page 144).

Compression of the aqueduct of Sylvius
– *obstructive hydrocephalus* with *signs and symptoms of raised intracranial pressure.*

EFFECTS FROM THIRD VENTRICULAR SPREAD

e.g. germinoma
– *hypothalamic damage, diabetes insipidus, hypo/hyperphagia, precocious puberty, hypopituitarism.*
– *optic chiasmal involvement, visual field defects.*

Pineal Region Tumours

Investigations:

CT scan shows a mass projecting into the posterior aspect of the third ventricle with associated dilatation of the third and lateral ventricles.

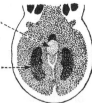

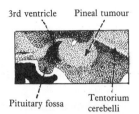

3rd ventricle   Pineal tumour

Pituitary fossa   Tentorium cerebelli

Sagittal CT reconstruction clarifies the exact tumour relationship to the third ventricle.

Pineocytomas – may appear calcified.
Teratomas – may contain mixed densities from fat to calcification.

CSF cytology: occasionally reveals malignant cells and may indicate the tumour type.

Serum human chorionic gonadotrophin
Serum alpha fetoprotein } may arise in patients with germinoma.

Management:

Hydrocephalus often requires urgent treatment with a *ventriculo-peritoneal* or *atrial shunt*. Large tumours may obstruct the foramen of Munro, making bilateral ventricular drainage necessary.

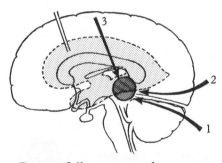

The site of pineal region tumours makes operative approach difficult. Although modern techniques considerably diminish the risk of a direct operation, most neurosurgeons advocate initial treatment with *radiotherapy* (without tissue diagnosis). About 70% of tumours are radiosensitive and show a dramatic reduction in size. Failure to respond indicates the need for tissue diagnosis; most then proceed either to *stereotactic biopsy* or to *direct operative exploration*.

Routes of direct approach
1. Infratentorial.
2. Supratentorial.
3. Transventricular.

Patients undergoing a CSF shunt followed by radiotherapy, survive 4 years on average.

329

Tumours of the Ventricular System

EPENDYMOMA

Intracranial ependymomas originate from cells lining the ventricular cavities. Most arise in the 4th ventricle and in this site occur predominatly in children. Both low grade and malignant forms are found and tumour cells may seed throughout CSF pathways.

In the *4th ventricle*, ependymomas present with cerebellar signs or, more commonly, with signs and symptoms of raised intracranial pressure from CSF obstruction. *Vomiting* is often an early feature.

CT scanning shows an isodense mass, with or without calcification, lying within the 4th ventricle and usually enhancing with contrast.

Management:

The aim is complete operative removal, although infiltration of the floor of the 4th ventricle may prevent this. Most clinicians advise radiotherapy postoperatively, but its value is limited in the low grade tumours.

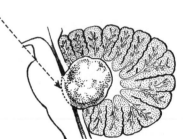

Prognosis:

Despite relatively slow growth, results are often disappointing with 5 year survival ranging from 20–50%.

CHOROID PLEXUS PAPILLOMA

Rare, benign tumour with a granular surface and a gritty texture.

They develop from the choroid plexus – in the *4th ventricle – adults,*
– in the *lateral ventricle – children.*

Malignant forms occasionally occur in children.

Most patients present with hydrocephalus, either due to obstruction or to excessive CSF secretion from the tumour.

CT scanning shows a hyperdense mass within the ventricular system.

Operative removal gives good results.

COLLOID CYST OF THE THIRD VENTRICLE

A benign cyst, containing a mucoid fluid may arise from embryological remnants in the roof of the third ventricle. When of sufficient size (about 2cm) it occludes CSF drainage from both lateral ventricles through the foramen of Munro.

Clinical features: Symptoms may be intermittent, possibly due to a ball-valve effect, with episodes of loss of consciousness or sudden weakness of legs.

CT scan shows a small round mass of increased density, lying level with the foramen of Munro, causing lateral ventricular dilatation. Operative removal through the right lateral ventricle carries little risk.

MENINGIOMA: rarely arises in the *lateral* ventricles. Often symptoms are mild and long standing. Operative removal only becomes necessary when symptoms and signs appear.

GERMINOMA
TERATOMA   see Pineal Region Tumours, page 328

Tumours of the Orbit

The orbital cavity is bounded –

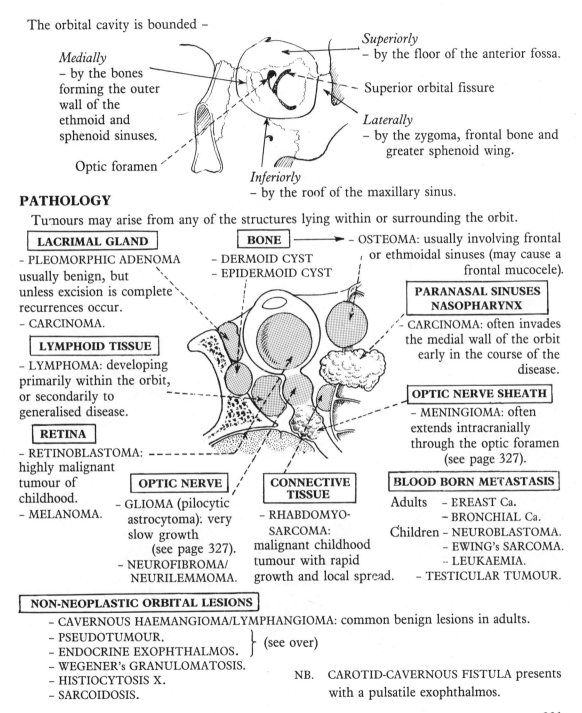

Medially
– by the bones forming the outer wall of the ethmoid and sphenoid sinuses.

Optic foramen

Superiorly
– by the floor of the anterior fossa.

Superior orbital fissure

Laterally
– by the zygoma, frontal bone and greater sphenoid wing.

Inferiorly
– by the roof of the maxillary sinus.

PATHOLOGY

Tumours may arise from any of the structures lying within or surrounding the orbit.

LACRIMAL GLAND
– PLEOMORPHIC ADENOMA usually benign, but unless excision is complete recurrences occur.
– CARCINOMA.

LYMPHOID TISSUE
– LYMPHOMA: developing primarily within the orbit, or secondarily to generalised disease.

RETINA
– RETINOBLASTOMA: highly malignant tumour of childhood.
– MELANOMA.

BONE ⟶
– DERMOID CYST
– EPIDERMOID CYST

– OSTEOMA: usually involving frontal or ethmoidal sinuses (may cause a frontal mucocele).

PARANASAL SINUSES NASOPHARYNX
– CARCINOMA: often invades the medial wall of the orbit early in the course of the disease.

OPTIC NERVE SHEATH
– MENINGIOMA: often extends intracranially through the optic foramen (see page 327).

OPTIC NERVE
– GLIOMA (pilocytic astrocytoma): very slow growth (see page 327).
– NEUROFIBROMA/ NEURILEMMOMA.

CONNECTIVE TISSUE
– RHABDOMYO-SARCOMA: malignant childhood tumour with rapid growth and local spread.

BLOOD BORN METASTASIS
Adults   – EREAST Ca.
          – BRONCHIAL Ca.
Children – NEUROBLASTOMA.
          – EWING's SARCOMA.
          – LEUKAEMIA.
          – TESTICULAR TUMOUR.

NON-NEOPLASTIC ORBITAL LESIONS
– CAVERNOUS HAEMANGIOMA/LYMPHANGIOMA: common benign lesions in adults.
– PSEUDOTUMOUR.
– ENDOCRINE EXOPHTHALMOS. } (see over)
– WEGENER's GRANULOMATOSIS.
– HISTIOCYTOSIS X.
– SARCOIDOSIS.

NB. CAROTID-CAVERNOUS FISTULA presents with a pulsatile exophthalmos.

331

Tumours of the Orbit

Clinical Symptoms and Signs

Orbital pain: prominent in rapidly growing malignant tumours, but also a characteristic feature of benign 'pseudotumour' and carotid-cavernous fistula.

Proptosis: forward displacement of the globe is a common feature, progressing gradually and painlessly over months or years (benign tumours) or rapidly (malignant lesions).

Lid swelling: may be pronounced in pseudotumour, endocrine exophthalmos or carotid-cavernous fistula.

Palpation: may reveal a mass causing globe or lid distortion – especially with lacrimal gland tumours or with a mucocele. *Pulsation* indicates a vascular lesion – carotid-cavernous fistula or arteriovenous malformation – listen for a bruit.

Eye movements: often limited for mechanical reasons, but if marked, may result from an endocrine ophthalmoplegia or from III,IV or VI nerve lesions in the orbital fissure (e.g. Tolosa Hunt syndrome) or cavernous sinus.

Visual acuity: may diminish due to direct involvement of the optic nerve or retina, or indirectly from vascular damage.

Investigations

X-ray of the orbit: may reveal local erosion (malignancy), dilatation of the optic foramen (meningioma, optic nerve glioma) and occasionally calcification (retinoblastoma, lacrimal gland tumours). A meningioma often causes local sclerosis.

CT scan of the orbits demonstrates the precise site of intraorbital pathology and shows the presence of any intracranial extension.

Transverse view showing an optic nerve glioma. Coronal views are also possible.

Orbital venography may help.

Management

BENIGN tumours: require excision, but if visual loss would inevitably result, the clinician may adopt a conservative approach.

MALIGNANT tumours: require biopsy plus radiotherapy. Lymphomas may also benefit from chemotherapy. Occasionally localised lesions (e.g. carcinoma of the lacrimal gland) require radical resection.

OPERATIVE APPROACH

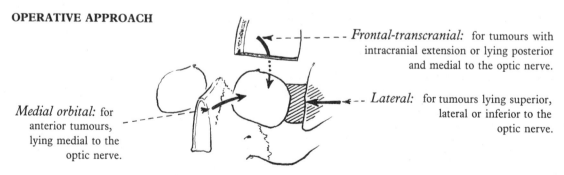

Frontal-transcranial: for tumours with intracranial extension or lying posterior and medial to the optic nerve.

Lateral: for tumours lying superior, lateral or inferior to the optic nerve.

Medial orbital: for anterior tumours, lying medial to the optic nerve.

Non-Neoplastic Orbital Lesions

PSEUDOTUMOUR (Orbital granuloma)

Sudden onset of *orbital pain* with *lid oedema, proptosis* and *chemosis* due to a diffuse granulomatous infiltrate of lymphocytes and plasma cells involving multiple structures within the orbit.

This condition usually occurs in middle age and seldom occurs bilaterally. CT scanning shows a diffuse orbital lesion, although one structure may be predominantly involved e.g. optic nerve, extraocular muscles or the lacrimal gland. If diagnostic doubt remains, a biopsy is required. Most patients show a dramatic response to high dose *steroid therapy*. If symptoms persist, the lesion should respond well to radiotherapy.

ENDOCRINE EXOPHTHALMOS

The thyrotoxic patient with bilateral exophthalmos presents no diagnostic difficulty, but endocrine exophthalmos, with marked lid oedema, lid retraction and ophthalmoplegia *may occur unilaterally and with normal serum thyroxine and triiodothyronine.* If suspect, thyroid releasing hormone (TRH) stimulation tests may help establish the diagnosis.

In some patients the disease progresses, causing corneal ulceration, papilloedema and even blindness. In these circumstances orbital decompression may benefit.

Tumours of the Skull Base

MALIGNANT

CARCINOMA

Carcinoma of the nasopharynx, paranasal sinuses or ear may extend intracranially either via direct erosion or through the skull foramina. It frequently penetrates the dura (in contrast to metastatic carcinoma of the spinal cord) and may involve almost any cranial nerve. Spread to the CSF pathways leads to *carcinomatous meningitis* and may cause multiple cranial nerve palsies.

Skull X-ray or *CT scan* shows an osteolytic lesion of the skull base.

Treatment is usually restricted to retropharyngeal biopsy plus radiotherapy.

CHORDOMA

Chordoma – sites of intracranial origin

Rare tumours of notochordal cell rests arising predominantly in the sphenoido-oc-cipital and sacrococcygeal regions. Although growth begins in the midline, they often expand asymmetrically into the intracranial cavity. Chordomas may present at any age, but the incidence peaks in the 4th decade. Metastases rarely occur.

Clinical: most patients develop nasal obstruction. Cranial nerve palsies usually follow and depend on the exact tumour site.

Skull X-ray shows a soft tissue mass with an osteolytic lesion of the sphenoid, basi-occiput or petrous apex.

CT scan confirms the presence of a partly calcified mass causing marked bone destruction and extending into the nasopharyngeal space.

Management: the tumour site prevents complete removal. Usually extensive debulking (sometimes through the transoral route) is combined with radiotherapy. Most patients die within 10 years of the initial presentation.

BENIGN

GLOMUS JUGULARE TUMOUR: rare tumour arising from chemoreceptor cells in the jugular bulb or from similar cells in the middle ear mucosa. This tumour extensively erodes the jugular foramen and petrous bone; many patients present with cranial nerve palsies, especially IX–XII.

X-ray and *CT scan* demonstrate an osteolytic lesion expanding the jugular foramen.

Angiography reveals a vascular tumour, usually only filling from the external carotid artery, but occasionally from vertebral branches.

Management: unless completely restricted to the ear, attempted excision causes considerable risk. As the external carotid artery supplies most tumours, the recent technique of selective embolisation appears to provide the safest approach.

OSTEOMA: rare tumours, usually occurring in the frontal sinus and eroding into the orbit, nasal cavity or anterior fossa. If sinus drainage becomes obstructed, a *mucocele* develops, often with infected contents. These lesions require excision, either through an ethmoidal approach or through a frontal craniotomy.

Intracranial Abscess

The advent of antibiotics and improved treatment of ear and sinus infection has led to a reduction in intracranial abscess formation but the incidence still lies at 2–3 patients per million per year.

Pus may accumulate in:
- the extradural space - - - - - - -
  EXTRADURAL ABSCESS
- the subdural space - - - - - -
  SUBDURAL EMPYEMA
- the brain parenchyma - - - - -
  CEREBRAL ABSCESS

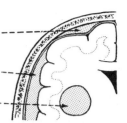

CEREBRAL ABSCESS
Source of Infection

Haematogenous
- subacute bacterial endocarditis.
- congenital heart disease (especially right to left shunt).
- bronchiectasis or pulmonary abscess.

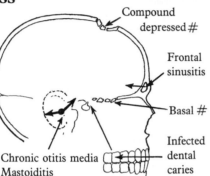

Compound depressed #

Frontal sinusitis

Basal #

Infected dental caries

Chronic otitis media
Mastoiditis

Intracranial spread

direct penetration of the dura.

indirect —— extension of an infected thrombus.
embolic spread along a vein.

Abscess *site* depends on the source e.g. frontal sinusitis
→ frontal lobes.
mastoiditis → temporal lobe
↘ or cerebellum.

Organisms: Streptococcus (especially strep. viridens).

Anaerobic streptococcus ⎱
Bacteroides fragilis ⎰ Improved anaerobic culture techniques have demonstrated the frequent occurrence of these organisms in intracranial abscesses. Prior to this, 50% of cultures appeared 'sterile'.

Staphylococcus aureus.   Haemophilis.
E.coli.   Proteus.

Pathogenesis:

Infection source

Local   Haematogenous

Small vessel occlusion or surface thrombophlebitis may precede parenchymal involvement (bacteria appear to favour damaged brain).

↓

Parenchymal bacterial invasion.

↓

Polymorphonuclear infiltrate and impaired vascular permeability. → Zone of granulation tissue 'CEREBRITIS' → Thin capsule of fibroblasts and reticular fibres forms.

Risk of rupture into adjacent ventricle - -

'Mass' + surrounding oedema → *raised ICP*

Extension to cortical surface → *purulent meningitis*

ABSCESS

'*Daughter*' *loculi* may form

Mature capsule forms with central zone of necrotic tissue, inflammatory cells and necrotic debris.

↑

335

Intracranial Abscess

CEREBRAL ABSCESS *(continued)*

Clinical effects:
Symptoms and signs usually develop over 2–3 weeks although occasionally the onset is more insidious. Clinical features arise from:

1. Toxicity – *pyrexia, malaise.*
2. Raised intracranial pressure – *headache, vomiting* ⟶ *deterioration of conscious level.*
3. Focal damage – *hemiparesis, dysphasia, ataxia, nystagmus.*
   epilepsy – partial or generalised, occurring in over 30%.
4. Infection source – *tenderness over mastoid* or *sinuses, discharging ear.*
   bacterial endocarditis – *cardiac murmurs, petechiae, splenomegaly.*

N.B. Beware attributing patient's deteriorating clinical state to the primary condition e.g. otitis media, thus delaying essential investigations.

Investigations:
X-ray of the sinuses and mastoids: opacities indicate infection.

CT scan: in the stage of 'cerebritis' the CT scan may appear normal or only show an area of low density. With mature abscess formation a characteristic appearance emerges:

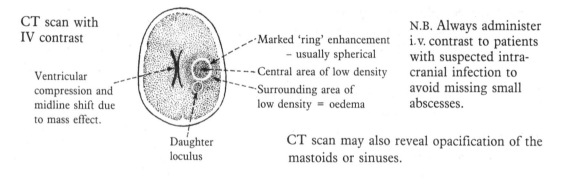

CT scan with IV contrast

Ventricular compression and midline shift due to mass effect.

Marked 'ring' enhancement – usually spherical

Central area of low density

Surrounding area of low density = oedema

Daughter loculus

N.B. Always administer i.v. contrast to patients with suspected intra-cranial infection to avoid missing small abscesses.

CT scan may also reveal opacification of the mastoids or sinuses.

⎡ Prior to the availability of CT scanning, *isotope scans* accurately identified the lesion site, but did not confirm its nature. ⎤

Peripheral blood – may show ↑ESR, leucocytosis, or positive blood culture.

CSF – ↑protein e.g. 1g/l, ↑white cell count (several hundred/ml) – polymorphs or lymphocytes.

N.B. Do not perform lumbar puncture in the presence of a suspected mass lesion.

Intracranial Abscess

CEREBRAL ABSCESS *(continued)*

Management:

1. Antibiotics

Commence i.v. antibiotics on establishing the diagnosis (prior to determining the responsible organism or its sensitivities). Antibiotics are selected for their ability to cross the blood-brain barrier. The ease with which they penetrate the abscess capsule remains uncertain.

Use combined therapy:
- PENICILLIN 4 megaunits q.i.d.
- CHLORAMPHENICOL 1g q.i.d.
- METRONIDAZOLE 500mg q.i.d.

Penicillin covers streptococcus, metronidazole covers anaerobic organisms.

Later determination of the organism and its sensitivities permits alteration to more specific drugs. Antibiotic medication should continue for 4–6 weeks.

2. Abscess drainage

Various methods exist:

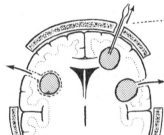

Burr hole aspiration of pus, with repeated aspirations as required.

Primary excision of the whole abscess including the capsule (standard treatment of cerebellar abscess)

Evacuation of the abscess contents under direct vision, leaving the capsule remnants.

Burr hole aspiration is simple and relatively safe. Persistent reaccumulation of pus despite repeated aspiration requires secondary excision. Primary excision removes the abscess in a single procedure, but carries the risk of damage to surrounding brain tissue. Open evacuation of the abscess contents requires a craniotomy, but avoids damaging surrounding brain.

3. Treatment of the infection site

Mastoiditis or sinusitis requires prompt operative treatment, otherwise this acts as a persistent source of infection.

Steroids help reduce associated oedema but they may also reduce antibiotic penetration. Their value in management remains controversial.

Conservative management: In some situations the risks of operative intervention outweigh its benefits. In those patients, treatment depends on i.v. antibiotics.

Indications: – small deep abscesses e.g. thalamic.
             – multiple abscesses.

Prognosis:

The use of CT scanning in the diagnosis and management of intracranial abscesses and the recognition and treatment of pathogenic anaerobic organisms have led to a reduction in the mortality rate from 40% to 10%. In survivors, focal deficits usually improve dramatically with time.

Intracranial Abscess

SUBDURAL EMPYEMA

Subdural empyema occurs far less frequently than intracerebral abscess formation. Infection usually spreads from infected sinuses or mastoids, but may arise from any of the aforementioned sources. Similarly organisms and clinical features match those of intracerebral abscess but since rapid extension occurs across the subdural space, symptoms often develop suddenly.

CT scan shows a low density extracerebral collection with mass effect; occasionally isodense lesions make identification difficult.

Management: Intravenous antibiotic treatment is combined with evacuation of pus either through multiple burr holes or a craniotomy flap. Despite active treatment, the mortality rate still runs at approximately 20%.

Granuloma

TUBERCULOMA

Although tuberculomas still constitute an important cause of mass lesions in underdeveloped countries (20% in India) they are now rare in Britain. The lesions may be single or multiple. They often lie in the cerebellum, especially in children.

Clinical features are those of any intracranial mass; alternatively tuberculoma may present in conjunction with tuberculous meningitis.

CT scan clearly demonstrates an enhancing lesion – but this often resembles astrocytoma or metastasis; tuberculomas have no distinguishing features.

Other investigations: ESR, chest X-ray and Manteoux often fail to confirm the diagnosis.

Management: When tuberculoma is suspected, a trial of antituberculous therapy is worthwhile. Follow up CT scans should show a reduction in the lesion size. Other patients require an exploratory operation and biopsy followed by long term drug treatment.

SARCOIDOSIS

When sarcoid infiltrates the nervous system, it involves the meninges or peripheral nerves. In some patients mass lesions may develop from the dura, but more commonly signs and symptoms relate to an adhesive arachnoiditis involving the skull base, cranial nerves and pituitary stalk. If suspect, a positive Kveim test may obviate the need for biopsy.

Management: Long term steroids.

Dementias

GENERAL

Definition:
Progressive deterioration of intellect, behaviour and personality as a consequence of diffuse or disseminated disease of the cerebral hemispheres.

Distinguish from *delirium* which is an acute disturbance of cerebral function with impaired conscious level, hallucinations and autonomic overactivity as a consequence of toxic, metabolic or infective conditions.

Dementia may occur at any age but is more common in the elderly, accounting for 40 per cent of long term psychiatric in-patients over the age of 65 years. Dementia is a symptom of disease rather than a single disease entity. When occurring under the age of 65 years it is labelled 'pre-senile' dementia. This term is artificial and does not advance diagnosis.

Clinical Course: The rate of progression depends upon the underlying cause.

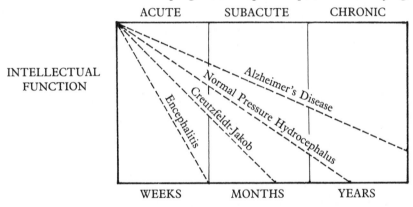

The duration of history helps establish the cause of dementia; Alzheimer's disease is slowly progressive over years, whereas encephalitis may be rapid over weeks. Dementia due to cerebrovascular disease appears to occur 'stroke by stroke'.

All dementias show a tendency to be accelerated by change of environment, intercurrent infection or surgical procedures.

Development of Symptoms:

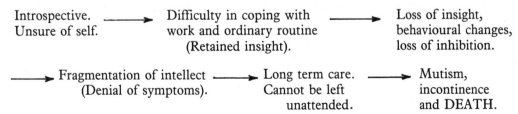

The initial phase of dementia may be inseparable from the *pseudoretardation* of *depressive illness*.

Dementias – Classification

Based on cause:

(i) Dementia with clinical or laboratory evidence of systemic disease
  Hypothyroidism.
  Cushing's syndrome.
  Dietary deficiency:
    Thiamine (alcoholic dementia).
    B_{12}.
    Folic acid.
  Liver disease.
  Hypoparathyroidism and
    pseudohypoparathyroidism.
  Drug abuse.

(ii) Dementia with other neurological signs
  Multi-infarction dementia.
  Tumour.
  Infection:
    Virus ———— Herpes simplex.
    Slow virus —— Creutzfeldt-Jakob.
    Specific ——— Neurosyphilis.
    Opportunistic – Cryptococcal meningitis.
  Degenerative— Huntingdon's chorea.
  Trauma.
  Normal pressure hydrocephalus.

(iii) Dementia as a single entity
  Pick's disease.
  Alzheimer's disease.

It is important to fully investigate all patients with dementia as many causes are treatable; in practice 10–15 per cent can be reversed.

Based on site:

A further useful clinical classification is based upon the part of the cerebral hemisphere initially affected.

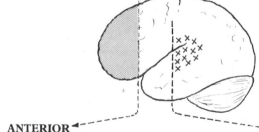

ANTERIOR
(Frontal pre-motor cortex)

Behavioural changes/loss of inhibition,
antisocial behaviour,
facile and irresponsible.

Normal pressure hydrocephalus.
Huntingdon's chorea.
Metabolic disease.

POSTERIOR
(Parietal and temporal lobes)

Disturbance of cognitive function
(memory and language)
without marked changes
in behaviour.

ALZHEIMER's DISEASE

Alzheimer's disease is practically the only cause of posterior dementia though vascular (multi-infarct) dementia may show early posterior features. *Posterior and anterior dementias will eventually merge.*

340

Dementias – Clinical Examination

Clinical examination should include a full assessment of higher cortical function (see chapter 1), also examination for other neurological signs as well as signs of general medical disease.

In dementia *primitive reflexes* may be obtained. These are:

1. Pout Reflex

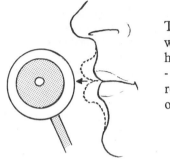

Tap lips with tendon hammer - a pout response is observed.

2. Glabellar Reflex

Patient cannot inhibit blinking in response to stimulation (tapping between the eyes).

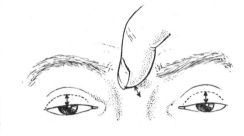

3. Grasp Reflex

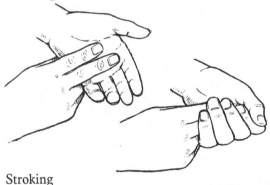

Stroking palm of hand induces 'grasp'.

4. Palmo-mental Reflex

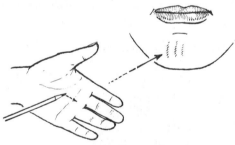

Quick scratch on palm of hand induces sudden contraction of mentalis muscle in face.

Primitive reflexes are present in infancy and return in adult life in cases of frontal or diffuse cerebral damage.

Dementias – Specific Diseases

1. ALZHEIMER's DISEASE

Accounts for 50 per cent of all dementias.
Generally synonymous with 'senile dementia'.
Posterior presentation.   Slowly progressive.
Focal neurological signs in under 5 per cent of cases.

Pathology

(i) Senile plaque

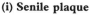

Aggregates of filaments
with a central core
of amyloid.
Found in cortex
and basal gangiia.

(ii) Neurofibrillary tangle

Helical strands of
protein close to
nuclei of neurones.
Mainly affecting
pyramidal cells of cortex.

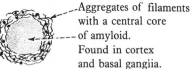

The brain is small (occasionally
below 1,000 grams in weight).
Atrophy is most evident in the
superior and middle
temporal gyri. - - - - - - - - - -

Diagnosis may be established during life
by slow progression, posterior presentation and normal metabolic investigation as well as absence
of focal neurological signs.

CT scanning aids diagnosis

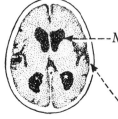

Shrunken walnut appearance - - -

(Through
ventricular
system)

- - - Mild to moderate ventricular
enlargement

(High 'cut'
over
cortex)

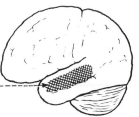

Enlarged cortical sulci

Large basal cisterns and
large Sylvian fissure.

Note the absence of multiple infarction or mass lesion.

Causation:

Normal ageing process (accelerated)?   Remain
Viral origin?   Heavy metal poisoning?   speculative

Treatment:

No specific treatment. Choline and lecithin (based on reduction of the enzyme choline acetyl
transferase (CAT) in post mortem material) given by mouth have not proved effective in reversing
or halting the dementing process.

342

Dementias – Specific Diseases

2. MULTI-INFARCT (Arteriosclerotic dementia)

This is an overdiagnosed condition which accounts for only 10 per cent of cases of dementia. Dementia occurs 'stroke by stroke' with progressive focal loss of function. Clinical features of stroke profile — hypertension, diabetes, etc. — are present.

It is estimated that 50—100ml of cerebral softening must be present before dementia is apparent.

Diagnosis is reached from history; confirmation obtained from CT scan.

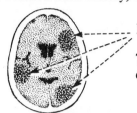

Low density areas of infarction.

These areas are not space-occupying and do not enhance after intravenous contrast.

Treatment: Maintain adequate blood pressure control.

3. METABOLIC DEMENTIA

Usually an anterior presentation.

General medical examination is important in suggesting underlying systemic disease.

B_{12} deficiency may produce dementia rather than subacute combined degeneration of spinal cord.

In alcoholics, consider not only vitamin deficiency but also CHRONIC SUBDURAL HAEMATOMA.

4. NORMAL PRESSURE HYDROCEPHALUS

Normal pressure hydrocephalus (NPH) is the term applied to the classical triad of:

Dementia
Gait disturbance
Urinary incontinence

occurring in conjunction with *hydrocephalus* and *normal* intracranial pressure.

Two types occur:

1. NPH with a *preceding cause* — Subarachnoid haemorrhage.
   — Meningitis.
   — Trauma.

(This must be distinguished from hydrocephalus with raised intracranial pressure associated with these causes.)

2. NPH with no known preceding cause — *Idiopathic*.

Dementias – Specific Diseases

Normal pressure hydrocephalus *(continued)*

Aetiology is unclear. It is presumed that at some preceding period, impedence to normal CSF flow causes raised intraventricular pressure and ventricular dilatation. Compensatory mechanisms permit a reduction in CSF pressure yet the ventricular dilatation persists and causes symptoms:

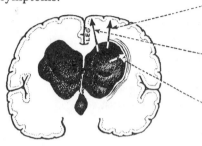

Pressure on frontal lobes   ⟶   Dementia.
(possibly related to decreased cerebral blood flow).

Pressure on the cortical centre   ⟶   Incontinence.
for bladder and bowel control in the paracentral lobe.

Pressure on the 'leg fibres' from   ⟶   Gait disturbance
the cortex passing around the   and pyramidal
ventricle towards the internal capsule.   signs in the legs.

Diagnosis is based on clinical picture plus CT scan evidence of ventricular enlargement.

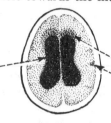

The lateral ventricles are often dilated more than the 3rd and 4th.

Note the presence or absence of periventricular lucency (PVL) and width of cortical sulci.

Normal pressure hydrocephalus must be differentiated from patients whose ventricular enlargement is merely the result of shrinkage of the surrounding brain e.g. Alzheimer's disease. These patients do not respond to CSF shunting, whereas a proportion of patients with NPH (but not all) show a definitive improvement with shunting.

Investigations are designed to identify patients most likely to benefit from operation.
Numerous predictive tests have been assessed including:

ISOTOPE CISTERNOGRAPHY — a radioisotope injected into the cervical subarachnoid space does not pass over the hemispheres as expected but enters the ventricular system.

CSF INFUSION STUDIES —— these note the intracranial pressure response to a volume of fluid infused into the ventricles or directly into the lumber theca.

SULCAL WIDTH on CT scan — theoretically, the wider the sulci, the greater the atrophy, the poorer the response — but not consistent in practice.

The most reliable guides to response appear to be:
1. The presence of PERIVENTRICULAR LUCENCY on CT scan.
2. The presence of BETA WAVES for more than 5 per cent of a 24 hour period of intraventricular pressure monitoring.

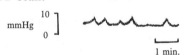

Beta waves

$$10 \rceil$$
mmHg
$$0$$

1 min.

Operation — Ventriculo-peritoneal or ventriculo-atrial shunt (see page 362).

Results — The best response occurs in patients with a known preceding cause (e.g. subarachnoid haemorrhage), PVL on CT scan and beta waves on ICP monitoring.

Dementias – Specific Diseases

5. TUMOUR presenting as dementia

Concern is always expressed at the possibility of dementia being due to intracranial tumour. This is rare, but may happen when tumours occur in certain sites.

Mental or behavioural changes occur in 50 –70 per cent of all brain tumours as distinct from dementia which is associated with **frontal lobe tumours** (and subfrontal tumours),
  III ventricle tumours and
  corpus callosum tumours.

Suspect in recent onset dementia with focal signs e.g. subfrontal lesions may be associated with loss of smell (I cranial nerve involvement) and optic atrophy (II cranial nerve involvement).

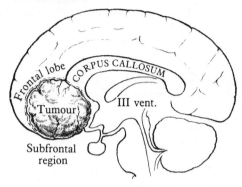

Other causes of dementia are considered in relevant chapters:

  Infection: Viruses.   Yeast/fungi.   Syphilis.
  Trauma.
  Slow virus disorders.
  Degenerative: Huntington's chorea.
  Multiple sclerosis.

Dementia – Investigation

Routine recommended biochemical investigation:

Full blood count — Polycythaemia.
Serology (VDRL, TPHA) — Neurosyphilis.
Thyroid function (T3,T4,TSH) — Hypothyroidism.
B_{12} folate and transketolase — Deficiency states.
Cortisols — Cushing's syndrome.
Liver function test — Liver disease.
Urea and electrolytes — Uraemia.
Calcium — Calcium disorders (Hypoparathyroidism, pseudohypoparathyroidism).
Barbiturate levels — Chronic barbiturate abuse suspected.

The Electroencephalogram may show generalised slow wave activity of a diffuse disorder or a focal abnormality suggesting a structural lesion.

Lumbar Puncture in suspected neurosyphilis or chronic meningitis may be vital in reaching diagnosis. First exclude a mass lesion.

CT Scanning is essential where structural brain disease is suspected. The incidence of dementia is such that this investigation cannot be universally applied and discrimination is essential.

Brain Biopsy may be necessary to diagnose rare disorders e.g. Creutzfeldt-Jakob disease. (Special precautions are necessary, see page 491).

SUMMARY

Common and increasing medical problem in ageing community.
Remedial causes not common but must be excluded.
PRIMARY INVESTIGATION — exclude metabolic causes.
SECONDARY INVESTIGATION — depends on clinical examination — should include EEG, isotope and CT brain scans.
SHORT HISTORY DEMANDS FULL INVESTIGATION.

Movement Disorders — Extrapyramidal System

The control of voluntary movement is effected by the interaction of the pyramidal, cerebellar and extrapyramidal systems interconnecting with each other as well as projecting to the anterior horn region or cranial nerve motor nuclei.

The extrapyramidal system is diffuse, consisting of paired subcortical masses or nuclei of grey matter.

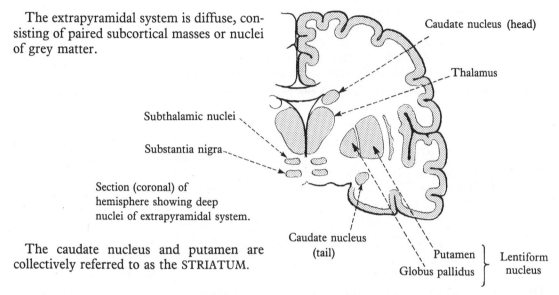

Section (coronal) of hemisphere showing deep nuclei of extrapyramidal system.

Caudate nucleus (head)

Thalamus

Subthalamic nuclei

Substantia nigra

Caudate nucleus (tail)

Putamen ⎤ Lentiform
Globus pallidus ⎦ nucleus

The caudate nucleus and putamen are collectively referred to as the STRIATUM.

Interconnections of the deep nuclei

These connections are complex with input from the motor cortex and the cerebellar cortex via dentate nucleus adding to the complexity.

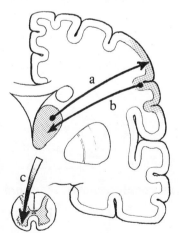

General observations can be made:

(a) The thalamus plays a vital rôle in projecting information from the basal nuclei and cerebellum to the motor cortex via *thalamocortical pathways* and exerts an influence on the *corticospinal pathway* at its origin.

(b) The cortical neurones project to the thalamus thus providing a feedback loop between these structures.

(c) Descending extrapyramidal fibres from deep nuclei project to the anterior horn region of the spinal cord.

Movement Disorders — Extrapyramidal System

NEUROTRANSMITTER FUNCTION

Knowledge that such drugs as Haloperidol can produce symptoms identical to known extrapyramidal disease – Parkinsonism – emphasises the role of neurotransmitter substances in the development of such disorders.

Neurotransmitters – e.g. ACETYLCHOLINE, DOPAMINE,
5-HYDROXYTRYPTAMINE,
HOMOVANILLIC ACID,
ɤAMINOBUTYRIC ACID (GABA),
NORADRENALINE, – are present in the deep nuclei.

The Dopamine/Acetylcholine system is the best understood. This system is *balanced*.

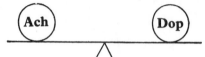

Both neurotransmitters have excitatory and inhibitory actions.
Acetylcholine is found in highest concentration in the *putamen* and *caudate nucleus* (the striatum).

Dopamine is a catecholamine within the metabolic pathways —

Tyrosine ⟶ Dopa ⟶ Dopamine ⟶ Noradrenaline ⟶ Adrenaline.

As well as being a step in the production of noradrenaline and adrenaline, dopamine has its own function as a neurotransmitter and is broken down to homovanillic acid (HVA).

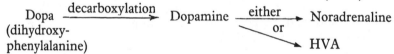

Dopa (dihydroxy-phenylalanine) ──decarboxylation──▶ Dopamine ──either / or──▶ Noradrenaline / HVA

Dopamine is found in highest concentration in the *substantia nigra*.

Imbalance –

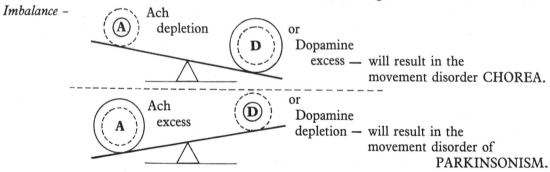

Ach depletion (A) or Dopamine excess (D) — will result in the movement disorder CHOREA.

Ach excess (A) or Dopamine depletion (D) — will result in the movement disorder of PARKINSONISM.

Drugs may produce movement disorders by interfering with neurotransmission in the following ways:

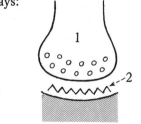

1. By reducing transmitter at nerve terminal e.g. tetrabenazine reduces dopamine.
2. By blocking the receptor site post-synaptically – as phenothiazines do to dopamine receptors.

Both reduce effective dopamine and create a relative excess of acetylcholine
↓
Parkinsonism

Movement Disorders — Extrapyramidal Diseases

CLINICAL FEATURES

The effects of disease of the extrapyramidal system on movement can be regarded as *positive* and *negative*.

> *Positive:*   Involuntary movements.
>   Rigidity.
>
> *Negative:*   Slowness of voluntary movement (BRADYKINESIA).
>   Loss of postural reflexes resulting in imbalance.

In Parkinson's disease both positive features e.g. tremor, and negative features e.g. bradykinesia, occur.

In Huntington's chorea positive features, e.g. chorea, predominate.

POSITIVE FEATURES

(a) *Types of involuntary movement* in extrapyramidal disease:

> Tremor,   Athetosis,   Hemiballismus.
> Chorea,   Dystonia,

Chorea and athetosis may merge into one another – choreoathetosis.

(b) *Rigidity* – a feature of Parkinson's disease.

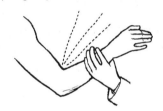

Stiffness felt by the examiner when passively moving a limb. This 'resistance' is present to the same degree throughout the full range of movement and is described as PLASTIC or LEAD PIPE rigidity.

When tremor is superimposed upon rigidity it produces a COGWHEELING quality.

NEGATIVE FEATURES

(a) *Bradykinesia:* – A loss or slowness of voluntary movement.

This is a major feature of Parkinson's disease and produces:

- reduced facial expression (mask-like).
- reduced blinking.
- reduced adjustments of posture when seated.

When agitated the patient will move swiftly – *'Kinesia paradoxica'*.

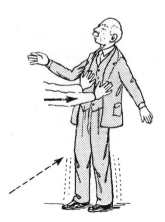

(b) *Postural Disturbance*

When postural reflexes are disturbed, the patient becomes unsteady and assumes an abnormal stance (usually of flexion) with difficulty in maintaining balance when pushed.

Parkinson's Disease

Described by James Parkinson (1817) "An essay on the shaking palsy".
Recognised as an extrapyramidal disorder by Kinnier Wilson (1912).

Incidence: 1 : 1000.

Sex incidence: equal.

Age of onset: 50 years upwards. (May occur in a younger age group but less commonly.)

Familial incidence occurs in 5%.

Aetiology   Parkinson's disease must be distinguished from Parkinsonism caused by drugs, toxins and trauma.

The cause of Parkinson's disease is unknown but certain points merit attention:

The presence of Parkinsonism in *degenerative disorders* e.g. Alzheimer's disease, progressive supranuclear palsy, suggests a similar aetiology.

Many patients have *arteriosclerotic vascular disease,* but this possibly coexists with rather than causes Parkinson's disease.

Any relationship with *antecedent viral infection* remains unproven (with the exception of Encephalitis Lethargica).

A disorder indistinguishable from Parkinson's disease occurs in drug abusers taking an intravenous pethidine analogue. From this analogue, MPTP (1 methyl 4 phenyl 1,2,5,6 tetrahydropyridine) has been isolated. When given to primates, this produces an animal model of Parkinson's disease, allowing examination of the pathophysiology and evaluation of various therapies.

In view of the unclear aetiology of Parkinson's disease it is referred to as *Idiopathic Parkinson's Disease* as opposed to *Parkinsonism* where the causation is clear e.g.:

> *Drugs* — phenothiazines,
> reserpine,
> haloperidol.
>
> *Toxic substances* — manganese,
> carbon monoxide.
>
> *Trauma* — single or repetitive head injury.

PATHOLOGY of Idiopathic Parkinson's Disease

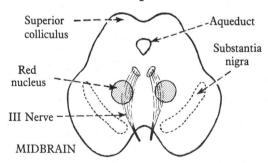

The substantia nigra contains pigmented cells (neuromelanin) which give it a characteristic 'black' appearance (macroscopic). These cells are lost in Parkinson's disease and the substantia nigra becomes pale. Remaining cells contain atypical eosinophilic inclusions in the cytoplasm – *Lewy bodies.*

Minor changes are seen in other basal nuclei – striatum and globus pallidus.

In Parkinsonism these structural changes do not occur. In all patients the common feature, irrespective of cause, is Dopamine deficiency.

Parkinson's Disease

CLINICAL FEATURES

Initial symptoms are vague, the patient often complains of aches and pains.

1. A coarse TREMOR at a rate of 4 per second usually develops early in the disease. It begins unilaterally in the upper limbs and eventually spreads to all four limbs. The tremor is termed *'Pill rolling'*, the thumb moving rhythmically backwards and forwards on the palm of the hand. It occurs at rest, improves with movement and disappears during sleep.

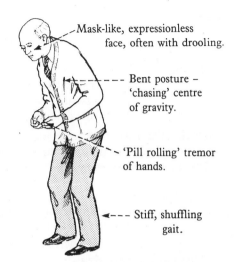

Mask-like, expressionless face, often with drooling.

Bent posture – 'chasing' centre of gravity.

'Pill rolling' tremor of hands.

Stiff, shuffling gait.

2. RIGIDITY is detected by examination. It predominates in the flexor muscles of the neck, trunk and limbs and results in the typical *'flexed posture'*.

3. BRADYKINESIA: This slowness or paucity of movement affects facial muscles of expression (mask-like appearance) as well as muscles of mastication, speech, voluntary swallowing and muscles of the trunk and limbs.
    Dysarthria, dysphagia and a slow deliberate gait with little associated movement (e.g. arm swinging) result.

Tremor, rigidity and bradykinesia deteriorate simultaneously, affecting every aspect of the patient's life:
Handwriting reduces in size.
The gait becomes shuffling and festinant (small rapid steps to 'keep up with' the centre of gravity) and the posture more flexed.
Rising from a chair becomes laborious with progressive difficulty in initiating lower limb movement from a stationary position.
Eye movements may be affected with loss of ocular convergence and upward gaze.
Tremor (bletharoclonus) or spasm (bletharospasm) of the eyelids occurs.
Excessive sweating and greasy skin (seborrhoea) can be troublesome.
Postural hypotension with syncope results from sympathetic (autonomic) nervous system involvement.
Depression, drug induced confusional states and even dementia occur in a proportion of patients.

Post-encephalic Parkinson's disease (Encephalitis Lethargica) is characterised by an earlier age of onset and oculogyric crises (acute ocular deviation).

Parkinson's Disease

DIAGNOSIS

When tremor, rigidity and bradykinesia coexist, distinguish Parkinson's disease from Parkinsonism by the absence of a relevant drug history/toxic exposure.

Distinguish TREMOR from

senile tremor
essential tremor } all are absent at rest and more pronounced
metabolic tremor   on voluntary movement.

Distinguish RIGIDITY from spasticity – with passive limb movement, spasticity is felt towards the end rather than through the full range of movement.

Distinguish BRADYKINESIA from – depression, dementia, multi-infarct state.

TREATMENT is symptomatic and does not halt the pathological process.

It aims at restoring the dopamine/acetylcholine balance (dopamine deficiency) by:

1. reducing acetylcholine.
2. increasing dopamine.

1. Anti-cholinergic drugs

Synthetic anticholinergics e.g. benzhexol – useful in control of tremor but effect on rigidity and bradykinesia is often minimal.

Side effects:

Central { confusions / hallucinations / chorea   *Peripheral* { dry mouth / blurred vision / urinary retention

2. Increase dopamine

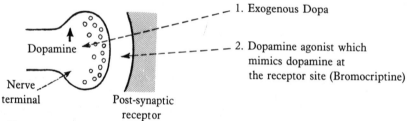

1. Exogenous Dopa

2. Dopamine agonist which mimics dopamine at the receptor site (Bromocriptine)

Exogenous Dopa

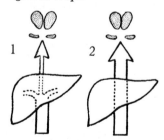

Given as 1. Levodopa or 2. Levodopa + decarboxylase inhibitor which prevents peripheral breakdown in the liver allowing a higher concentration of dopa to reach the blood brain barrier; also the peripheral side effects (nausea, vomiting, hypotension) are diminished.

Central side effects: Confusion, depression, choreiform movements and following long-term treatment – *'On/Off'* phenomenon (see later).

Exogenous dopa improves bradykinesia, rigidity, and to a lesser extent tremor, but in 30% the response is poor. 'Good' responders often develop central side effects later – especially the 'on/off' phenomenon.

Parkinson's Disease

Treatment *(continued)*

> *Dopamine agonists* (e.g. bromocriptine) mimic dopamine at the receptor site. Central side effects are similar to those of levodopa. Bromocriptine is an ergot derivative and peripheral side effects are those of ergotism. When central side effects of exogenous levodopa become problematical it may be used in combination with a reduced dosage of levodopa. Similarly selegiline hydrochloride, a selective monoamine oxidase inhibitor, may benefit when combined with levodopa.
>
> Amantidine, an antiviral drug, may help rigidity. The mode of action is not known.

Advances in drug treatment in recent years have reduced the need for stereotactic surgery (see page 369) but in young patients with intractable tremor this is still of benefit. A stereotactic lesion in the globus pallidus or ventrolateral nucleus of the thalamus (contralateral to the tremor) may produce dramatic results.

Regime of Treatment

> *Early* Parkinson's disease – Anticholinergics
> ± amantadine

> *Established moderate disease* – Levodopa,
> Levodopa + decarboxlase inhibitor
> ± amantidine
> and/or anticholinergics.

> *Established severe disease* —— Small, frequent doses of levodopa + decarboxylase inhibitor
> *with central side effects* with consideration of low dose bromocriptine.

The early use of bromocriptine awaits evaluation.

For details of drug dosage the reader should consult a pharmacology text.

'On/Off' phenomenon – a consequence of prolonged levodopa treatment in which signs of Parkinson's disease (undertreatment) and drug overdosage (overtreatment) alternate rapidly as though being turned on and off. These changes may bear no relationship to the time of drug medication.

Treatment is difficult, the patient having mild chorea at one moment and marked bradykinesia, tremor and rigidity the next. Reduce exogenous levodopa and consider bromocriptine.

Conclusion

Prior to the introduction of levodopa, patients survived nine years on average from diagnosis. Present treatment has improved the quality and duration of life. The development of more specific dopamine agonists and sustained release forms of levodopa should result in further improvement in the future.

Chorea

Definition: (From the Greek – 'Dance')

An involuntary, irregular, jerking movement affecting the limbs and trunk. Normally this movement is complex and resembles voluntary movement e.g. crossing and uncrossing legs. It is termed 'semi-purposeful'.

Dopamine excess (overtreatment of Parkinson's disease) or acetylcholine deficiency is regarded as the biochemical basis of these abnormal movements.

Chorea is a characteristic of several disorders:

HUNTINGTON's CHOREA

Huntington's chorea is an autosomal dominant inherited disorder with onset in middle life and progression to death within 10–12 years.

It may occur in young persons (juvenile form); here chorea is less apparent and rigidity predominates.

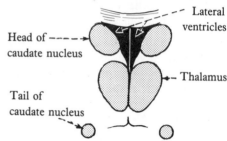

Pathology

The caudate nucleus (head) shrinks as a result of neuronal loss and no longer 'indents' the lateral ventricle. The putamen is affected to a lesser degree. Neuronal loss also occurs in the frontal lobes. Cells remaining in the caudate nucleus appear to have increased sensitivity to dopamine and are deficient in enzymes required for acetylcholine and GABA synthesis.

Symptoms

Chorea — may be the initial symptom. Progresses from mere fidgetiness to gross involuntary movements which interrupt voluntary movement and make feeding and walking impossible.

Dementia — anterior in type with behavioural changes progressing to disinhibition, antisocial behaviour and incontinence. Intellect will eventually suffer, with disturbance of memory.

Hypotonicity often accompanies fidgety, choreiform movements. Primitive reflexes – grasp, pout and palmomental – are usually elicited.

Diagnosis

Most have a family history. Distinguish from benign hereditary chorea in which intellect is preserved. Sporadic cases are rare but cause diagnostic difficulties:

Exclude *senile chorea* by older age of onset; and absence of dementia.

Exclude other causes of chorea (see over).

Prediction of disease

Because the disease manifests usually after child-bearing age, relatives should seek genetic advice before starting a family.

A genetic marker (recombinant DNA) offers predictive possibilities and awaits full evaluation.

A levodopa challenge test – 3 grams daily for 1 month to precipitate chorea in potential sufferers – is unreliable.

Treatment

Phenothiazines, haloperidol or tetrabenazine, may control the chorea in the preliminary stages of the disease.

Chorea

SYDENHAM's CHOREA

Acute onset. Associated with streptococcal infection. Remits in weeks.

Pathology: Necrotising arteritis in thalamus, caudate nucleus and putamen.
Diagnosis is confirmed by elevated ESR and ASO (antistreptolysin) titre.
Treatment: Sedation, phenothiazines.

The condition may become recurrent – during pregnancy, intercurrent infection.

CHOREA GRAVIDARUM

Acute onset in pregnancy, usually the first trimester.
Restricted to face or generalised. Perhaps caused by reactivation of Sydenham's chorea.

Pathology: Unknown.
Treatment: Haloperidol.

OTHER CAUSES OF CHOREA

Drug induced – Levodopa.
Polycythaemia rubra vera.
Lupus erythematosus.
Wilson's disease.

Tricyclic antidepressants.
Alcohol abuse.
Senile chorea.
Oral contraceptive.

Dystonia

DYSTONIA manifests as a prolonged
abnormal posture produced by spasms
of large trunk and limb muscles e.g.
                    sustained head retraction....

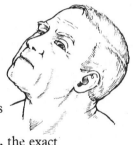

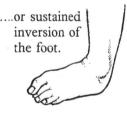

....or sustained
inversion of
the foot.

Dystonias may be:
generalised – dystonia musculorum deformans
or *partial* e.g. spasmodic torticollis.
Although considered extrapyramidal in origin, the exact
anatomical basis of dystonias remains unknown.

DYSTONIA MUSCULORUM DEFORMANS

Onset in childhood often with autosomal recessive inheritance.
Initially, a flexion deformity of leg develops when walking.
Movements then become generalised with posturing of the head, trunk and
limbs. They are initially intermittent but ultimately constant. Despite
eventual gross contortion the postures disappear during sleep.

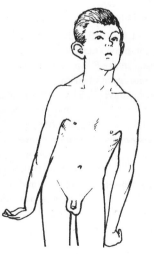

Diagnosis is made on clinical grounds and by exclusion.
 – Normal perinatal history.
 – No laboratory evidence of Wilson's disease.

Pathology: unknown.

Treatment: Levodopa or carbamezapine may be of benefit in some;
anticholinergics in others.
Stereotactic surgery – a lesion in the region of the ventrolateral nucleus of
the thalamus may reduce the dystonia in the contralateral limb.

Dystonias — Partial

SPASMODIC TORTICOLLIS (Wry neck)

Unilateral deviation of the head.

Aetiology is unknown, but a viral cause has been suggested.

Psychogenic factors are involved but it is not a purely psychiatric disorder.

Dystonic contraction of the *left* sternomastoid produces head turning to the *right*.

Pressure of the index finger on the *right* side of the chin may turn the head back to the neutral position.

Turning of the head is specially noticeable when the patient is walking.

Eventually hypertrophy of the sternomastoid occurs.

Pathology: unknown.   **Diagnosis** is based on clinical findings.

Treatment: anticholinergics and phenothiazines produce degrees of benefit in 50% of patients.

Operative techniques: – Myotomy.

– Section of spinal accessory and upper cervical anterior roots.

(Results from these procedures are unpredictable and varied.)

Prognosis: Remission occurs in 20% of patients. Dystonia may spread into other muscle groups. In the long term, psychological disturbance often occurs.

WRITER's CRAMP Variable age of onset.

Muscles of the hand and forearm tighten on attempting to write and pain may occur in the forearm muscles.

Previously regarded as an 'occupational neurosis' but now classified as a partial dystonia.

May be associated with other signs of extrapyramidal disease e.g. tremor.

Treatment: Benzodiazepines and anticholinergics are of limited value.

OROMANDIBULAR DYSTONIA

Constant involuntary prolonged tight eye closure (blepharospasm) is associated with dystonia of mouth, tongue or jaw muscles. Response to treatment is poor though phenothiazines should be tried. Section of the nerves to orbicularis oculi muscles will relieve blepharospasm.

DRUG INDUCED DYSTONIA

Acute adoption of abnormal dystonic posture – usually head and neck or oculogyric crisis (upward deviation of eyes) – caused by phenothiazines, butyrophenones e.g. haloperidol, metoclopramide.

Anticholinergics e.g. benztropine for 24–48 hours helps symptoms settle.

PROGRESSIVE SUPRANUCLEAR PALSY

A condition characterised by gaze palsies, Parkinsonian features and *axial dystonia* (truncal dystonia).

Onset in the 5th to 6th decade.

Aetiology: unknown.

Pathology: Neuronal loss is evident in periaqueductal grey matter, brain stem nuclei, subthalamic nuclei and the superior colliculi.

Neurofibrillary tangles as seen in Alzheimer's disease are also found.

Symptoms: Downward eye movement is initially impaired followed by all other voluntary eye movement.

Pseudobulbar signs develop (see page 536).

The head then hyperextends (dystonia) and tremor and rigidity ensue in the limbs.

Treatment: Levodopa and anticholinergics give disappointing results.

The course is relentless and progression more rapid than Parkinson's disease, with eventual death in 2–5 years.

Other Extrapyramidal Movement Disorders

HEMIBALLISMUS

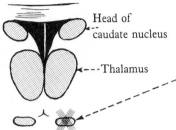

Head of caudate nucleus

Thalamus

This is a movement disorder characterised by unilateral, violent flinging of the limbs. This involuntary movement is occasionally severe enough to throw the patient off balance or even from his bed.

The anatomical basis is a lesion of the *subthalamic nuclei* contralateral to the abnormal movement. It usually results from vascular disease (posterior cerebral artery territory), but occasionally occurs in multiple sclerosis.

Drug treatment is ineffective. The condition often settles spontaneously.

ATHETOSIS

Athetosis presents in childhood and appears as a slow writhing movement disorder with a rate of movement between that of chorea and dystonia. It usually involves the digits, hands and face on each side.

These abnormal movements may result from:
- Hypoxic neonatal brain damage,
- Kernicterus,
- Lipid storage diseases.

Response to anticholinergics is variable and occasionally dramatic.

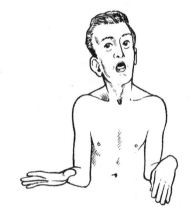

TARDIVE DYSKINESIA

This is a consequence of long term drug treatment – phenothiazines, butyrophenones.

Involuntary movements in the face, mouth and tongue (oro-facial dyskinesia) as well as limb movements of a *choreoathetoid nature* appear.

This movement disorder may commence even after stopping the responsible drug and can persist indefinitely.

Response to treatment is poor.

Prevention

The incidence may be reduced by:

(1) Drug 'holidays' (periods of rest from causative drug).

(2) Early recognition and drug withdrawal.

The practice of increasing the dose of the offending drug when movements occur should be avoided. This will improve movements initially but they will 'break through' later.

357

Other Extrapyramidal Movement Disorders

WILSON's DISEASE

An autosomal recessive disorder of copper metabolism in which extrapyramidal features are evident.
Syn. Hepatolenticular degeneration.

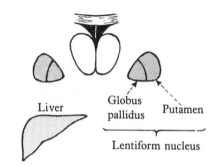

Liver   Globus pallidus   Putamen

Lentiform nucleus

Pathology

Cavitation and neuronal loss occurs within the putamen and the globus pallidus.

The liver shows the appearance of coarse cirrhosis. Copper accumulates in all organs, especially in Descemet's membrane in the eye, nail beds and kidney.

Biochemistry

There is deficiency of $\alpha_2$globulin – Ceruloplasmin – which normally binds 98% of copper in the plasma. This results in an increase in loosely bound copper/albumin, and deposition occurs in all organs. Urinary copper is increased.

Clinical features   There are two clinical forms:

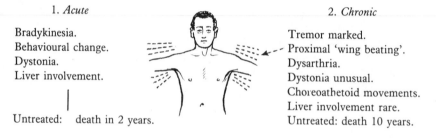

1. Acute

Bradykinesia.
Behavioural change.
Dystonia.
Liver involvement.

Untreated: death in 2 years.

2. Chronic

Tremor marked.
Proximal 'wing beating'.
Dysarthria.
Dystonia unusual.
Choreoathetoid movements.
Liver involvement rare.
Untreated: death 10 years.

The deposition of copper in Descemet's membrane produces the golden brown *Kayser-Fleischer* ring which is seen by the naked eye and is diagnostic.

Diagnosis

Clinical findings supported by biochemical evidence:

1. Low ceruloplasmin.
2. Low serum copper.
3. High urinary copper.

Treatment

Low copper diet and d.penicillamine, a copper chelating agent.

With treatment, the Kayser-Fleischer rings will disappear.

Treatment is necessary for the rest of the patient's life. Adequate treatment is compatible with normal life expectancy.

Hydrocephalus

Definition:

Hydrocephalus is an increase in cerebrospinal fluid (CSF) volume, usually resulting from impaired absorption, rarely from excessive secretion.

This definition excludes ventricular expansion secondary to brain shrinkage from a diffuse atrophic process (hydrocephalus ex vacuo).

CSF formation and absorption

CSF forms at a rate of 500 ml/day (0.35ml/min), secreted predominantly by the choroid plexus of the lateral, third and fourth ventricles. CSF flows in a caudal direction through the ventricular system and exits through the foramina of Luschka and Magendie into the subarachnoid space. After passing through the tentorial hiatus and over the hemispheric convexity, absorption occurs through the arachnoid granulations into the venous system.

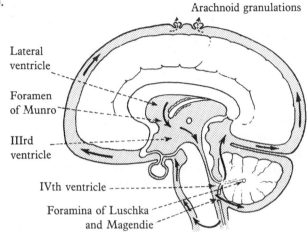

Arachnoid granulations

Lateral ventricle

Foramen of Munro

IIIrd ventricle

IVth ventricle

Foramina of Luschka and Magendie

Classification:

'Obstructive' hydrocephalus —— obstruction to CSF flow *within* the ventricular system.

'Communicating' hydrocephalus — obstruction to CSF flow *outwith* the ventricular system i.e. ventricular CSF 'communicates' with the subarachnoid space.

Causes of hydrocephalus:

Obstructive	Communicating

Congenital – Aqueduct stenosis or forking.
 – Dandy-Walker syndrome (atresia of foramina of Magendie and Luschka).
 – Arnold-Chiari malformation.
 – Vein of Galen aneurysm.
	Thickening of the leptomeninges and/or involvement of the arachnoid granulations
	 – infection (pyogenic, T.B., fungal).
	 – subarachnoid haemorrhage
	     – spontaneous
	     – trauma
	     – post-operative.
	 – carcinomatous meningitis.

Acquired – Acquired aqueduct stenosis (adhesions following infection or haemorrhage).
 – Intraventricular haematoma.
 – Tumours – ventricular e.g. colloid cyst.
      – pineal region.
      – posterior fossa.
 – Abscesses/granuloma.
 – Arachnoid cysts.
	Increased CSF viscosity e.g. high protein content.
	Excessive CSF production – choroid plexus papilloma (rare).
	Supratentorial masses causing tentorial herniation.

359

Hydrocephalus

Pathological effects:

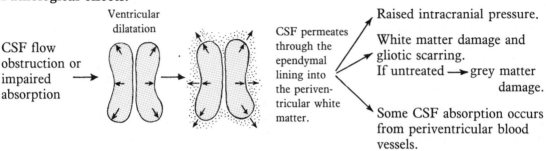

CSF flow obstruction or impaired absorption → Ventricular dilatation → CSF permeates through the ependymal lining into the periventricular white matter.

Raised intracranial pressure.

White matter damage and gliotic scarring.
If untreated → grey matter damage.

Some CSF absorption occurs from periventricular blood vessels.

In the infant, prior to suture fusion, head expansion and massive ventricular dilatation may occur, often leaving only a thin rim of cerebral 'mantle'. Untreated, death usually results, but in many cases the hydrocephalus *'arrests'*. Although the ventricles remain dilated, intracranial pressure (ICP) returns to normal and CSF absorption appears to balance production. When hydrocephalus arrests, normal developmental patterns resume, although pre-existing mental or physical damage may leave a permanent handicap. In these patients, the rapid return of further pressure symptoms following a minor injury or infection suggests that the CSF dynamics remain in an unstable state.

Clinical features:

Infants and young children

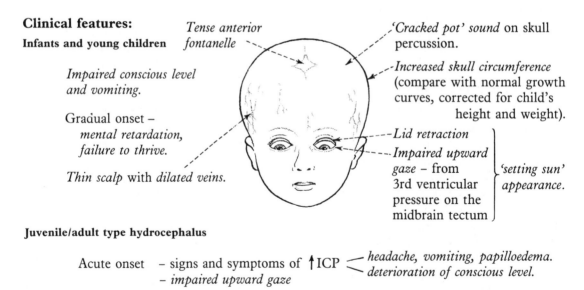

Tense anterior fontanelle

'Cracked pot' sound on skull percussion.

Impaired conscious level and vomiting.

Increased skull circumference (compare with normal growth curves, corrected for child's height and weight).

Gradual onset – *mental retardation, failure to thrive.*

Lid retraction

Impaired upward gaze – from 3rd ventricular pressure on the midbrain tectum

'setting sun' appearance.

Thin scalp with *dilated veins.*

Juvenile/adult type hydrocephalus

Acute onset – signs and symptoms of ↑ICP — *headache, vomiting, papilloedema.*
— *deterioration of conscious level.*
– *impaired upward gaze*

Gradual onset – *dementia*
– *gait ataxia*
– *incontinence*

This triad of symptoms may occur despite an apparently 'normal' CSF pressure i.e. normal pressure hydrocephalus (see page 343).
The condition often relates to previous trauma, meningitis or subarachnoid haemorrhage.

Hydrocephalus

Investigations:

Skull X-ray: Note: – skull size and suture width.
– evidence of chronic raised pressure – erosion of the posterior clinoids.
– associated defects – platybasia, basilar invagination.

CT scan

The *pattern of ventricular enlargement* helps determine the cause i.e.

lateral + *3rd ventricular dilatation* 〈 *normal 4th ventricle* — suggests aqueduct stenosis.

deviated or absent 4th ventricle — suggests a posterior fossa mass.

generalised dilatation — suggests a communicating hydrocephalus.

The presence of *periventricular lucency* (and absent sulci) suggests raised CSF pressure.

The absence of periventricular lucency and prominent sulci suggests appearances resulting from an atrophic process.

-- Dilated 3rd ventricle
-- Dilated lateral ventricle
-- Normal 4th ventricle

Ultrasonography through the anterior fontanelle, usefully demonstrates ventricular enlargement in infants but provides less precise information than CT scanning.

Isotope cisternography/CSF infusion studies/ ICP monitoring: investigations in patients with suspected normal pressure hydrocephalus designed to predict the likelihood of a beneficial response to shunting.

Developmental assessment and **psychometric analysis** detect impaired cerebral function and provide a baseline for future comparison.

Management:

Acute deterioration 〈 Ventricular drainage or
Ventriculo-peritoneal (VP) or ventriculo-atrial (VA) shunt
Lumbar puncture – if communicating hydrocephalus e.g. following sub-arachnoid haemorrhage.

Gradual deterioration 〈 VP or VA shunt (lumbo-peritoneal shunts are occasionally used for communicating hydrocephalus).
Removal of a mass lesion if present – this may obviate the need for a shunt.

'Arrested' hydrocephalus — Symptomless ventricular dilatation requires no treatment, but regular developmental or psychometric assessment ensures no ill effects develop from this potentially unstable state.

Hydrocephalus

Shunt techniques:

A *reservoir* permits CSF aspiration for analysis.

A *valve* is incorporated in the system, either proximally
– ball or diaphragm type (Hakim, Pudenz, Spitz-Holter)
or distally
– slit valve at distal tip (Pudenz).
Valve opening pressures range from 5–150mmH$_2$O.

[*Lumbo-peritoneal shunt* – catheter inserted into the lumbar theca either directly at open operation or percutaneously through a Tuohy needle. The distal end is sited in the peritoneal cavity.]

A *ventricular catheter* is inserted through the occipital (or frontal) horn. The tip lies at the level of the foramen of Munro.

Ventriculo-atrial shunt – distal catheter inserted through the internal jugular vein to the right atrium (T6/7 level on chest X-ray).

Silastic tubing tunnelled subcutaneously.

Ventriculo-peritoneal shunt – distal catheter inserted into the peritoneal cavity. In children, redundant coils permit growth without revision.

Complications of shunting:

Infection: results in meningitis, peritonitis or inflammation extending along the subcutaneous channel. In patients with a V-A shunt, bacteraemia may lead to shunt 'nephritis'. Staphylococci epidermis or aureus are usually involved, with infants at particular risk. Prophylactic antibiotics may minimise the risk of infection, but when established, irradication usually requires shunt removal.

Subdural haematoma: sudden ventricular collapse pulls the cortical surface from the dura leaving a subdural CSF collection or causing subdural haemorrhage. Lying the patient supine for 24–48 hours after shunting helps reduce the risk.

Shunt obstruction: blockage of the shunt system with choroid plexus, debris, high CSF protein, omentum or blood clot results in intermittent or persistent recurrence of symptoms and indicates the need for shunt revision. Demonstration of an increase in ventricular size compared to a previous baseline CT scan confirms shunt malfunction. In children, growth pulls the distal tip of a ventriculo-atrial shunt out of the right atrium, resulting in thrombus formation and occlusion. Ventriculo-peritoneal shunting avoids this complication.

Low pressure state: following shunting, some patients develop headache and vomiting on sitting or standing. This low pressure state usually resolves with a high fluid intake and gradual mobilisation. If not, conversion to a high pressure valve is required.

Prognosis: Provided treatment precedes irreversible brain damage, results are good with most children attaining normal I.Q's. Repeated complications, however, particularly prevalent in infancy and in young children carry a significant morbidity.

Benign Intracranial Hypertension

Benign intracranial hypertension (pseudotumour cerebri) is a term applied to patients with raised intracranial pressure and no evidence of any 'mass' lesion or of hydrocephalus.

Aetiology: This condition is related to a variety of clinical problems:

Some clearly demonstrate a direct causal link –

VENOUS OUTFLOW OBSTRUCTION TO CSF ABSORPTION

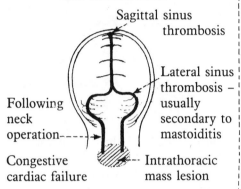

Sagittal sinus thrombosis

Lateral sinus thrombosis – usually secondary to mastoiditis

Following neck operation----

Congestive cardiac failure

Intrathoracic mass lesion

In the majority, the causal relationship remains obscure – **'Idiopathic'** group –

DIET – obesity.
    – hyper/hypovitaminosis A.
ENDOCRINE – pregnancy, menarche, menstrual irregularities, Addison's disease.
HAEMATOLOGICAL – iron deficiency anaemia.
    – polycythaemia vera.
DRUGS – oral contraceptives.
    – steroid withdrawal.
    – tetracycline.
    – nalidixic acid.

In the idiopathic group various mechanisms have been postulated.

– BRAIN SWELLING
– ↓ CSF ABSORPTION
– ↑ CSF SECRETION

Different studies support different mechanisms. The close relationship with obesity suggests an underlying endocrine basis, but with the exception of patients with Addison's disease, endocrine assessment has failed to reveal abnormalities.

Clinical features:

Age: any age, but predominantly 10–15 years.
Sex: female > male – especially in the idiopathic group.

Symptoms	Signs	Investigations
Headache and vomiting	Obesity	
Visual obscurations		
Impaired visual acuity } ←Papilloedema		
Diplopia ←	VI nerve palsy	

CT scan negative – ventricles usually small.
Visual field charting –
{ Enlarged blind spot (often used to monitor progress).
{ Peripheral field constriction.
Lumbar puncture and pressure measurement.
ICP monitoring – if diagnostic doubt persists.

Treatment:
Treat the underlying cause if known.
Weight reduction diet.
Drugs – acetazolamide (reduces CSF production).
    – thiazide diuretics.
    – steroid therapy.
If above fail ⟶ *lumbo-peritoneal shunt*
(subtemporal decompression, now rarely required).
Optic nerve decompression – if progressive impairment of visual acuity despite treatment.

Prognosis:
Most patients respond rapidly to short term treatment, but up to one third develop recurrent attacks. In 10%, visual impairment persists.

Arnold-Chiari Malformation

Although the names of two authors are linked to the description of malformations at the medullary-spinal junction, Chiari must take most credit for providing a detailed description of this condition.

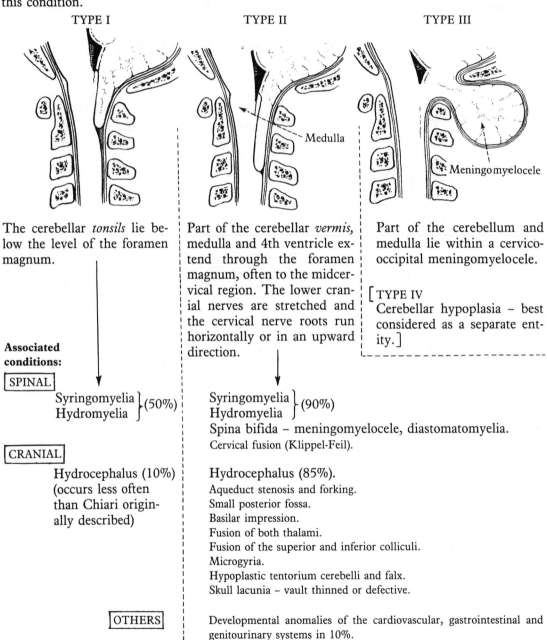

TYPE I   TYPE II   TYPE III

Medulla

Meningomyelocele

The cerebellar *tonsils* lie below the level of the foramen magnum.

Part of the cerebellar *vermis,* medulla and 4th ventricle extend through the foramen magnum, often to the midcervical region. The lower cranial nerves are stretched and the cervical nerve roots run horizontally or in an upward direction.

Part of the cerebellum and medulla lie within a cervico-occipital meningomyelocele.

[TYPE IV
Cerebellar hypoplasia – best considered as a separate entity.]

Associated conditions:

SPINAL

Syringomyelia } (50%)
Hydromyelia

Syringomyelia } (90%)
Hydromyelia
Spina bifida – meningomyelocele, diastomatomyelia.
Cervical fusion (Klippel-Feil).

CRANIAL

Hydrocephalus (10%)
(occurs less often than Chiari originally described)

Hydrocephalus (85%).
Aqueduct stenosis and forking.
Small posterior fossa.
Basilar impression.
Fusion of both thalami.
Fusion of the superior and inferior colliculi.
Microgyria.
Hypoplastic tentorium cerebelli and falx.
Skull lacunia – vault thinned or defective.

OTHERS

Developmental anomalies of the cardiovascular, gastrointestinal and genitourinary systems in 10%.

Arnold-Chiari Malformation

Pathogenesis:

Several hypotheses have been proposed to explain the pathological findings of these malformations. Gardner suggested that downward pressure from *hydrocephalus* played an important role in displacing the posterior fossa structures, and when associated with a patent central canal explained the high incidence of syringomyelia (page 386). Others supposed that *traction* from a tethered spinal cord (dysraphism) or a *CSF leak* through a myelocele into the amniotic sac in fetal life resulted in caudal displacement of the posterior fossa structures. Of these theories, none provides an entirely satisfactory explanation; a more realistic view attributes the hindbrain deformity to *maldevelopment* during early fetal life. This would explain the presence of other developmental anomalies.

Clinical presentation:

Depends on age

INFANCY — Severe type II (or III) deformities present with *respiratory difficulties* and *lower cranial nerve palsies*. Death may result from *aspiration pneumonia* or *apnoeic attacks,* or from complications of associated malformations e.g. *spina bifida*. In milder forms, *nystagmus* (horizontal), *retrocollis* (neck extension) and *spasticity* predominate.

CHILDHOOD — With increasing age, *gait ataxia* may become evident. Features of an associated syringomyelia – *dissociated sensory loss* and *spastic quadraparesis* often contribute to the clinical problems.

ADULT — Only patients with a type I or a mild type II deformity present in adult life –
occipital headaches are induced by coughing or straining.
nystagmus – downbeat or rotatory (on looking down) (on lateral gaze) } may result from medullary compression or from an associated syringomyelia.
ataxia.
spastic quadraparesis.
Progression may eventually lead to severe bulbar symptoms – *lower cranial nerve palsies, respiratory difficulties.*

Investigations:

Straight X-rays
— *Skull:* note the presence of platybasia, basilar impression or lacuniae (vault defects).
— *Cervical spine:* note increased canal width or fusion of vertebrae (especially C2,3) – Klippel Feil syndrome.
— *Lumbosacral spine:* note spina bifida.

Myelography

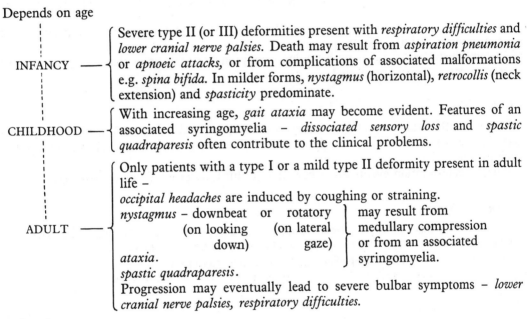

Contrast run up to the foramen magnum with the patient in the supine position outlines a posteriorly situated filling defect.

CT scan – preferably with contrast in the theca demonstrates cerebellar tissue lying within the cervical canal.

Arnold-Chiari Malformation

Management:

(see also syringomyelia, page 387)

In patients with hydrocephalus and signs and symptoms of raised intracranial pressure. $\longrightarrow$ *Ventriculo-peritoneal* or *atrial shunt* may significantly improve signs and symptoms attributed to the Chiari malformation.

In patients with other symptoms and signs $\longrightarrow$ *Posterior fossa decompression* – by removing the posterior rim of the foramen magnum and the arch of the atlas. The dura is opened and a dural graft inserted. Attempts at freeing tonsillar adhesions should be resisted.

NB: An apnoea monitor in the initial postoperative period helps prevent potentially fatal apnoea, especially during sleep.

[In some instances, patients with minimal symptoms or with no evidence of progression may warrant a conservative approach.]

Prognosis:

Patients with mild symptoms and signs often respond well to operation, but those with long standing neurological deficits rarely improve. Treatment should aim at preventing further progression.

Further deterioration eventually occurs in one third, despite operative measures.

SYRINGOBULBIA

Extension of a syringomyelic cavity upwards into the medulla may produce signs and symptoms which are difficult to distinguish from those of medullary compression in the Arnold-Chiari syndrome:
- difficulty in swallowing, dysphonia, dysarthria, vertigo, facial pain.
- nystagmus, palatal and vocal cord weakness, occasional facial and tongue weakness.

The Dandy-Walker Syndrome

This rare developmental anomaly comprises:

1. Dilatation of the lateral and third ventricles (but to a lesser extent than the fourth ventricle)

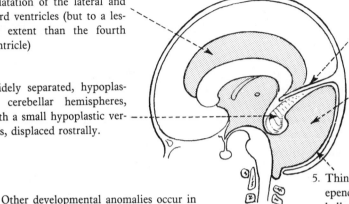

3. Enlarged posterior fossa with high tentorium cerebelli and transverse sinuses.

4. Cystic dilatation of the 4th ventricle – *usually* related to congenital absence of the foramina of Luschka and Magendie.

2. Widely separated, hypoplastic cerebellar hemispheres, with a small hypoplastic vermis, displaced rostrally.

5. Thin, transparent membrane containing ependymal cells and occasionally cerebellar tissue.

Other developmental anomalies occur in 65% of patients.

Clinical presentation:

INFANCY —— Symptoms and signs of hydrocephalus (page 360) combined with a prominent occiput.

CHILDHOOD —— Signs of cerebellar dysfunction with or without signs of hydrocephalus.

Investigations:

Skull X-ray: —— usually shows elevation of the transverse sinuses and occipital bulging, confirming the presence of an enlarged posterior fossa.

CT scan:

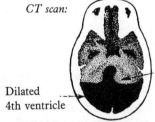

Dilated 4th ventricle

Confirms dilatation of the 4th ventricle with lateral displacement of hypoplastic cerebellar tissue.

Differentiate from:
– midline arachnoid cyst.
– enlarged cisterna magna.

distinguish from Dandy-Walker by identifying cerebellar tissue or septum between the cyst and the 4th ventricle.

Management

– excision of the cyst membrane, 'marsupialising' the 4th ventricle.
Alternatively, and more simply:
– cysto-peritoneal shunt.

Prognosis

Marked neurological impairment prior to treatment carries a poor outlook. In less impaired patients, the prognosis relates more to the presence of other developmental anomalies.

Craniosynostosis

In normal childhood development, the cranial sutures allow passive skull enlargement as the brain grows. *Premature fusion of one or more sutures* results in restricted growth of bone alongside the suture and excessive compensatory growth at the non-united joints. The effect depends on the site and number of sutures involved. Sagittal synostosis is the most frequently occurring deformity (80%).

Sagittal synostosis

Lateral growth is restricted, resulting in a long narrow head with a pronounced sagittal suture (scaphocephaly).

Treatment is by excision of the sagittal suture. Lining the bone edges with a silicon film helps prevent reossification.

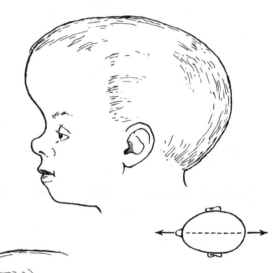

Coronal synostosis

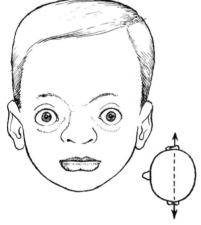

Bilateral or unilateral.

Expansion occurs in a superior and lateral direction (brachiocephaly). This produces a short anterior fossa, shallow orbits and hypertelorism (widening of the interocular distance). Exophthalmos, visual impairment and elevated ICP may result. Bilateral coronal synostosis commonly occurs as one of several congenital defects incorporated in *Crouzon's* and *Apert's syndromes*.

Treatment involves extensive craniofacial surgery correcting both cranial and orbital deformities.

Involvement of all sutures (oxycephaly) results in skull expansion towards the vertex, the line of least resistance.

Indication for operative treatment is primarily cosmetic when only one suture is involved, but with involvement of two or more sutures operation is also aimed at prevention of visual and cerebral damage during growth.

Stereotactic Surgery

Stereotactic techniques developed initially for lesion making, enable accurate placement of a cannula or electrode at a predetermined target site within the brain.

Many different stereotactic frames have been developed e.g. Leksell, Todd-Wells, Guiot. These, combined with radiological landmarks (usually ventriculography) and a brain atlas, provide anatomical localisation to within ± 1 mm. Since some functional variability occurs at each anatomical site, electrode localisation is also based on the recorded neuronal activity and on the effects of electrical stimulation.

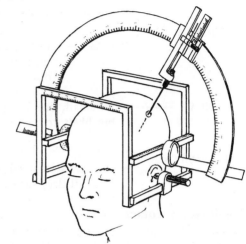

Methods of lesion making:

- *heat* — radiofrequency current delivered through a fine electrode. ⎱ lesion size determined by temperature change
- *cooling* — with a cryogenic probe. ⎰ and duration.
- *radiation* — implantation of a radioactive seed e.g. yttrium^{90}.
  — focussed beam from cobalt^{60} rods (sited on a specially adapted Leksell frame).

Uses of Stereotactic Surgery:

Movement disorders

- tremor ⎱
- dystonia ⎰ lesions in thalamic nuclei
- spasmodic torticollis
- spasticity — lesion in dentate nucleus or pulvinar.

Pain — especially intractable head or neck pain in malignancy.

- Lesion in thalamic relay and intralaminar nuclei, or descending tract of the trigeminal nucleus.

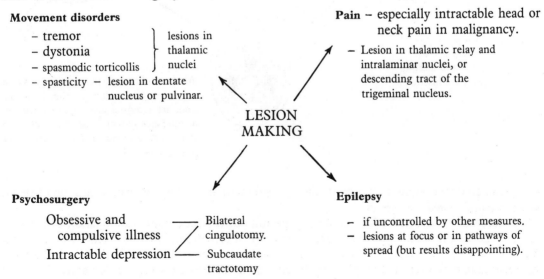

LESION MAKING

Psychosurgery

Obsessive and compulsive illness —— Bilateral cingulotomy.

Intractable depression —— Subcaudate tractotomy

Epilepsy

- if uncontrolled by other measures.
- lesions at focus or in pathways of spread (but results disappointing).

369

Stereotactic Surgery

Uses of Stereotactic Surgery *(continued)*

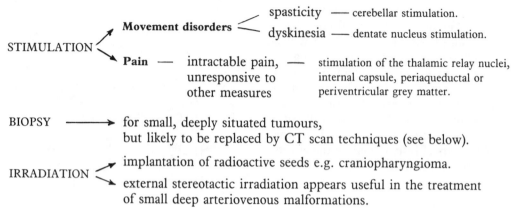

STIMULATION

Movement disorders
- spasticity — cerebellar stimulation.
- dyskinesia — dentate nucleus stimulation.

Pain — intractable pain, unresponsive to other measures — stimulation of the thalamic relay nuclei, internal capsule, periaqueductal or periventricular grey matter.

BIOPSY ⟶ for small, deeply situated tumours, but likely to be replaced by CT scan techniques (see below).

IRRADIATION
- implantation of radioactive seeds e.g. craniopharyngioma.
- external stereotactic irradiation appears useful in the treatment of small deep arteriovenous malformations.

CT guided stereotactic system

Several CT compatible stereotactic systems are now available which allow cannula insertion to any point selected on the CT image. The Brown-Robert-Wells (BRW) system is based on a new concept:

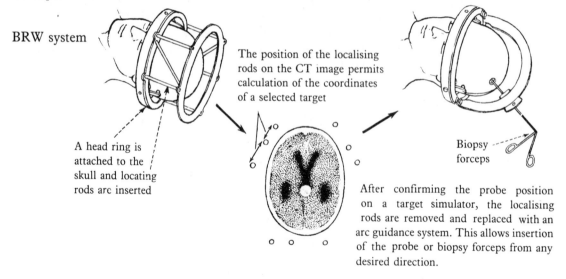

BRW system

The position of the localising rods on the CT image permits calculation of the coordinates of a selected target

A head ring is attached to the skull and locating rods are inserted

Biopsy forceps

After confirming the probe position on a target simulator, the localising rods are removed and replaced with an arc guidance system. This allows insertion of the probe or biopsy forceps from any desired direction.

CT scan guidance techniques provide the optimal method for the biopsy or aspiration of *small, deeply situated tumours or abscesses.*

CT stereotaxy combined with craniotomy permits direct endoscopic examination of a lesion and may aid localisation, e.g. a small arteriovenous malformation. The improved resolution now available with CT scanning may lead to sufficient anatomical localisation for lesion making and this technique may eventually replace traditional methods based on ventriculography.

Psychosurgery

In 1935, observations of behavioural changes in chimpanzees following bilateral ablation of the frontal association area, led to the introduction of lesion making for psychiatric disease (Moniz). The operation of *prefrontal leucotomy* was perfected and used on patients with a wide variety of problems. In Britain, between 1940–1955, neurosurgeons performed over 10,000 operations. It became evident that patients with affective problems – depression, anxiety and obsessional neurosis – showed better results than those with schizophrenia.

As a consequence of the introduction of *chlorpromazine* in the 1950's, and the operative complications and results, perhaps limited by poor case selection, prefrontal leucotomy fell into disrepute. The need for a surgical procedure persisted however in those patients where drugs had little effect. Despite pharmacological improvements, some patients developed chronically disabling conditions requiring continual hospital care; in others with acute depressive illness, the suicide rate was high.

Stereotactic surgery provided a method of lesion making which was virtually risk free and this is now generally accepted as a suitable treatment in *selected patients where drug treatment has failed.*

Indications for Stereotactic surgery and Lesion site

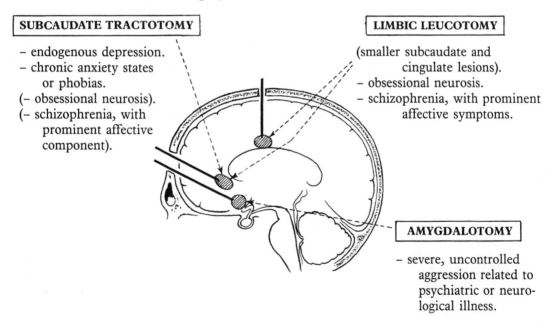

SUBCAUDATE TRACTOTOMY

– endogenous depression.
– chronic anxiety states
  or phobias.
(– obsessional neurosis).
(– schizophrenia, with
  prominent affective
  component).

LIMBIC LEUCOTOMY

(smaller subcaudate and
  cingulate lesions).
– obsessional neurosis.
– schizophrenia, with prominent
  affective symptoms.

AMYGDALOTOMY

– severe, uncontrolled
  aggression related to
  psychiatric or neuro-
  logical illness.

Results:

Depression/anxiety states – up to two thirds benefit from subcaudate tractotomy.
Obsessional neurosis   – 80% improve following limbic leucotomy.
Schizophrenia   – poor results, unless operation is restricted to those patients with concurrent depression, anxiety or obsession, where some benefit may occur.

SECTION IV

**Localised Neurological Disease
and its Management**

B. Spinal Cord and Roots

The Spinal Cord and Roots

Pathologies localised to the spinal cord or nerve roots are detailed below, but note that many diffuse neurological disease processes also affect the cord (see Section V, e.g. demyelination, Freidreich's ataxia).

SPINAL CORD and ROOT COMPRESSION

As the spinal canal is a rigidly enclosed cavity, an expanding disease process will eventually cause cord or root compression.

Causes:

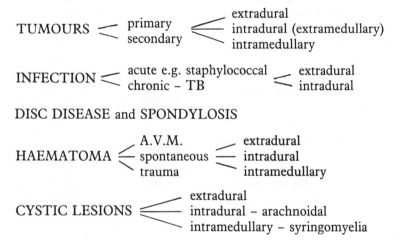

TUMOURS — primary, secondary — extradural, intradural (extramedullary), intramedullary

INFECTION — acute e.g. staphylococcal, chronic – TB — extradural, intradural

DISC DISEASE and SPONDYLOSIS

HAEMATOMA — A.V.M., spontaneous, trauma — extradural, intradural, intramedullary

CYSTIC LESIONS — extradural, intradural – arachnoidal, intramedullary – syringomyelia

Manifestations of cord or root compression depend upon the following:

Site of lesion within the spinal canal: an expanding lesion outside the cord produces signs and symptoms from root and segmental damage.

ROOT – lower motor neurone (l.m.n.) and sensory impairment appropriate to the distribution of the damaged root.

SEGMENTAL – l.m.n. and sensory impairment appropriate to segmental level.

interruption of ascending sensory and descending motor tracts produces sensory impairment and an upper motor neurone (u.m.n.) deficit below the level of the lesion.

Lesions within the cord (intramedullary) produce segmental signs and symptoms.

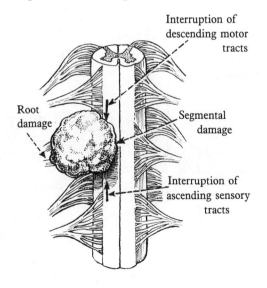

Interruption of descending motor tracts

Root damage

Segmental damage

Interruption of ascending sensory tracts

Spinal Cord and Root Compression

Level of the lesion: – a lesion above the L1 vertebral body may damage both the cord and its roots. Below this, only roots are damaged.

Vascular involvement: – whether neuronal damage results from mechanical stretching or is secondary to ischaemia remains uncertain. On occasions, clinical findings indicate cord damage well beyond the level of the compressive lesion; this implies a distant ischaemic effect due to blood vessel compression at the lesion site.

Speed of onset: – speed of compression affects the clinical picture. Despite producing upper motor neurone damage, a rapidly progressive cord lesion often produces a 'flaccid paralysis' with loss of reflexes and absent plantar responses. This state is akin to 'spinal shock' seen following trauma. Several days or weeks may elapse before tone returns accompanied by the expected 'upper motor neurone' signs.

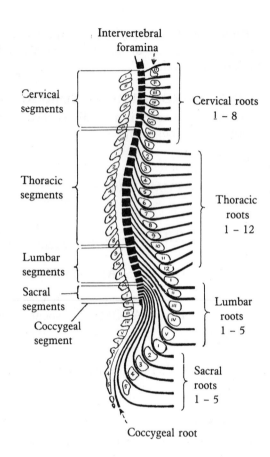

(After BING)

CLINICAL FEATURES

These depend on the site and level of the compressive lesion.

Pain:

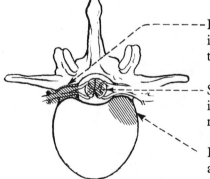

ROOT – severe, sharp, shooting, burning pain radiating into the cutaneous distribution or muscle group supplied by the root; aggravated by movement, straining or coughing.

SEGMENTAL – continuous, deep aching pain radiating into whole leg or one half of body; not affected by movement.

BONE – continuous, dull pain and tenderness over the affected area; may or may not be aggravated by movement.

376

Spinal Cord and Root Compression — Neurological Effects

LATERAL COMPRESSIVE LESION

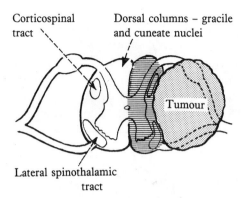

Corticospinal tract

Dorsal columns – gracile and cuneate nuclei

Tumour

Lateral spinothalamic tract

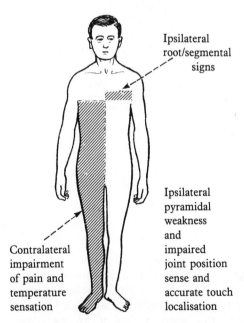

Ipsilateral root/segmental signs

Ipsilateral pyramidal weakness and impaired joint position sense and accurate touch localisation

Contralateral impairment of pain and temperature sensation

Root/Segmental damage

MUSCLE WEAKNESS in groups supplied by the involved root and segment with
LOWER MOTOR NEURONE (l.m.n.) signs:
– wasting; – loss of tone; – fasciculation;
– diminished or absent reflexes.
N.B. motor deficit is seldom detected in roots above C5 and from T2 to L1.

SENSORY DEFECT of all modalities or hyperaesthesia in area supplied by the root, but overlap from adjacent roots may prevent detection.

Long Tract damage –
Partial lesion (Brown-Séquard syndrome)

MOTOR DEFICIT – difficulty in walking due to stiffness. The legs may 'jump' at night. In high cervical lesions weakness of finger movements is noted on the side of the lesion.
Upper motor neurone (u.m.n.) signs:
(maximal on side of lesion).
– increased tone, clonus; – increased reflexes;
– extensor plantar response.

SENSORY DEFICIT – numbness may occur on the same side as the lesion and a burning dysaesthesia on the opposite side.
– joint position sense and accurate touch localisation (two point discrimination) impaired on side of lesion.
– pinprick and temperature sensation impaired on opposite side.

In practice, cord damage is seldom restricted to one side. Usually a mixed picture occurs, with an asymmetric distribution of signs and symptoms.

Damage to sympathetic pathways in the T1 root or cervical cord causes an ipsilateral *Horner's syndrome* (page 132).

BLADDER symptoms are infrequent and only occur when cord damage is bilateral. Precipitancy or difficulty in starting micturition may precede retention.

Spinal Cord and Root Compression — Neurological Effects

Lateral Compressive Lesion (*continued*)

Long tract damage – Complete lesion

MOTOR DEFICIT: the speed of cord compression affects the clinical picture. Slowly growing lesions are usually detected before bilateral damage occurs. If not bilateral, u.m.n. signs predominate. Rapidly progressive lesions produce 'spinal shock' – the limbs are flaccid, power and reflexes diminished or absent and plantar responses are absent or extensor.

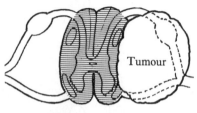

Tumour

SENSORY DEFICIT: involves all modalities and occurs up to the level of the lesion.

BLADDER: patient first notices difficulty in initiating micturition. Retention follows, associated with incontinence as automatic emptying occurs.
Constipation is only noticed after a few days. Some patients develop *priapism* (painful erection).

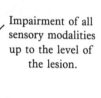

Impairment of all sensory modalities up to the level of the lesion.

Power and reflexes diminished or absent

Bladder dilated

Limbs flaccid

CENTRAL CORD LESION

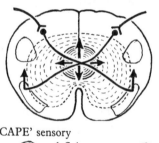

'CAPE' sensory deficit

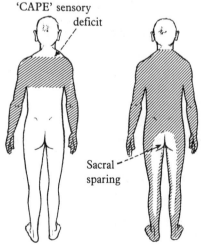

Sacral sparing

Segmental damage: a central lesion initially damages the second sensory neurone crossing to the lateral spinothalamic tract; pain and temperature sensations are impaired in the distribution of the involved segment. As the lesion expands, anterior horn cells are also involved and a l.m.n. weakness occurs.

Long tract damage: further lesion expansion damages the spinothalamic tract and corticospinal tracts, the most medially situated fibres being involved first. With lesion in the cervical region, the sensory deficit to pain and temperature extends downwards in a 'CAPE'-like distribution. As the sacral fibres lie peripherally in the lateral spinothalamic tract, SACRAL SPARING can occur, even with a large lesion. Involvement of the corticospinal tracts produces u.m.n. signs and symptoms in the limbs below the level of the lesion. The bladder is usually involved late.

In the cervical cord, sympathetic involvement may produce a unilateral or bilateral *Horner's syndrome*.

Spinal Cord and Root Compression — Neurological Effects

CAUDA EQUINA LESION

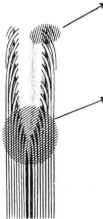

Root or segmental lesions may involve the upper part of the cauda equina and produce root/segmental and long tract signs as described on the previous page, e.g. an expanding L4 root lesion causes weakness and wasting of the foot dorsiflexors, sensory deficit over the inner calf, an increased ankle jerk and an extensor plantar response. Bladder involvement tends to occur late.

The lower sacral roots are involved early, producing loss of motor and sensory bladder control with detrusor paralysis. Overflow incontinence ensues. Impotence and faecal incontinence may be noted. A l.m.n. weakness is found in the sacral root muscles (foot plantarflexors and evertors), the ankle jerks are absent or impaired and a sensory deficit occurs over the *'saddle'* area.

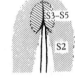

'Saddle' area

VERTEBRAL COLUMN

If a spinal cord or root lesion is suspected look for:

Scoliosis, loss of lordosis or *limitation of straight leg raising* } – suggests root irritation.

Paravertebral swelling *Tenderness* on bone percussion } – suggests malignant disease or infection.

Restricted spinal mobility – suggests bone, disc or root involvement.

Sacral *dimple* or *tuft of hair* – suggests spina bifida oculta/dermoid.

379

Spinal Cord and Root Compression — Investigations

Straight X-ray

On the ANTERO-POSTERIOR views, look for:

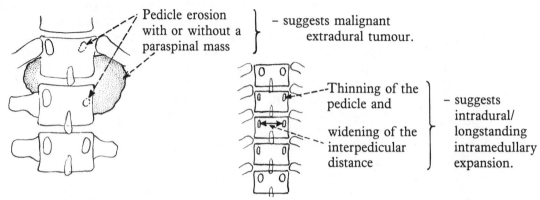

Pedicle erosion
with or without a
paraspinal mass

} – suggests malignant
extradural tumour.

Thinning of the
pedicle and

widening of the
interpedicular
distance

} – suggests
intradural/
longstanding
intramedullary
expansion.

On the LATERAL view

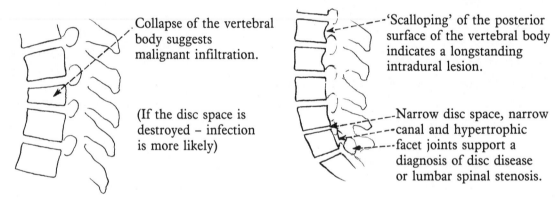

Collapse of the vertebral
body suggests
malignant infiltration.

(If the disc space is
destroyed – infection
is more likely)

'Scalloping' of the posterior
surface of the vertebral body
indicates a longstanding
intradural lesion.

Narrow disc space, narrow
canal and hypertrophic
facet joints support a
diagnosis of disc disease
or lumbar spinal stenosis.

On OBLIQUE views

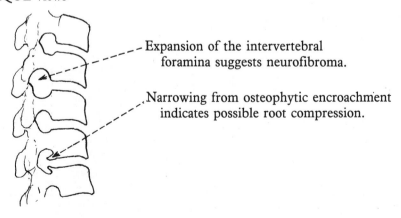

Expansion of the intervertebral
foramina suggests neurofibroma.

Narrowing from osteophytic encroachment
indicates possible root compression.

Spinal Cord and Root Compression — Investigations

MYELOGRAPHY

Myelography identifies the level of the compressive lesion and its site e.g. intradural, extradural.

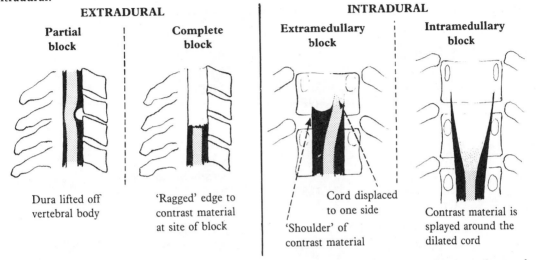

EXTRADURAL

Partial block

Dura lifted off vertebral body

Complete block

'Ragged' edge to contrast material at site of block

INTRADURAL

Extramedullary block

'Shoulder' of contrast material

Cord displaced to one side

Intramedullary block

Contrast material is splayed around the dilated cord

If the clinical signs do not correspond to the level of the block or if it is necessary to know the longitudinal extent of the lesion, then contrast medium is also inserted from above through a lateral cervical puncture.

Radio-opaque markers on the skin surface at the site of the block are a useful operative guide.

CSF ANALYSIS

This is of limited value in cord compression. Abnormalities frequently occur, but *lumbar puncture may precipitate neurological deterioration,* presumably due to the creation of a pressure gradient. *If cord compression is suspect then lumbar puncture and CSF analysis should await myelography.*

CSF Protein: often increased, especially below a complete block.

CSF Cell Count: a marked leucocyte count suggests an infective cause – abscess or tuberculosis.

Queckenstedt's Test: absence of pressure transmission during lumbar puncture when the neck veins are compressed or during coughing indicates a complete block.

CT SCAN

It is impractical to use this as a screening investigation for cord compression, but if the level is known, CT scan can provide additional information. It is of particular value in.

1. demonstrating the extraspinal extent of intraspinal lesion e.g. neurofibroma.
2. demonstrating laterally situated disc protrusions.
3. demonstrating the diameter of the bony canal and size of the facet joints.

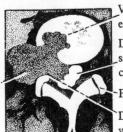

Neurofibroma.

Vertebral body eroded by tumour.

Displaced thecal sac containing contrast medium.

Facet joint.

Dilated intra-vertebral foramen.

Spinal Cord and Root Compression

TUMOUR INCIDENCE

The table shows the number of patients with histologically confirmed tumours admitted to the Institute of Neurological Sciences, Glasgow, over a 5 year period (population 2.7 millions). Tumour types differ in adults and children and are considered separately.

Adults

EXTRADURAL
Metastasis	118	
Myeloma	19	
Neurofibroma	15	**(78%)**
Lymphoma	14	
Others	7	

INTRADURAL
Meningioma	22	
Schwannoma	13	**(18%)**
Others	4	

INTRAMEDULLARY
Astrocytoma	8	**(4%)**
Others	1	

Children

EXTRADURAL
Mestastasis	1	**(18%)**
Lymphoma	1	

INTRADURAL
Dermoid/epidermoid	6	**(64%)**
Others	1	

INTRAMEDULLARY
Astrocytoma	2	**(18%)**

(Table adapted from Adams, Graham and Doyle: Brain Biopsy, 1982.)

Pathology: the pathological features of spinal tumours match those of their intracranial counterparts (see page 285).

METASTATIC TUMOUR

Primary site: Usually breast, lung, prostate or kidney.

Metastatic site: Thoracic vertebrae most often involved, but metastasis may occur at any site and may be multiple.

Clinical features: Bone pain and tenderness are common features usually preceding limb and autonomic dysfunction.

Investigations: Osteolytic lesions or vertebral collapse are often present. Myelography confirms the presence of an extradural block, identifies its level and helps exclude multiple lesions.

Management: Standard methods.

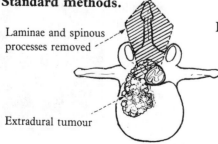

Laminae and spinous processes removed

Extradural tumour

DECOMPRESSIVE LAMINECTOMY

The laminae overlying the site of cord compression are removed along with accessible tumour tissue lying posteriorly to the dura.

382

Spinal Cord and Root Compression

Management: Standard methods (*continued*)

RADIOTHERAPY is routinely used to supplement laminectomy. Some tumours are particularly radiosensitive (e.g. lymphoma) but the more frequently occurring carcinomas show a less dramatic response.

Note: — Patients with flaccid limbs and urinary retention of more than 48 hours duration seldom walk again or regain bladder control. Cord compression therefore requires *urgent treatment.*

— *It is essential to establish the cause of the cord compression.* When laminectomy is not justified (e.g. prolonged flaccid paraplegia) NEEDLE BIOPSY of a paraspinous mass or of infiltrated bone will exclude a benign lesion.

— *Instability* may contribute towards the disappointing results in this condition. Infiltrating tumour often involves the vertebral body. Laminectomy may remove any residual support. Some surgeons therefore combine decompressive laminectomy with a FIXATION procedure using metallic bars. Others claim that this does not decompress the spinal cord, stretched around an anterior mass; they recommend an anterior approach to the vertebral body, removal of all infiltrated bone and replacement and fusion with bone strut grafts. Benefits from these advanced techniques still require confirmation.

— Some studies suggest that radiotherapy alone is as effective as decompressive laminectomy combined with radiotherapy, but the evidence is by no means conclusive.

Prognosis: Metastatic cord compression is a depressing problem. Only about $\frac{1}{3}$ improve after treatment; of those who survive the primary lesion, only $\frac{1}{2}$ can still walk at one year.

Poor prognostic features include:

– complete loss of power and automatic function of more than 48 hours duration.

– rapid progression of cord dysfunction.

MYELOMA

This malignant condition tends to occur in older age groups. It is usually multifocal, involving the spine, pelvis, ribs and skull, but tumours may occur in isolation ('plasmacytoma').

If suspect, look for characteristic changes in the plasma proteins and for Bence-Jones protein in the urine. An isotope bone scan may be less informative than a radiological skeletal survey.

Management is as for metastatic tumour and the prognosis is similar.

MENINGIOMA

Spinal meningiomas tend to occur in elderly patients and are more common in females than in males. They usually arise in the thoracic region and are almost always intradural. Slow growth often permits considerable cord flattening to occur before symptoms become evident.

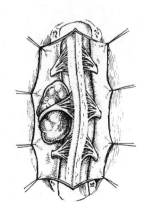

The operative aim is complete removal. Results are usually good, but if the tumour arises anteriorly to the cord, the dural/arachnoid origin cannot be excised and recurrence is possible.

Spinal Cord and Root Compression

SCHWANNOMA / NEUROFIBROMA

Schwannomas are slowly growing benign tumours occurring at any level and arising from the posterior nerve roots. They lie either entirely within the spinal canal or 'dumbbell' through the intervertebral foramen, on occasions presenting as a mass in the thorax or posterior abdominal wall.

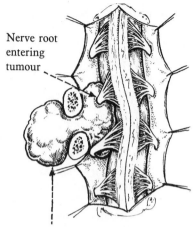

Nerve root entering tumour

Neurofibromas are identical apart from their microscopic appearance (page 286) and their association with multiple neurofibromatosis (Von Recklinghausen' disease) – look for café au lait patches in the skin.

Schwannomas tend to occur in the 30–60 age group. Typically they present with root pain, but in contrast to the pain from root compression, this is often worse at night. Root signs and/or signs of cord compression may follow.

Myelography identifies an intradural/extramedullary lesion. Oblique X-rays may show foraminal enlargement;

Neurofibroma 'dumb-belling' through intervertebral foramen

CT scan will delineate any extraspinal extension (see page 381). Complete operative removal is feasible but the nerve root of origin is inevitably sacrificed. Overlap from adjacent nerve roots usually minimises any resultant neurological deficit.

INTRAMEDULLARY TUMOURS

Intrinsic tumours of the spinal cord occur infrequently. In the Glasgow series (Table, page 382) almost all were slowly growing *astrocytomas* (grades I and II) although other series report an equal incidence of *ependymomas*.

Clinical features:

The onset is usually gradual. Segmental pain is common. Interruption of the decussating fibres to the lateral spinothalamic tract causes loss of pain and temperature sensation at the level of the involved segments.

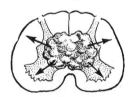

Tumour expansion and involvement of the anterior horn cells produces a lower motor neurone weakness of the corresponding muscle groups; long tract involvement produces an upper motor neurone weakness below the level of the lesion. The sensory deficit spreads downwards bilaterally, the sacral region being the last to become involved.

Investigations:

Straight X-rays occasionally show widening of the interpedicular distance or 'scalloping' of the vertebral bodies. Myelography confirms the presence of an intramedullary lesion. Failure of the expanded segment to collapse with the introduction of air into the thecal sac, a high definition CT scan or nuclear magnetic resonance may help to differentiate an intrinsic tumour from syringomyelia.

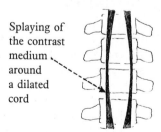

Splaying of the contrast medium around a dilated cord

Spinal Cord and Root Compression

Intramedullary tumours *(continued)*

Management:

When an intrinsic cord tumour is suspect, an explanatory laminectomy is required. An attempt is made to obtain a diagnosis either by needle biopsy or through a longitudinal midline cord incision. Cystic cavities within a tumour or an associated syringomyelia may benefit from aspiration. Rarely benign lesions (e.g. tuberculoma, epidermoid tumour, lipoma) are found. Further management is usually restricted to radiotherapy, but with some ependymomas a plane of cleavage is evident and partial or even total removal is possible.

EPENDYMOMA of the CAUDA EQUINA

More than half of the spinal ependymomas occur around the roots of the cauda equina. They present predominantly with pain and features of a central cauda equina syndrome (page 379). Myelography may show a complete block or an intradural filling defect. The operative aim is to remove the tumour without causing significant root damage. Inevitably, small tumour particles remain, but when the operation is combined with radiotherapy long term results are good.

If the clinical symptoms and signs suggest a more disseminated lesion than demonstrated on myelography, suspect metastatic seeding.

SPINAL CYSTIC LESIONS

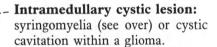

Enterogenous cysts: cysts with a mucoid content are occasionally found lying ventral or dorsal to the cord. They are often associated with vertebral malformation or other congenital abnormality, and are thought to arise from remnants of the neuroenteric canal.

Epidermoid/Dermoid cysts: may be of developmental origin or may follow implantation from a preceding lumbar puncture procedure.

Intramedullary cystic lesion: syringomyelia (see over) or cystic cavitation within a glioma.

Arachnoid cysts: the incidental finding of arachnoid pouches filling with contrast medium are occasionally seen during myelography. These may seal off, producing CSF filled cysts. They occur predominantly in the thoracic region and sometimes cause cord compression. Children with extradural arachnoid cysts frequently develop kyphosis; the causal relationship remains unknown.

Spinal Cord and Root Compression

SYRINGOMYELIA

Syringomyelia is the development of a cystic cavity within the spinal cord, either involving the central canal (hydromyelia), or resulting from cavitation within the cord substance. The lower cervical segments are usually affected; extension may occur into the brain stem – syringobulbia (page 366). Syringomyelia should be distinguished from cystic intramedullary tumours, although both pathologies may coexist. Two types occur:

(1) CONGENITAL: where the syringomyelia is associated with craniovertebral anomalies, in particular the Arnold-Chiari malformation (page 364).
(2) ACQUIRED: the syringomyelia occurs secondarily to trauma or arachnoiditis.

Pathogenesis:

The exact cause of this condition remains unknown but theories abound. In 1965, Gardner proposed the *'hydrodynamic theory'*, suggesting that the craniovertebral anomaly may impair CSF outflow from the 4th ventricle to the cisterna magna. This in turn may result in transmission of a CSF arterial pulse wave through a patent central canal, dilating the canal below the level of compression. This theory however does not explain the occurrence of syringomyelia in patients with non-patent canals. It is possible that the syrinx may itself be a congenital defect rather than a secondary effect. In the acquired type, syringomyelia probably follows intramedullary necrosis and reabsorption.

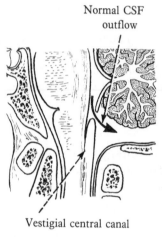

Normal CSF outflow

Vestigial central canal

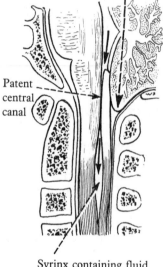

Arnold-Chiari malformation with cerebellar tonsils impacted in the foramen magnum.

Patent central canal

Syrinx containing fluid identical to CSF

Clinical features:

Clinical features are those of a central cord lesion – dissociated sensory loss (i.e. loss of pain and temperature sensation with retention of joint position sense) occurring in a 'cape-like' distribution. Painless cigarette burns in the fingers are a classical sign. Weakness and wasting of the small muscles of the hand are common. Long tract signs follow.

An associated Arnold-Chiari malformation may produce brain stem and cerebellar signs and symptoms.

Hydrocephalus occurs in 25% of patients but is usually symptomless.

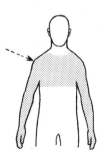

Spinal Cord and Root Compression

Syringomyelia *(continued)*

Investigations:

MYELOGRAPHY demonstrates dilatation of the spinal cord. With coexisting Arnold-Chiari malformation, screening in the *supine* position will show the cerebellar tonsils descending below the foramen magnum. The introduction of air into the CSF space – AIR MYELOGRAPHY, may cause 'collapse' of the dilated segment thereby excluding an intrinsic cord tumour. A CT-scan, six hours after injection of intrathecal contrast or nuclear magnetic resonance may demonstrate the syrinx. These techniques may replace myelography as they become more readily available. Puncture of the syrinx is occasionally possible and subsequent injection of contrast shows its exact extent.

Management:

Operative techniques are only of limited benefit. The approach depends on the presence or absence of an associated Arnold-Chiari malformation.

(a)
    If Arnold-Chiari malformation is present – *decompression* by removing the posterior rim of the foramen magnum and posterior arch of the atlas results in improvement in approximately 30%. Progression is halted in a further 40%. These benefits are probably due to relief of hind brain pressure, rather than an alteration of the hydrodynamics of the syrinx.

    If deterioration in the above patients continues or if no associated Arnold-Chiari malformation exists, attempt either:

(b)   Syringostomy   or   (c)   Filum terminale division

The syrinx is drained via a silastic tube into the surrounding CSF space.

    Alternatively, a syringo-peritoneal shunt is performed. Some patients benefit from this procedure but in $\frac{1}{3}$, progressive deterioration continues.

To CSF space
or peritoneum

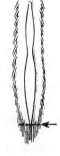

In some patients the syrinx or a patent central canal extends down to the conus medullaris; in these, division of the filum terminale permits syrinx drainage. Although a relatively safe technique, it is difficult to ascertain whether the central canal is patent to this level. The benefits of this technique still require to be confirmed.

Syringomyelia remains a difficult condition to treat. Despite all efforts, at least $\frac{1}{3}$ of patients suffer progressive deterioration.

Spinal Cord and Root Compression

SPINAL INFECTION

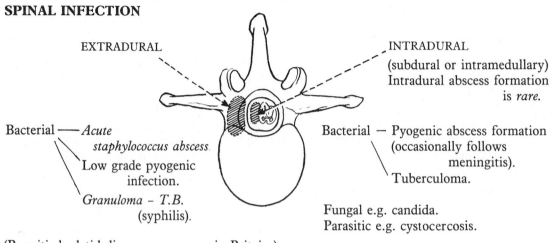

EXTRADURAL

INTRADURAL
(subdural or intramedullary)
Intradural abscess formation
is *rare.*

Bacterial —— *Acute
staphylococcus abscess.*
Low grade pyogenic
infection.
Granuloma – T.B.
(syphilis).

Bacterial — Pyogenic abscess formation
(occasionally follows
meningitis).
Tuberculoma.

Fungal e.g. candida.
Parasitic e.g. cystocercosis.

(Parasitic-hydatid disease – very rare in Britain.)

ACUTE EXTRADURAL ABSCESS

Organism: —— Invariably *staphylococcus aureus.*

Spread: —— Haematogenous (e.g. from a boil) or from osteitis of the neural arch or pedicle.

Site: —— Usually thoracic, but may affect any level. Cord damage occurs either from direct compression or secondary to a thrombophlebitis and venous infarction.

Clinical —— May mimic a rapidly progressive extradural tumour or haematoma with
features: bilateral leg weakness, a sensory level and urinary retention, but distinguishing features are:
– very severe pain and tenderness over the involved site.
– toxaemia – pyrexia, malaise, increased pulse rate.
– rigidity of neck and spinal column, with marked resistance to flexion.
As the abscess extends upwards, the sensory level may rise.

Investigations:– *Straight X-ray* may or may not show an associated osteitis.
A *myelogram* confirms the site of the extradural lesion.
CSF may show an increased white cell count, usually polymorphonuclear, but may be normal.
A *leucocytosis* is usually present and the *ESR* raised.

Management:– Urgent decompressive laminectomy and abscess drainage combined with intravenous antibiotic therapy provides the best chance of recovery of function.

Spinal Cord and Root Compression

SPINAL TUBERCULOSIS (Pott's disease of the spine)

In developing countries, spinal TB is mostly a disease of childhood or adolescence. In Britain it usually affects the middle aged and is particularly prevalent in immigrant populations.

The lower thoracic spine is commonly involved and the disease initially affects two adjacent vertebral bodies.

Clinical features:

The classical systemic features of night fever and cachexia are often absent.

Pain occurs over the affected area and is only relieved by rest.

Symptoms and signs of cord compression occur in approximately 20 per cent of cases.

The onset may be gradual as pus, caseous material or granulation tissue accumulate, or sudden as vertebral bodies collapse and a kyphosis develops.

STRAIGHT X-RAYS are characteristic.

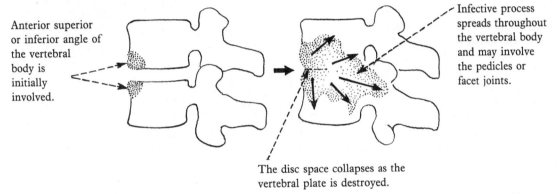

Anterior superior or inferior angle of the vertebral body is initially involved.

Infective process spreads throughout the vertebral body and may involve the pedicles or facet joints.

The disc space collapses as the vertebral plate is destroyed.

Management:

Every effort is made to establish the diagnosis. A *needle biopsy* is often sufficient, but occasionally an exploratory operation (costotransversectomy) is required. Long term *antituberculous therapy* is commenced.

If signs of cord compression develop, decompression is required.

Anterolateral approach

Several ribs are resected medially, along with the transverse processes allowing removal of all pus and caseous debris, without retraction of the spinal cord.

A posterior decompression, removing the remaining unaffected bone, is likely to cause instability. An *anterolateral decompression* is therefore the operation of choice.

Disc Prolapse and Spondylosis

Intervertebral discs act as shock absorbers for the bony spine.

A tough outer layer — the annulus fibrosis — surrounds a softer central nucleus pulposus.

Discs degenerate with age, the fluid within the nucleus pulposus gradually drying out. Disc collapse produces excessive strain on the facet joints i.e. the superior and inferior articulatory processes of each vertebral body, and leads to degeneration and hypertrophy.

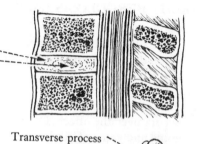

Lumbar Disc Prolapse

An *acute disc prolapse* occurs when the soft nucleus herniates through a tear in the annulus and may result from a single or repeated traumatic incidents. Herniation usually occurs laterally and compresses adjacent nerve roots, but may occasionally occur centrally, compressing the cauda equina.

A 'free fragment' of the nucleus pulposus may extrude and lie above or below the level of the disc space.

Associated hypertrophy of degenerated facet joints is often a further source of back and leg pain and is an important cause of root compression.

Transverse process

Superior articular facet

Facet joint · Compressed nerve root

Inferior articular facet · Spinous process

Lateral disc protrusion

Compressed roots within cauda equina

Central disc protrusion

Hypertrophied facet joint

Compressed nerve root

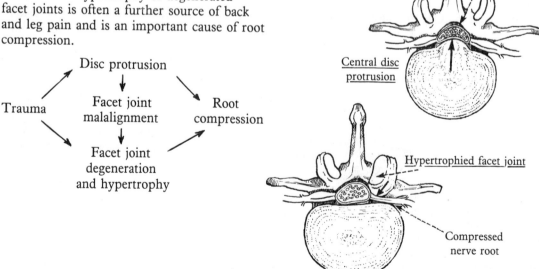

```
                  Disc protrusion
                ↗               ↘
Trauma        Facet joint        Root
              malalignment      compression
                ↓              ↗
              Facet joint
              degeneration
              and hypertrophy
```

Lumbar Disc Prolapse

A *congenitally narrowed spinal canal* increases susceptibility to the development of nerve root compression. Here the spinal canal diameter is considerably diminished and minor disc protrusion or mild joint hypertrophy may readily compress the nerve root.

Lateral disc herniations usually compress the nerve root exiting through the foramen below the affected level, e.g an L3/4 disc lesion will compress the L4 nerve root, but large disc protrusions or a free fragment may compress any adjacent root.

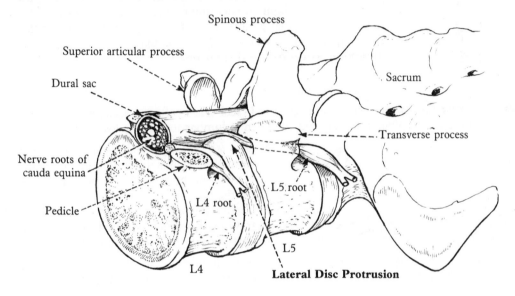

Lumbar disc lesions may occur at any level but L4/5 and L5/S1 are the commonest sites (95%).

Lumbar Disc Prolapse

CLINICAL FEATURES
Lateral Disc Protrusion

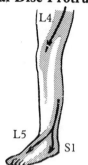

Injury: A history of falling, or lifting heavy weights often precedes the onset of symptoms.

Leg pain: Root irritation or compression produces pain in the distribution of the affected root and this usually extends below the mid-calf. Coughing, sneezing or straining aggravates the leg pain which is usually more severe than any associated backache. If compression causes severe root damage the leg pain may disappear as neurological signs develop.

Paraesthesia: Numbness or tingling occurs in the distribution of the affected root.

'Mechanical' signs: Spinal movements are restricted, scoliosis is often present and is related to spasm of the erector spinae muscles, and the normal lumbar lordosis is lost.

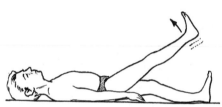

Straight leg raising: L5 and S1 root compression causes limitation to less than 60° from the horizontal and produces pain down the back of the leg. Dorsiflexion of the foot while the leg is elevated (Lasegue's test) aggravates the pain. Elevation of the 'good' leg may produce pain in the other leg.

(If in doubt about the veracity of a restricted straight leg raising deficit, sit the patient up on the examination couch with the legs straight. This is equivalent to 90° straight leg raising.)

Reverse leg raising (Femoral stretch)

Tests for irritation of higher nerve roots (L4 and above)

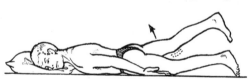

Neurological deficit: Depends on the root involved

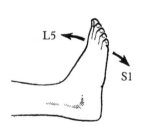

L4 — Quadriceps wasting and weakness;
sensory impairment over medial calf;
impaired knee jerk.

L5 — Wasting and weakness of dorsiflexors of foot, extensor digitorum longus and extensor hallucis longus;
sensory impairment over lateral calf and dorsum of foot.

S1 — Wasting and weakness of plantar flexors;
sensory impairment over lateral aspect of foot and sole;
impaired ankle jerk.

Root signs cannot reliably localise the level of disc protrusion due to variability of the anatomical distribution.

Lumbar Disc Prolapse

CLINICAL FEATURES *(continued)*

Central Disc Protrusion

Symptoms and signs of central disc protrusion are usually bilateral, although one side is often worse than the other.

Leg pain: Extends bilaterally down the back of the thighs. Pain may disappear with the onset of paralysis.

Paraesthesia: Occurs in the same distribution.

Sphincter paralysis: Loss of bladder and urethral sensation with intermittent or complete retention of urine occurs in most patients. Anal sensation is usually impaired and accompanies constipation.

Severe pain associated with lateral disc protrusion may inhibit micturition. In this instance, strong analgesia should allow normal micturition, and the presence of normal perineal sensation excludes root compression as the cause of the retention.

Sensory loss: Extends over all or part of the sacral area ('saddle' anaesthesia) and confirms a neurogenic cause for the sphincter disturbance.

Motor loss: Usually presents as foot drop with complete loss of power in the dorsiflexors and plantarflexors of both feet.

Reflex loss: The ankle jerks are usually absent on each side.

INVESTIGATION

Straight X-ray of lumbo-sacral spine is of limited benefit in the investigation of lumbar disc disease — it may show loss of a disc space or an associated spondylolisthesis (see page 395). Straight X-rays are *important in excluding other pathology* such as metastatic carcinoma.

Radiculography outlines the thecal sac and nerve roots. Disc protrusion may cause:

(i) a filling defect in the theca on the A.P. or lateral view of the appropriate disc level.

(ii) obliteration or displacement of the nerve root sleeve.

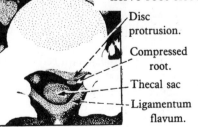

Disc protrusion.
Compressed root.
Thecal sac.
Ligamentum flavum.

Oblique view:
L5 root
Occluded S1 root
Filling defect L5/S1 disc protrusion

Spinal CT scan may detect small laterally placed disc protrusions occasionally missed on radiculography.

In addition, it clearly shows hypertrophied facet joints and the diameter of the spinal canal.

393

Lumbar Disc Prolapse

MANAGEMENT   **(a) Lateral Disc Protrusion**

CONSERVATIVE MANAGEMENT: Most bouts of leg pain settle spontaneously by taking simple measures:

   (i) *bed rest* for 2-3 weeks on an orthopaedic mattress or with a hard board under mattress;

   (ii) *traction* applied to skin may help, but pain may return when traction is removed;

   (iii) *plaster jacket* or *spinal brace* is of benefit in some patients and provides rest yet retains mobility.

When the pain settles, the patient is advised to *avoid heavy lifting.* Even picking up objects from the floor should be accompanied by bending the knees and keeping the back straight.

INDICATIONS FOR OPERATION

   (i) Severe *unremitting leg pain* despite conservative measures.

   (ii) *Recurrent attacks* of pain, especially when causing repeated time loss from work.

   (iii) The development of a *neurological deficit.*

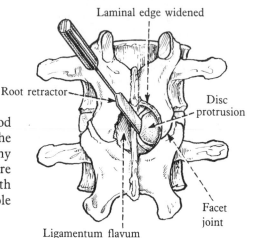

TECHNIQUE: Fenestration usually provides good access. Retraction of the root and dural sac exposes the disc protrusion and allows removal with rongeurs. Any protuberance from the facet joint causing root pressure or narrowing of the root canal is also removed. With large disc lesion, some prefer removal of the whole lamina.

RESULTS: Approximately 70 per cent of patients obtain good results after operation. The remainder may have recurrent problems due to a further disc protrusion at the same or another level. Occasionally bony instability complicates the operation. Now that a water-soluble contrast medium is used for investigation (instead of oil-based 'myodil'), arachnoiditis rarely occurs.

After disc operation, patients are advised to avoid heavy lifting, preferably for an indefinite period. Persistance in a heavy manual job may lead to further trouble.

In general, patients with clear-cut indications for operation do well, whereas those with dubious clinical or radiographic signs tend to have a high incidence of recurrent problems.

(b) Central Disc Protrusion

In contrast to lateral disc protrusion, *compression of the cauda equina from a central disc constitutes a neurosurgical emergency.* Delay in root decompression results in a reduced chance of motor and sphincter recovery.

A full laminectomy at the appropriate level rather than fenestration is usually required to obtain adequate exposure.

Motor, sensory and sphincter function should gradually recover over a two year period but results are often disappointing. For example, although most regain bladder control, few have completely normal function.

Lumbar Spinal Stenosis

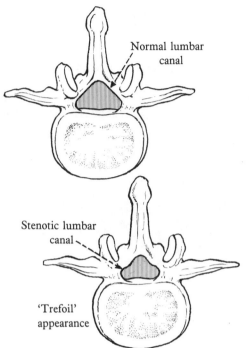

Normal lumbar canal

Stenotic lumbar canal

'Trefoil' appearance

Congenital narrowing of the lumber spinal cord, or secondary narrowing due to hypertrophic facet joints, may predispose to root compression from a herniated disc, but in addition may produce 'neurogenic claudication'. Symptoms of root pain, paraesthesia or weakness develop after standing or walking and may be relieved by sitting or lying down. Straight leg raising is seldom impaired, in contrast to patients with disc protrusion.

Objective neurological findings may only appear after exercise. Plain X-rays and radiculography may suggest lumbar spinal stenosis but CT scanning is required to establish the diagnosis.

Treatment: A wide laminectomy with root decompression usually produces good results with complete relief of symptoms.

Spondylolisthesis

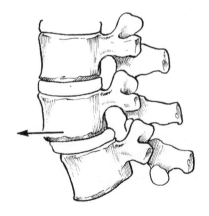

Spondylolisthesis is a forward shift of one vertebral body on another (usually L4 or L5). Slip occurs due either to defective facet joints (degenerative or congenital) or to a break or elongation of the lamina. Sponylolisthesis is often symptomless but the resultant narrowing in canal width may accentuate symptoms of root compression from disc protrusion or joint hypertrophy.

Treatment: usually conservative, but if signs of root compression are present, then decompression of the root canal is necessary. Occasionally fusion is required especially if back pain predominates.

Thoracic Disc Prolapse

This occurs rarely (0.2% of all disc lesions) due to the relative stability of the thoracic spine.

PRESENTATION: – root pain and/or cord compression
$$or$$
progressive or fluctuating paraparesis (may lead to mistaken diagnosis).

INVESTIGATION: Myelography, although difficult in the thoracic spine, demonstrates an anterior filling defect at the level of the disc space. Clinical signs may extend above the level of the disc protrusion suggesting vascular impairment.

MANAGEMENT
Root pain — may settle with bed rest.
Cord compression — a posterior approach
  to the disc carries an unacceptably
  high risk of paraplegia. This risk
  is minimised by *antero-lateral decompression.*

An *intrathoracic* approach to the vertebral bodies and disc spaces provides a useful alternative route.

Cervical Spondylosis

The mobile cervical spine is particularly subject to osteoarthritic change and this occurs in more than half the population over 50 years of age; of these approximately 20 per cent develop related symptoms.

Pathogenesis

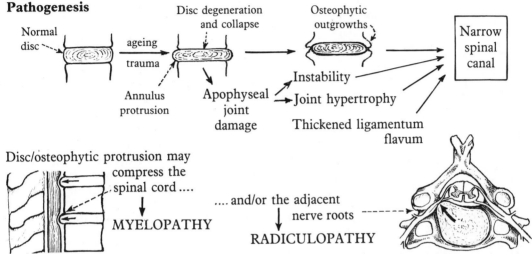

Resultant damage to the spinal cord may arise from direct pressure or may follow vascular impairment. The onset is usually gradual. Trauma may or may not predispose to the development of symptoms.

Acute cervical disc prolapse: In contrast to cervical spondylosis cervical 'soft' disc protrusion is uncommon. This tends to occur acutely in younger patients and may be related to a specific incident such as a sudden twist or injury to the neck. The protrusion usually occurs postero-laterally, causing a radiculopathy rather than a myelopathy.

CLINICAL FEATURES
Radiculopathy

Pain: a sharp stabbing pain, worse on coughing, may be superimposed on a more constant deep ache radiating over the shoulders and down the arm.

Paraesthesia: Numbness or tingling follows a dermatomal distribution.

Root signs:
Sensory loss i.e. pin prick deficit in the appropriate dermatomal distribution.
Muscle (l.m.n.) weakness and wasting in appropriate muscle groups e.g. C5...biceps, deltoid: C7...triceps.
Reflex impairment/loss e.g. C5,6...biceps, supinator jerk: C7...triceps jerk.
Trophic change: in long-standing root compression, skin becomes dry, scaly, inelastic, blue and cold.

Cervical Spondylosis

CLINICAL FEATURES *(continued)*
Myelopathy

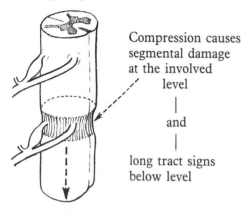

Compression causes segmental damage at the involved level

|

and

|

long tract signs below level

N.B. Involved segments may extend above or below the level of compression if the vascular supply is also impaired.

Arms: l.m.n. signs and symptoms as above at the level of the lesion

and/or

u.m.n. signs and symptoms below the level of the lesion

e.g. C5 lesion $\left\{\begin{array}{l}\text{biceps weakness, wasting:}\\ \text{diminished biceps jerk:}\\ \text{increased finger jerks.}\end{array}\right.$

Legs: u.m.n. signs and symptoms i.e. difficulty in walking due to stiffness; 'pyramidal' weakness, increased tone, clonus and extensor plantar responses; sensory symptoms and signs are variable and less prominent.

Sphincter disturbance is seldom a prominent early feature.

INVESTIGATION

Straight X-ray of cervical spine
Look for:
— congenital narrowing of canal, loss of lordosis.
— disc space collapse and osteophyte protrusion (foraminal encroachment is best seen in oblique views).
— subluxation. Flexion/extension views may be required.

Cervical myelogram

Lateral view: Identifies anterior disc bars compressing the cord.

Antero-posterior view: Shows root obliteration/filling defect due to disc protrusion. The extent of cord flattening at disc level often reflects the degree of cord compression.

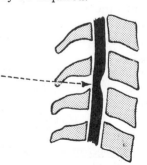

Cervical Spondylosis

MANAGEMENT
CONSERVATIVE
- — Analgesics
- — Cervical collar
- — Traction

Symptoms of radiculopathy, whether acute or chronic, usually respond to conservative measures. Progression of a disabling neurological deficit however demands surgical intervention. A myelopathy may also respond to conservative treatment, but undue delay (i.e. more than 3 months) may reduce the chance of recovery.

INDICATIONS FOR OPERATION
1. Progressive neurological deficit – myelopathy or radiculopathy.
2. Intractable pain, when this fails to respond to conservative measures. This is rarely the sole indication for operation and usually applies to acute disc protrusions rather than chronic radiculopathy.

OPERATIVE TECHNIQUES

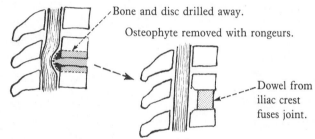

1. *Anterior approach,*
   Cloward's anterior fusion
   A core of bone and disc is
   drilled out allowing removal
   of the osteophytic projection.
   Insertion of a bone dowel from
   the iliac crest fuses the joint.

Bone and disc drilled away.

Osteophyte removed with rongeurs.

Dowel from iliac crest fuses joint.

   Suitable for root or cord compression from an anterior protrusion at one level, although two and even three levels may be fused.

2. *Posterior approach*

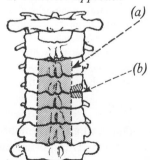

(a) *Laminectomy:*   a wide decompression, usually from C3-C7 is carried out. Suitable for multilevel cord compression especially when superimposed on a congenitally narrow spinal canal.

(b) *Foraminotomy:*   the nerve root at one or more levels may be decompressed by drilling away overlying bone.

Results:
Operative results vary widely in different series and probably depend on patient selection. Improvement occurs in 50–60 per cent of patients. Operation should be aimed at preventing progression rather than curing all symptoms.

Spinal Trauma

Approximately 2 per 100,000 of the population per year sustain a spinal injury.

At impact, *spinal cord damage* may or may not accompany the *bony or ligamentous damage.* After impact, stability at the level of injury plays a crucial part in further management. Injudicious movement of a patient with an unstable lesion may precipitate spinal cord injury or aggravate any pre-existing damage.

MECHANISMS of INJURY

The mechanism of injury helps determine the degree of stability:

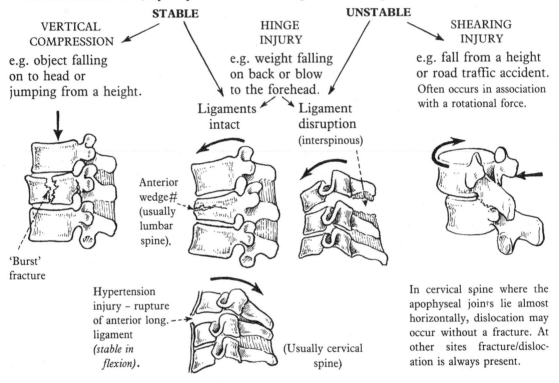

STABLE

VERTICAL COMPRESSION

e.g. object falling on to head or jumping from a height.

'Burst' fracture

HINGE INJURY

e.g. weight falling on back or blow to the forehead.

Ligaments intact

Anterior wedge# (usually lumbar spine).

Hypertension injury – rupture of anterior long. ligament (*stable in flexion*).

Ligament disruption (interspinous)

(Usually cervical spine)

UNSTABLE

SHEARING INJURY

e.g. fall from a height or road traffic accident. Often occurs in association with a rotational force.

In cervical spine where the apophyseal joints lie almost horizontally, dislocation may occur without a fracture. At other sites fracture/dislocation is always present.

Initial assessment

The possibility of spinal injury must be considered at the scene of the accident and all movements and transportation of the patient undertaken with extreme caution. This is especially important in the unconscious patient who cannot complain of *pain, numbness or difficulty with limb movements.*

Examination may reveal *tenderness over the spinous processes, paraspinal swelling* or a *gap between the spinous processes,* indicating rupture of an interspinous ligament.

Neurogenic paradoxical ventilation (indrawing of the chest on inspiration due to absent intercostal function) may occur with cervical cord damage.

Bilateral absence of limb reflexes in flaccid limbs, unresponsive to painful stimuli, indicates spinal cord damage (unless death is imminent from severe head injury).

Urinary retention or *priapism* may also occur.

Spinal Trauma — Investigations

STRAIGHT X-RAYS

- LATERAL VIEW

In the *cervical spine*
- note evidence of
soft tissue swelling
between the pharynx
and the vertebrae.

- ensure *C6 and C7*
are included in the film.
If not, repeat with gentle
downward arm traction.

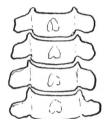

- note any *malalignment* of the anterior or
posterior margins of the vertebral body or of
the lamina i.e. subluxation.

- note any undue *widening of the interspinous
distance or of the disc space.*

- note *damage to the vertebral body, apophyseal joints, lamina or spinous process* e.g.
anterior wedge collapse,
'burst' fracture.

[In the upper thoracic spine
only **TOMOGRAPHY** may
satisfactorily demonstrate
the lateral view.]

- ANTERO-POSTERIOR VIEW

- note the
alignment and
the *width of
the apophyseal
joints.*

- ANTERO-POSTERIOR 'OPEN MOUTH' VIEW

- required to
demonstrate a
*fracture of
the odontoid
peg.*

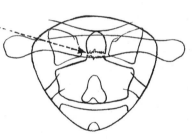

If doubt remains –
take **OBLIQUE VIEWS** to demonstrate
the intervertebral foramina.

CERVICAL
SPINE

Disruption of the
foraminal outline
suggests malalignment

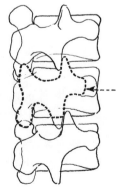

In the LUMBAR spine look for
the normal *'scotty dog'*
appearance – if misshapen,
suggests a fracture/dislocation.

If in doubt about stability, take **FLEXION/EXTENSION VIEWS,** but only with expert
supervision.

MYELOGRAPHY and **CT SCANNING** show the extent to which bone fragments indent the spinal
cord, but these investigations only help if operative decompression is considered.

Spinal Trauma — Management

Management depends on the site and stability of the lesion, but basic principles apply.
1. An *unstable* lesion risks further damage to the spinal cord and roots and requires either –
    – *operative fixation* or
    – *immobilisation* e.g. skull traction, Halo or plaster jacket.
2. There is no evidence that 'decompressing' the cord lesion (either anteriorly or posteriorly) improves the neurological outcome, but –
3. If a patient with normal cord function or with an incomplete cord lesion (i.e. with some residual function) *progressively deteriorates,* then *operative decompression* is required.

Many additional therapies and techniques (e.g. steroids, cord cooling, hyperbaric oxygen) are employed with the aim of improving neurological outcome; as yet none have been shown to produce any significant benefit.

Management of injury at specific sites:

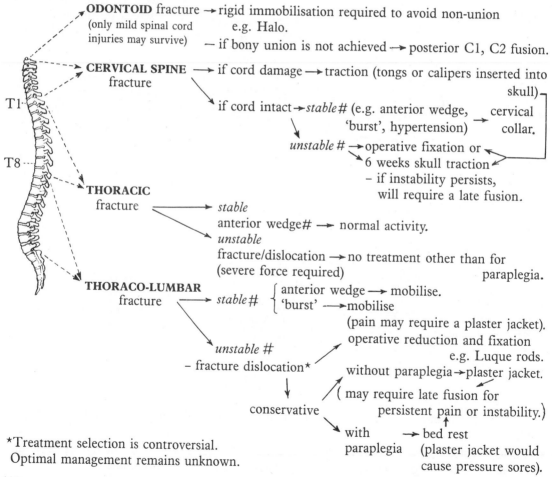

ODONTOID fracture → rigid immobilisation required to avoid non-union
(only mild spinal cord   e.g. Halo.
injuries may survive)   – if bony union is not achieved → posterior C1, C2 fusion.

CERVICAL SPINE → if cord damage → traction (tongs or calipers inserted into
fracture   skull)
            if cord intact → *stable* # (e.g. anterior wedge,   cervical
                                    'burst', hypertension)   →   collar.
                        unstable # → operative fixation or
                                        6 weeks skull traction
                                        – if instability persists,
                                            will require a late fusion.

THORACIC
fracture   → *stable*
            anterior wedge# → normal activity.
            unstable
            fracture/dislocation → no treatment other than for
            (severe force required)   paraplegia.

THORACO-LUMBAR
fracture   → *stable* # { anterior wedge → mobilise.
                            { 'burst' → mobilise
                                    (pain may require a plaster jacket).
                                    operative reduction and fixation
                                                    e.g. Luque rods.
            unstable #   without paraplegia → plaster jacket.
            – fracture dislocation*
                                    (may require late fusion for
                    conservative   persistent pain or instability.)
                                    with   → bed rest
                                    paraplegia (plaster jacket would
                                                cause pressure sores).

T1

T8

*Treatment selection is controversial.
Optimal management remains unknown.

402

Spinal Trauma — Management

Management of the Paraplegic Patient

After spinal cord injury, transfer to a spinal injury centre with medical and nursing staff skilled in the management of the paraplegic patient, provides optimal daily care and rehabilitation. Important features include:

1. *Skin care* – requires meticulous attention. Two hourly turning should prevent pressure sores. Attempt to avoid contact with bony prominences or creases in the bed sheets. Air or water beds or a sheepskin may help.
2. *Urinary tract* – long term catheter drainage is required (a supra-pubic catheter is ideal). Infection requires prompt treatment. Eventually, training may permit automatic reflex function (in cord lesions) or micturition by abdominal compression (in root lesions). In some, urodynamic studies may indicate possible benefit from bladder neck resection.
3. *Limbs* – intensive physiotherapy helps prevent flexion contractures (in cord injury) and plays an essential rôle in rehabilitation.

Outcome following spinal cord or root injury

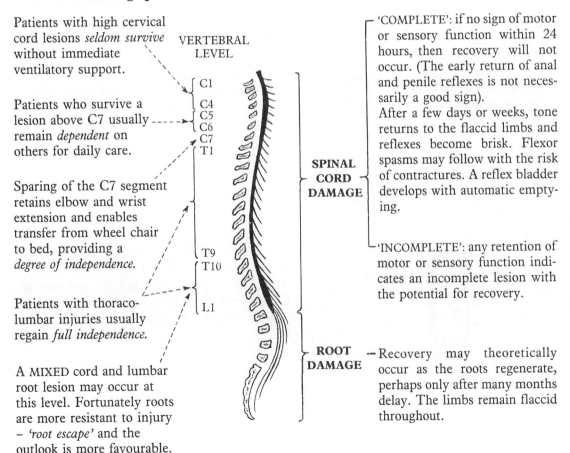

Patients with high cervical cord lesions *seldom survive* without immediate ventilatory support.

Patients who survive a lesion above C7 usually remain *dependent* on others for daily care.

Sparing of the C7 segment retains elbow and wrist extension and enables transfer from wheel chair to bed, providing a *degree of independence*.

Patients with thoraco-lumbar injuries usually regain *full independence*.

A MIXED cord and lumbar root lesion may occur at this level. Fortunately roots are more resistant to injury – *'root escape'* and the outlook is more favourable.

VERTEBRAL LEVEL

C1
C4
C5
C6
C7
T1

T9
T10

L1

SPINAL CORD DAMAGE

ROOT DAMAGE

'COMPLETE': if no sign of motor or sensory function within 24 hours, then recovery will not occur. (The early return of anal and penile reflexes is not necessarily a good sign).
After a few days or weeks, tone returns to the flaccid limbs and reflexes become brisk. Flexor spasms may follow with the risk of contractures. A reflex bladder develops with automatic emptying.

'INCOMPLETE': any retention of motor or sensory function indicates an incomplete lesion with the potential for recovery.

Recovery may theoretically occur as the roots regenerate, perhaps only after many months delay. The limbs remain flaccid throughout.

403

Vascular Diseases of the Spinal Cord

Blood supply to the spinal cord is complex; the main vessels are the anterior and posterior spinal arteries.

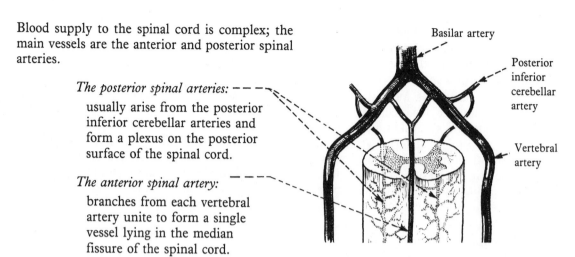

The posterior spinal arteries: – – –

usually arise from the posterior inferior cerebellar arteries and form a plexus on the posterior surface of the spinal cord.

The anterior spinal artery: – – –

branches from each vertebral artery unite to form a single vessel lying in the median fissure of the spinal cord.

Both anterior and posterior spinal arteries run the length of the spinal cord and receive anastomotic vessels.

The posterior spinal artery is joined on average by 12 *unpaired* radicular feeding arteries. This rich collateral circulation protects the posterior part of the spinal cord from vascular disease.

The anterior spinal artery has a much less efficient collateral supply and is thus more liable to damage as a consequence of vascular disease. It is joined on average by 8 *unpaired* radicular branches.

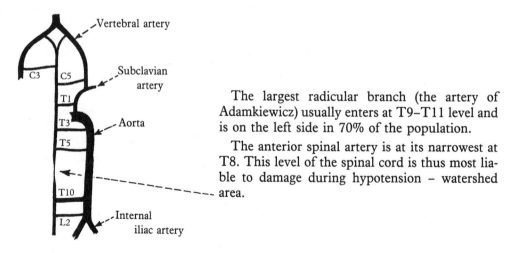

The largest radicular branch (the artery of Adamkiewicz) usually enters at T9–T11 level and is on the left side in 70% of the population.

The anterior spinal artery is at its narrowest at T8. This level of the spinal cord is thus most liable to damage during hypotension – watershed area.

Anterior radicular branches joining anterior spinal artery.

Vascular Diseases of the Spinal Cord

Posterior spinal artery territory

– Posterior $\frac{1}{3}$ of spinal cord.
– Dorsal column.

Virtually no anastomotic communication

Anterior spinal artery territory

Penetrating branches – anterior and part of posterior grey matter.

Circumferential branches – anterior white matter.

– Anterior $\frac{2}{3}$ of spinal cord.

Posterior spinal artery

Posterior radicular artery

Anterior radicular artery

Anterior spinal artery

Segmental artery

Aorta

Most radicular vessels only supply the root. On average 12 posterior radicular branches and 8 anterior radicular branches supply the spinal cord.

Atherosclerosis of spinal arteries is rare. When infarction occurs in the anterior spinal artery territory it is often a consequence of disease in the vessels of origin of the segmental arteries i.e. atheroma or dissection of the aorta.

Rich anastomotic network occurs between each segmental artery through the vertebral body and across the extradural space.

Section through spinal cord in thoracic region.

405

Vascular Diseases of the Spinal Cord

The ANTERIOR SPINAL ARTERY SYNDROME

Sudden onset of leg weakness and sensory loss (pin prick/temperature) with preservation of vibration and joint position sensation – *Dissociate sensory loss.*

Bladder and bowel functions are also affected.

Sensory level with pin prick and temperature lost.

Flaccid areflexic weakness

Days or weeks →

Spastic hyperactive reflexes. Total or partial paraglegia.

Spinal bladder/bowel

When only penetrating branches are involved, long tract damage may be selective and sensory loss may not occur.

The spinal cord symptoms due to aortic atheroma may be slowly progressive and need not be acute.

The blood supply to the spinal cord may be affected in:

1. Neurosyphilis.
2. Polyarteritis nodosa.
3. Systemic lupus erythematosus.
4. Compression of spinal arteries – Disc fragments, extradural mass – abscess or tumour.
5. Compression of segmental arteries – Posterior mediastinal mass, abdominal paravertebral mass.
6. Endarteritis secondary to local infection – Tuberculous meningitis, pneumococcal meningitis.
7. Dissecting aortic aneurysm.
8. Aortic surgery.
9. Aortic arteriography.

The posterior spinal arteries are rarely affected.

Vascular Diseases of the Spinal Cord

SPINAL ARTERIO-VENOUS MALFORMATION (Angiomatous Malformation)

Arterio-venous malformations (AVM's) are congenital abhormalities of blood vessels rather than neoplastic growths. Arteries communicating directly with veins bypass the capillary network and create a 'shunt'. The AVM appears as a mass of convoluted dilated vessels.

Site:

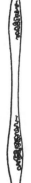

Cervical: uncommon site (∼15%). Arises from the anterior spinal artery and usually lies within the cord substance (intramedullary).

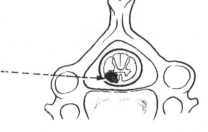

Thoraco-lumbar: this is the commonest site (∼85%). It may be extra- or intradural or within both compartments. Intramedullary lesions at this site are less common.

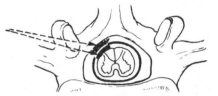

Spinal AVM's may present clinically at any age in either sex, but are most common in males in the 6th or 7th decade.

Clinical features:

SUDDEN ONSET (10–15%)

Due to – subarachnoid haemorrhage: headache, neck stiffness, back and leg pain.
– extradural haematoma.
– subdural haematoma.
– intramedullary haematoma (haematomyelia). } : signs of acute cord compression.

GRADUAL ONSET (85–90%)

Probably due to ↑ *venous pressure* but other factors may play a part:
– venous thrombosis.
– 'steal' phenomenon.
– venous bulk.
– arachnoiditis (if previous bleed).

Progressive deterioration of all spinal modalities simulating cord compression. Pain is common. With thoraco-lumbar lesions a mixed u.m.n./l.m.n. weakness in the legs is typical.
Intramedullary AVM's may cause fluctuating signs and symptoms and may mimic intermittent claudication.

A bruit may be heard overlying a spinal AVM and occasionally midline cutaneous angiomas are found. (Note that cutaneous angiomas are not uncommon and do not necessarily imply an underlying lesion.)

Vascular Diseases of the Spinal Cord

Spinal arterio-venous malformation *(continued)*

Investigation:

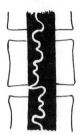

> *Myelography:* Contrast material outlines
> 'serpent-like' vessels on the cord surface.
> If the myelogram is positive,
> *spinal angiography* is required to delineate the
> extent of the AVM and the exact site of
> the shunt and feeding vessel.

Management:

Untreated, 50% of patients with gradual onset of symptoms would be unable to walk within 3 years.

Operation should prevent progression and may well improve a gait or bladder disturbance. Operative delay may result in irreversible cord damage.

Techniques: It is important to identify and divide the feeding vessel and excise the shunt. Total excision of all the dilated veins is probably unnecessary and would increase the operative hazards. A decompressive laminectomy alone is of no benefit. Intramedullary AVM's and/or AVM's lying ventral to the cord cannot be excised and embolisation of the feeding vessel may be tried. The long term benefits of this procedure are unknown.

Intraspinal haematoma: If the patient presents with signs of a rapid onset of spinal cord compression, and myelogram confirms an extra- or intradural block, then urgent laminectomy and decompression is required (without waiting for angiography). Examination of the haematoma whether extra- or intradural may reveal angiomatous tissue. In some patients there is no evident cause and the bleed is designated as 'spontaneous'.

Spinal Dysraphism

SPINAL DYSRAPHISM: This term encompasses all defects (open or closed) associated with a failure of closure of the posterior neural arch.

Embryology

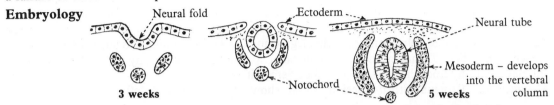

Neural fold / Ectoderm / Neural tube / Notochord / Mesoderm – develops into the vertebral column

3 weeks   5 weeks

Developmental errors may occur early in fetal life and lead to a variety of spinal defects:

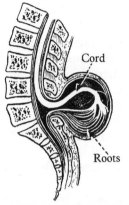

Cord

Roots

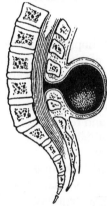

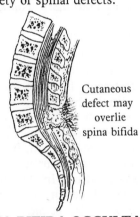

Cutaneous defect may overlie spina bifida

MYELOMEMINGOCELE

The spinal cord and roots protrude through the bony defect and lie within a cystic cavity, lined with meninges and/or skin. In most patients, the meningeal covering ruptures and the spinal cord and roots lie exposed to the air – myelodysplasia. CSF may leak from the open lesion.

Site: 80% occur in the lumbo-sacral region.

Incidence: 2/1000 births in Britain, but there is a geographical variation (0.2/1000 in Japan). A familial incidence increases the risk (5% if a sibling is affected). This suggests a genetic factor.

Associated abnormalities: *Hydrocephalus*
Arnold-Chiari, type II.
Aqueduct forking.

MENINGOCELE

Cystic CSF filled cavity – lined with meninges but devoid of neural tissue. The cavity communicates with the spinal canal through the bone defect (usually lumbosacral). Meningoceles occur far less frequently than myelomeningocele; they are rarely associated with other congenital anomalies.

SPINA BIFIDA OCCULTA

A bony deficit – present in 5–10% of the population and not clinically significant. Those who also have a lumbosacral cutaneous abnormality however (*tuft of hair, dimple, sinus or 'port wine' stain*) have a high incidence of related underlying defects:

- *diastomatomyelia*
- *lipoma*
- *dermoid cyst.*

These defects may cause symptoms of pain or neurological impairment after many years.

Spinal Dysraphism

Clinical Assessment

Myelomeningocele: This lesion should be carefully examined for the presence of neural elements. Transillumination of the sac may help. Observation of movement in the limbs and in specific muscle groups, occurring spontaneously and in response to pain applied both above and below the level of the lesion, helps determine the degree and level of neurological damage. Also note the presence of a dilated bladder and a patulous anal sphincter. Look for any associated congenital anomalies e.g. hydrocephalus, scoliosis, foot deformities.

Meningocele: Patients with this lesion seldom show any neurological deficit.

Investigations: Not required at the initial stage.

Management

Myelomenigocele: Advances in both orthopaedic and urological procedures have considerably improved the long-term management of the associated disabilities in most patients. Active treatment, however, in patients with gross hydrocephalus, complete paraplegia and other multiple anomalies as well as the spinal dysraphism, may merely prolong a painful existence. In these patients, many adopt a thoughtful conservative approach.

Immediate treatment requires closure and replacement of the neural tissues into the spinal canal to prevent infection. If necessary, this initial step provides more time to consider the wisdom of embarking on further active management.

Meningocele: In the presence of a CSF leak, urgent excision is performed; otherwise this is deferred, perhaps indefinitely if the lesion is small.

Spina bifida occulta: No treatment is required, although in patients with a cutaneous abnormality (and a higher incidence of an intraspinal anomaly), some recommend investigation with a view to prophylactic treatment.

Antenatal diagnosis

Screening the maternal serum and amniotic fluid for alpha-fetoprotein in high risk patients (e.g. with an affected sibling) provides an effective method of detecting neural tube defects and gives the parents the possibility of therapeutic abortion. In the long term this may reduce the incidence of this condition.

Spinal Dysraphism

DIASTOMATOMYELIA: a congenital splitting of part of the spinal cord usually at the upper lumbar vertebral level.

A *bony, fibrous* or *cartilagenous spur* often extends directly across the spinal canal in an antero-posterior direction. The split cord does not always reunite distal to the spur (diplomyelia). In most patients, the conus medullaris lies well below its normal level, *'tethered'* by the filum terminale. Since vertebral growth proceeds more rapidly than growth of the spinal cord, tethering may produce progressive back pain or neurological impairment as the spinal cord is stretched.

Spur

Low conus medullaris

'Tight' filum terminale

Straight X-ray
  └ may reveal associated congenital anomalies: spina bifida occulta, fused or hemivertebrae.
  └ tomography may demonstrate a bony spur.

Myelography combined with CT scan: provides more definitive evidence of diastomatomyelia and clearly demonstrates the presence of a bony spur and the level of the conus medullaris.

Management: Although some recommend prophylactic exploration – despite the absence of neurological impairment, most reserve operative treatment for those who present with a neurological deficit, especially if there is evidence of progression, or prior to the correction of any spinal deformity. At operation, any spur is removed and if tethering exists, the filum terminale and any fibrous bands are divided.

LIPOMENINGOCELE

Lipomas may occur in association with spinal dysraphism and range from purely intraspinal lesions to very large masses extending along with neural tissues through the bony defect. All are adherent to the conus and closely related to the lumbo-sacral roots, preventing complete removal and increasing operative hazards.

CONGENITAL DERMAL SINUS TRACT / DERMOID CYST

This congenital defect results from a failure of separation of neuronal from epithelial ectoderm and may occur with other midline fusion defects e.g. diastomatomyelia and a tethered cord. A tiny sinus in the lumbo-sacral region may represent the opening of a blind ending duct or may extend into the spinal canal. Dermoid cysts arise at any point along the sinus tract and often lie adjacent to the conus.

Clinical presentation varies from repeated attacks of unexplained meningitis to neurological deficits arising from the presence of an intraspinal mass. Treatment involves excision of the whole tract and any associated cyst (after treating any meningitic infection).

411

SECTION IV

**Localised Neurological Disease
and its Management**

C. Peripheral Nerve and Muscle

The Polyneuropathies — Functional Anatomy

The function of the peripheral nervous system is to carry impulses to and from the central nervous system. These impulses regulate motor, sensory and autonomic activities.

The peripheral nervous system is comprised of structures which lie outside the pial membrane of the brainstem and spinal cord and can be divided into cranial, spinal and autonomic components.

The STRUCTURE of the NERVE CELL and AXON

Each axon represents an elongation of the nerve cell – this lying within the central nervous system e.g. anterior horn cell, or in an outlying ganglion e.g. dorsal root ganglion. The cell body maintains the viability of the axon, being the centre of all cellular metabolic activity.

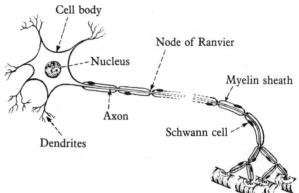

Many axons are surrounded by an insulation of myelin, which is enveloped by the Schwann cell membrane. Myelin is a protein-lipid complex. The membrane of the Schwann cell 'spirals' around the axon resulting in the formation of a multilayered myelin sheath.

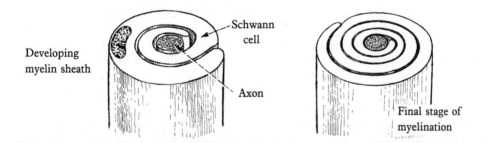

All axons have a cellular sheath – Schwann cell – but not all axons are myelinated.

Schwann cells with associated myelin are 250–1000 μm in length and separated from each other by the node of Ranvier. The axon is bare at this node and, during conduction, impulses jump from one node to the next – *saltatory* conduction. The rate of conduction is markedly increased in comparison with unmyelinated fibres. Myelin thus facilitates fast conduction. In unmyelinated fibres conduction depends upon the diameter of the nerve fibre; this determining the rate of longitudinal current flow.

415

The Polyneuropathies — Functional Anatomy

The SPINAL PERIPHERAL NERVOUS SYSTEM

Entry to and exit from the central nervous system is achieved by paired spinal nerve roots (31 in all).

These dorsal and ventral roots lie in the spinal subarachnoid space and come together at the intervertebral foramen to form the spinal nerve.

The dorsal root contains sensory fibres, arising from specialised sensory receptors in the periphery.

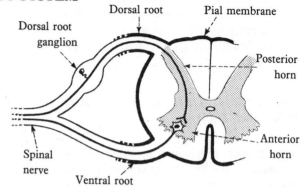

The dorsal root ganglia are collections of sensory cell bodies with axons extending peripherally as well as a central process which passes into the spinal cord in the region of the posterior horn of grey matter and makes appropriate central connections.

Sensation can be divided into:

Pain and Temperature
Simple Touch
Discriminatory Sensation – proprioception, vibration.

These different forms of sensation are carried from the periphery by axons with specific characteristics. The central connections and pathways vary also (see page 186).

The anterior horns of the spinal cord contain cell bodies whose axons pass to the periphery to innervate skeletal muscle – the alpha motor neurones. Smaller cell bodies also project into the anterior root and innervate the intrafusal muscle fibres of muscle spindles – the gamma motor neurones.

Each alpha motor neurone through its peripheral ramifications will innervate a number of muscle fibres. The number of fibres innnervated from a single cell varies from less than 20 in the eye muscles to more than 1000 in the large limb muscles (innervation ratio). The alpha motor neurone with its complement of muscle fibres is termed the *motor unit*.

PERIPHERAL NERVES

Peripheral nerves are composed of many axons bound together by connective tissue. A 'mixed' nerve contains motor, sensory and autonomic axons.

The blood supply to these bundles is by means of small nutrient vessels within the epineurium – the *vasa nervorum.*

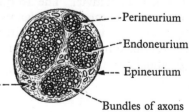

Cross section of nerve.

- Perineurium
- Endoneurium
- Epineurium
- Bundles of axons

The Polyneuropathies — Functional Anatomy

Peripheral Nerves *(continued)*

Nerve fibre type.

Axons within the peripheral nerve vary structurally. This is related to function.
Three distinct fibre types can be distinguished:

> **Type A** 2 – 20 μm in diameter.
> Myelinated.
> *Function:* Motor and sensory (vibration, proprioception).
> Conduction velocity: 10 – 70 metres/second.
>
> **Type B** 3 μm diameter.
> Thinly myelinated.
> *Function:* Mainly preganglionic autonomic, some pain and temperature.
> Conduction velocity: 7 – 15 metres/second.
>
> **Type C** < 1 μm diameter.
> Unmyelinated.
> *Function:* Sensory – pain and temperature.
> Conduction velocity: < 2 metres/second.

The structure of the spinal peripheral nervous system has been considered but the arrangement is also important. Spinal nerves, after emerging from the intervertebral foramen pass into the brachial plexus to supply the upper limbs and the lumbo-sacral plexus to supply the lower limbs.

The thoracic nerves supply skeletal muscles and subserve sensation of the thorax and abdomen.

The Autonomic Nervous System is described on page 442.

Patterns of Injury

Damage may occur to: axon, myelin sheath, cell body, supporting connective tissue, nutrient blood supply to nerves.

Three basic pathological processes occur:

WALLERIAN DEGENERATION	SEGMENTAL DEGENERATION	DISTAL AXONAL DEGENERATION

WALLERIAN DEGENERATION

Degeneration of axon distally following its interruption.

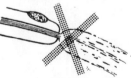

The axon disintegrates and the myelin breaks up into globules.

Regeneration of nerve is possible because the basement membrane of the Schwann cell survives and a new axon may grow down.

SEGMENTAL DEGENERATION

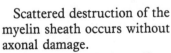

Scattered destruction of the myelin sheath occurs without axonal damage.

The primary lesion affects the Schwann cell.

DISTAL AXONAL DEGENERATION

Damage to the cell body or to the axon will affect the viability of the axon which will 'die back' from the periphery. Loss of the myelin sheath occurs as a secondary event.

Recovery is slow here because the axon must regenerate. When the cell body is destroyed no regrowth will occur.

417

The Polyneuropathies – Symptoms

Sensory:

Negative phenomena – loss of sensation.

Disease of large myelinated fibres produces loss of touch and joint position perception. Patients complain of difficulty in discriminating textures. Their hands and feet feel like cotton wool. Gait is unsteady, especially when in darkness where vision cannot compensate for loss of joint position sensation (proprioception).

Disease of small unmyelinated fibres produces loss of pain and temperature appreciation as a consequence of which painless burns/trauma result. Damage to joints without pain results in a 'neuropathic' joint (Charcot's joint) in which traumatic deformity is totally painless.

Positive phenomena

Disease of large myelinated fibres produces paraesthesia – a 'pins and needles' sensation with a peripheral distal distribution.

Disease of small unmyelinated fibres produces painful positive phenomena:

Burning extremities.

Dysaesthesia – when touching is painful.

Hyperalgesia – when threshold to pain appears lowered.

Hyperpathia – when threshold to pain appears elevated but, once reached, the painful stimulus is excessively felt.

Lightning pains take the form of sudden, very severe shooting pains and are virtually pathognemonic of tabes dorsalis.

Causalgia results from partial or incomplete nerve trauma and has an unpleasant diffuse burning quality to it.

Motor:

The patient notices weakness:

When distal e.g. difficulty in clearing the kerb when walking.

When proximal e.g. difficulty in climbing stairs or combing hair.

Cramps may be troublesome.

Twitching of muscles (fasciculation) may be felt.

The Polyneuropathies – Signs

Sensory examination:

All modalities are tested.
Light touch.
Two point discrimination. ⎫ Functions of large
Vibration sensation. ⎬ myelinated sensory
Joint position perception. ⎭ fibres.
Temperature perception. ⎫ Functions of small unmyelinated
Pain perception. ⎭ and thinly myelinated sensory fibres.

Initially the area of total sensory loss is defined. The test object e.g. a pin, should be moved from anaesthetic to normal area; it is more accurate to state when an object is felt rather than when it disappears.

In polyneuropathies, sensory loss is symmetrical and follows a characteristic stocking and glove distribution.

Examination of gait is important; with joint position impairment, sensory ataxia is evident. Rhomberg's test is positive (see page 178). Neuropathic burns/ulcers or joints may be present.

Trophic changes: Cold blue extremities.
Cutaneous hair loss.
Brittle finger/toe nails occasionally occur.

The Axon Reflex can be used to 'place' lesions in the sensory pathway.
Normally: The skin is scratched – local vasoconstriction (white reaction),
next – local oedema (red reaction)
and finally – surrounding vasodilatation or flare.

The flare is dependent upon the sensory axon.

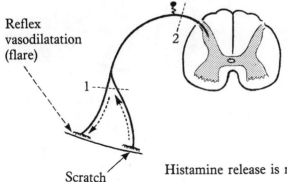

Reflex
vasodilatation
(flare)

Scratch

1. A distal sensory lesion will result in an absent flare response.

2. A proximal root lesion will not impair the response.

Histamine release is responsible for local vasodilatation/oedema.

The Polyneuropathies – Signs

Motor examination:

Muscle wasting is evident in subacute or chronic mixed or motor neuropathies. Oedema of immobile limbs may mask such a change. All muscle groups should be noted. The 1st dorsal interosseous muscle in the upper limbs and extensor digitorum brevis in the lower limbs are muscles which commonly show wasting in the neuropathies. The muscles should be examined for fasciculations – irregular twitches of groups of muscle fibres; this may be induced by exercise or muscle percussion and suggests anterior horn cell disease.

Muscle power is next to be tested. The pattern of weakness – proximal or distal, symmetrical or asymmetrical, flexors or extensors – must be properly analysed in order to locate the site of the cause of weakness (see Muscle weakness, page 180).   In the neuropathies, weakness is symmetrical generally and either distal or proximal in distribution.

The degree of weakness is 'scored' using the MRC (Medical Research Council) scale:

  Score 0 – No contraction.
  Score 1 – Flicker.
  Score 2 – Active movement/gravity eliminated.
  Score 3 – Active movement against gravity.
  Score 4 – Active movement against gravity and resistance.
  Score 5 – Normal power.

Weakness is proportional to the number of motor neurones acutely involved. It may develop suddenly or very slowly and, usually symmetrical, it is noticed at the extremities – usually lower limbs first – and gradually spreads or ascends into more proximal muscles.

The reason for the onset of symptoms distally is supposedly due to the 'dying back' of the axons towards their nerve cells – the longest ones being the most vulnerable.

Some neuropathies affect proximal muscle groups preferentially – Guillain Barre neuropathy and diabetic neuropathy – both are demyelinating neuropathies, whereas axonal neuropathies usually affect the longest axons initially and present with distal weakness.

In severe neuropathies, truncal and respiratory muscle involvement occurs. Respiratory muscle weakness may result in death.

The Tendon Reflexes:
  The tendon reflex is dependent upon:
    1. The gamma motor neurone activity.
    2. Intrafusal fibres of the muscle spindles.
    3. The spindle sensory nerves.
    4. The alpha motor neurone.

Reflexes commonly tested:

Deltoid ——— C5   – Circumflex nerve.   Triceps- C7,8 – Radial nerve.
Biceps ——— C5,6 – Musculocutaneous nerve.   Knee— L3,4 – Femoral nerve.
Brachioradialis- C5,6 – Radial nerve.   Ankle — S1,2 – Sciatic nerve.

The tendon reflexes are lost when any component of the reflex response is affected by disease. Reflexes are lost early in peripheral neuropathies when power and muscle bulk appear normal. Distal reflexes are generally lost before proximal ones.

The Polyneuropathies – Classification

There are several approaches to classification:

    by MODE of ONSET – Acute, subacute, chronic.
    by FUNCTIONAL DISTURBANCE – Motor, sensory, autonomic, mixed.
    by PATHOLOGICAL PROCESS – Axonal, demyelinating.
    by CAUSATION – e.g. infections; carcinomatous, diabetic, inflammatory, vascular.

Such a mixed classification has descriptive value and helps towards causative diagnosis. For instance, an acute motor demyelinating neuropathy usually denotes the post-infectious polyneuropathy of Guillain-Barré. Whereas the chronic mixed axonal neuropathy may indicate a search for underlying neoplasia.

Clinically it is of most value to classify the neuropathies according to mode of onset.

The following table is for reference. Certain neuropathies will be dealt with separately (see pages 425–429).

ACUTE	CAUSE	FUNCTIONAL DISTURBANCE	PATHOLOGY
A few days – 4 weeks	**Idiopathic** (Post-infectious Guillain-Barré)	Predominantly motor. Distal or proximal Autonomic disturbance.	Demyelination with perivascular lymphocytic infiltration.
	Diphtheria	Cranial nerve onset. Mixed motor/sensory.	Demyelinative. No inflammatory infiltration.
	Porphyria	Motor (may begin in arm). Autonomic disturbance. Minimal sensory loss.	Axonal.

SUBACUTE			
Develop over weeks	**Drug Induced** Isoniazid, Metronidazole, Phenytoin, Nitrofurantoin, Vincristine, etc.	Vincristine severe. Usually mild sensory, motor disturbance. Dapsone – pure motor involvement.	Axonal degeneration.
	Heavy Metals Solvents, Lead, Mercury, Arsenic, Thallium.	Usually sensory, motor disturbance; severity related to dose. Lead – severe, predominantly motor with arms involved first.	Lead – axonal degeneration with segmental demyelination. Other heavy metals and solvents produce axonal degeneration.
	Nutritional Deficiency B complex (includes alcoholic neuropathy)	Sensory disturbance with 'burning feet' and other painful dysaesthesiae. Motor component may be present and severe. Autonomic disturbance is common but only mild.	Axonal degeneration with segmental demyelination. (Demyelination is minimal in alcoholic neuropathy.)

The Polyneuropathies – Classification

CHRONIC	CAUSE	FUNCTIONAL DISTURBANCE	PATHOLOGY
Develop over months, years.	**Malignant disease** Carcinoma, Lymphoma, Myeloma.	Sensory or sensory/motor disturbance. May predate recognition of malignancy by some years.	Axonal degeneration.
	Paraproteinaemias Hypergamma-globulinaemia.	Sensory/motor disturbance.	Axonal or demyelinative degeneration.
	Collagenosis (Connective tissue disorders) Rheumatoid arthritis, Polyarteritis nodosa, Scleroderma, Systemic lupus erythematosis.	In rheumatoid arthritis multiple mononeuropathy is common. Motor/sensory disturbance is rare. Systemic lupus eryhtematosis – mild motor/sensory disturbance. Polyarteritis nodosa usually produces multiple mononeuropathy.	Occlusion of nutrient blood vessels to nerves (vasa nervorum).
	Amyloid disease Primary, familial or secondary	Motor/sensory disturbance with autonomic involvement. Also may develop 'entrapment' neuropathies.	Thickened nerves with amyloid deposition as well as small fibre axonal degeneration.
	Metabolic disorders Diabetes, Uraemia, Hypothyroidism.	Uraemic neuropathy is sensory/motor in type. Hypothyroidism produces mild sensory/motor disturbance. Diabetic neuropathy takes many forms.	Axonal degeneration.
	Hereditary neuropathies e.g. Peroneal muscular atrophy (Charcot-Marie-Tooth disease)	Mainly motor with some sensory features. Wasting is distal, peroneal muscles first. Dominant inheritance. Childhood onset usually.	Demyelinative type and axonal degenerative or neuronal type.
	Hypertrophic polyneuropathy (Dejerine-Sottas disease)	Onset in childhood with sensory symptoms followed by progressive distal weakness and wasting. Claw hand and foot deformity common. Autosomal recessive inheritance.	Recurrent demyelination and remyelination with Schwann cell hypertrophy.
	Refsum's disease	A phytanic acid storage disorder. Onset in first decade and slowly progressive. A severe sensorimotor neuropathy with associated cerebellar ataxia, ichthyosis, pigmentory retinal degeneration, deafness and cardiac abnormalities. Elevated serum phytanate.	Schwann cell hyperplasia – hypertrophic neuropathy.

Investigation of Neuropathy

Despite extensive investigation, the cause of chronic neuropathy cannot be identified in 30% of such cases.

The following conditions require exclusion before a chronic neuropathy is classified as idiopathic or of unknown aetiology: Diabetes, uraemia, deficiency states, connective tissue disorders, underlying malignancy, hereditary neuropathy. Toxic causes must be considered.

The cause of acute or subacute neuropathy can usually be defined. Here, CSF examination may prove a useful diagnostic investigation e.g. post-infectious polyneuropathy.

Special investigations

1. NERVE CONDUCTION STUDIES

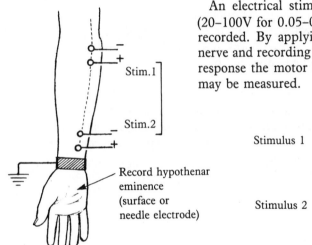

An electrical stimulus is applied at points along a nerve (20–100V for 0.05–0.1msec) and the evoked muscle response recorded. By applying a stimulus at various points along a nerve and recording the latency between stimulus and muscle response the motor conduction velocity of a particular nerve may be measured.

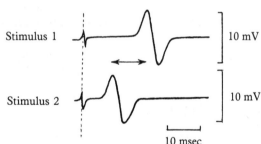

Motor conduction velocity can be measured in most motor peripheral nerves from the brachial plexus in the upper limbs and sciatic and femoral outlets in the lower limbs.

These studies not only aid in the diagnosis of generalised neuropathies but also in entrapments e.g. ulnar nerve at elbow or median nerve at wrist (carpal tunnel syndrome).

Investigation of Neuropathy

Sensory conduction can also be measured:

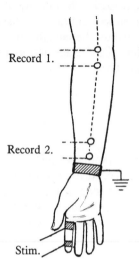

Record 1.

Record 2.

Stim.

The index finger is stimulated and the evoked sensory potential recorded at wrist and elbow. Measurements enable calculation to be made of the latencies and conduction velocity. Note the considerable difference in amplitude between sensory and motor evoked potentials.

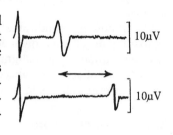

GENERAL OBSERVATIONS

Amplitude of response – a function of the number of axons which respond to stimulation.

Latency of response – a function of the speed at which the largest fibres in a nerve will conduct.

Distance travelled divided by time taken = CONDUCTION VELOCITY.

Axonal degeneration ⟶ *reduced amplitude or absence of response* to stimulation with mild slowing of conduction velocity.

Demyelinative disorders ⟶ marked *slowing of conduction velocity (30% at least reduced) with progressive reduction of amplitude.*

Localised compression of nerve ⟶ slowing of conduction in region of block e.g. over the elbow when ulnar nerve is compressed there.

2. ELECTROMYOGRAPHY

A fine needle is inserted into the muscle and the recorded activity displayed on an oscilloscope.

Electromyography is primarily of value in muscle disease but can also give indirect evidence of a neuropathic process.

If chronic denervation has occurred, re-innervation may be present with long duration high amplitude motor unit potentials.

Also, with voluntary effort, poor recruitment of motor units is seen on the oscilloscope screen.

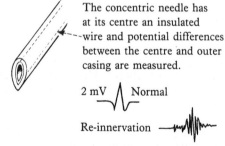

The concentric needle has at its centre an insulated wire and potential differences between the centre and outer casing are measured.

2 mV — Normal

Re-innervation —

Long duration, high amplitude, polyphasia.

3. NERVE BIOPSY

In neuropathies of uncertain cause, light and electron microscopy examination occasionally help diagnosis. The sural nerve is usually chosen for biopsy.

424

The Polyneuropathies – Specific Types

ACUTE IDIOPATHIC POST-INFECTIOUS POLYNEUROPATHY (syn. GUILLAIN-BARRÉ Syndrome)

Clinical features

50 per cent of patients describe an infectious illness in the 4 weeks prior to the onset of neuropathy.

Sensory symptoms prevail at the beginning with paraesthesia of feet, then hands. Pain, especially back pain, is an occasional initial symptom. Weakness next develops – this may be generalised, proximal in distribution or commence distally and ascend. In severe cases, respiratory and bulbar involvement occurs. Weakness is maximal three weeks after the onset of neurological symptoms. Tracheostomy/ventilation is required in 10 per cent of cases. Facial weakness is present to some extent in 50% of cases. Papilloedema may occur when CSF protein is markedly elevated (blocked arachnoid villi?). Autonomic involvement – tachycardia, fluctuating blood pressure, retention of urine – develops in some cases.

Sensory signs occur infrequently.

Investigations

CSF protein is elevated in most patients but may not be so until the second or third week of illness.

The γglobulin fraction is usually raised.

Cells are often absent but in 20% of cases up to 40 cells/mm^3 may be found.

Nerve conduction studies

When carried out early in the illness, these may be normal; this reflects the tendency initially for nerve root involvement with lesser distal damage. Later conduction velocities become prolonged.

Virological investigation

Viral studies occasionally reveal rising titres to specific viruses such as Ebstein Barr, cytomegalovirus.

Aetiology/Pathology

The condition occurs following virus infection but also with other infections e.g. mycoplasma, gram -ve infection, and following surgery or trauma.

The finding of decreased suppressor T cell response suggests a cell mediated immunological reaction directed at peripheral nerves.

Pathologically, segmental demyelination results with axonal damage if the process is severe. Perivascular infiltration with lymphocytes occurs around nerve roots. Lymphocytes probably release cytotoxic substances which damage Schwann cell/myelin. Macrophage infiltration then occurs with removal of myelin.

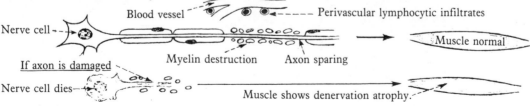

When axon damage and nerve cell death occur, regeneration cannot take place.

425

The Polyneuropathies – Specific Types

Acute Idiopathic Post-infectious Polyneuropathy *(continued)*

Treatment

Treatment is mainly supportive, with management of the paralysed patient and occasionally management of respiratory failure by ventilation.

The effectiveness of specific immunosuppressive therapy – steroids and cytotoxic drugs – is disappointing and anecdotal; indeed, steroids have been found ineffective in a controlled trial. Plasmapheresis is disappointing unless commenced very early in the clinical course.

Outcome

Mortality is 10 per cent of all cases.

Of those in respiratory failure, 20% are severely disabled for life and 10% moderately

In milder cases the outcome is excellent.   disabled.

Physical signs, e.g. areflexia, may persist despite return to normal function.

Of all patients, 5% develop a chronic relapsing course.

Cranial nerve variant

This presents with disproportionate involvement of cranial nerves – diplopia, facial weakness. Ataxia and areflexia also occur.

This variant of Guillain-Barré was described by Miller Fisher and bears his name.

A pure autonomic variant may also occur (see page 445).

CHRONIC RELAPSING POLYNEUROPATHY

A tendency to recurrent neuropathy is seen in the hereditary neuropathies and is characteristic of acute intermittent porphyria.

Idiopathic polyneuropathy also may become recurrent, each attack identical to the acute post-infectious presentation. With increasing episodes, neurological disability will ensue.

Pathologically, segmental demyelination with lymphocytic infiltration occurs. Eventually the nerves show hypertrophy with concentric Schwann cell proliferation reminiscent of an 'onion bulb'.

This condition is sometimes remarkably steroid responsive with relapse often on reduction of dosage. In the acute stage, plasmapheresis may be beneficial.

The Polyneuropathies – Specific Types

DIABETIC NEUROPATHY

Peripheral nerve damage is related to poor control of diabetes.

Pain and paraesthesia occur in up to 40 per cent of long standing diabetics but clinical signs are found in under 10 per cent. Neuropathy is uncommon in childhood and increases with age.

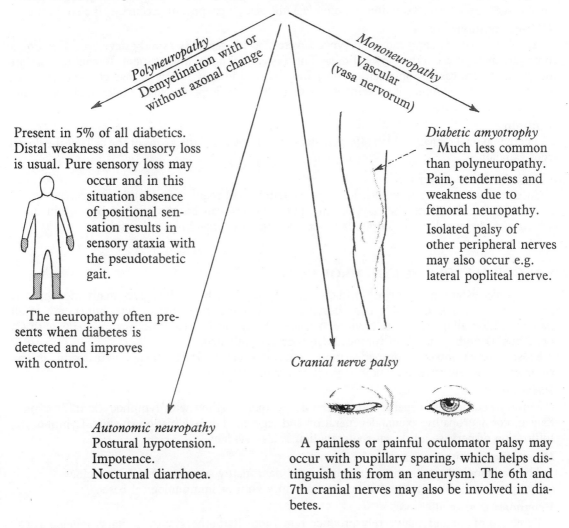

Polyneuropathy
Demyelination with or
without axonal change

Mononeuropathy
Vascular
(vasa nervorum)

Present in 5% of all diabetics. Distal weakness and sensory loss is usual. Pure sensory loss may occur and in this situation absence of positional sensation results in sensory ataxia with the pseudotabetic gait.

Diabetic amyotrophy
– Much less common than polyneuropathy. Pain, tenderness and weakness due to femoral neuropathy.

Isolated palsy of other peripheral nerves may also occur e.g. lateral popliteal nerve.

The neuropathy often presents when diabetes is detected and improves with control.

Cranial nerve palsy

Autonomic neuropathy
Postural hypotension.
Impotence.
Nocturnal diarrhoea.

A painless or painful oculomator palsy may occur with pupillary sparing, which helps distinguish this from an aneurysm. The 6th and 7th cranial nerves may also be involved in diabetes.

The prognosis is good in these complications of diabetes. Better control of diabetes should lead to improvement, though less so when autonomic features predominate. This is discussed on page 445.

The Polyneuropathies – Specific Types

PORPHYRIA
Acute intermittent porphyria is an autosomal dominant disorder in which symptoms of abdominal pain, psychosis, convulsions and peripheral neuropathy occur.

The metabolic fault occurs in the liver. An increased production of porphobilinogen is reflected by its increased urinary excretion. δ-amino laevulic acid, a porphyrin precursor, is also increased.

Clinical features
Acute in onset. Chiefly motor in type. Severe flaccid weakness rapidly develops. The upper limbs are more affected than lower limbs. There is cranial nerve involvement. Respiratory failure occurs in severe cases. Some sensory loss may occur and may follow a characteristic proximal distribution. Autonomic involvement with tachycardia/hypertension, abdominal pain and vomiting may occur.

Pathology
There is axonal damage which affects distal motor nerves and the axons of the cells of the dorsal root ganglion.

Clinical course is variable
Spontaneous recovery in weeks. Respiratory failure will require ventilation and carries a poor prognosis. Recurrent attacks may be anticipated. These can be precipitated by certain drugs which must be avoided e.g. sulphonamides, barbiturates, phenytoin, griseofulvin.

CARCINOMATOUS POLYNEUROPATHY
A chronic distal sensory or sensorimotor neuropathy which develops over many months.   It appears to be a non-metastatic complication of carcinoma, myeloma or lymphoma. 5% of all patients with malignant disease have such a neuropathy. 50% of cases occur in patients with Ca bronchus, though all types of tumour have been incriminated.

Sensimotor or mixed neuropathy most commonly occur. Pure sensory neuropathy is less common; here sensory ataxia may be profound and disabling.

Pathology
Sensory neuropathy: degeneration of the dorsal root ganglion with lymphocytic infiltration. Sensimotor neuropathy: axonal degeneration and segmental demyelination co-exist. Lymphocytic infiltration of nerves and dorsal root ganglion is also evident.

Causation remains unclear.
The pathological similarities with nutritional neuropathy suggest a similar aetiology.

Lymphocytic infiltrates suggest an inflammatory viral or immunological basis.

Prognosis is generally poor.
Resection of tumour may rarely produce remission. Radiotherapy to 'solitary' myeloma may result in excellent prognosis. Steroids occasionally are of benefit.

428

The Polyneuropathies – Specific Types

PERONEAL MUSCULAR ATROPHY – CHARCOT-MARIE-TOOTH DISEASE

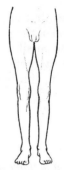

Characterised by distal wasting of lower limbs which usually stops at low thigh level, spreading to upper limbs. The legs resemble an inverted wine bottle. Pes cavus deformity of the feet develops. When the hands become involved, claw-like deformity is seen. Sensory signs are usually mild.

Age of onset varies from childhood to middle age.

Inheritance is usually autosomal dominant.

Progression is slow with periods of stability.

Clinical variants occur e.g. involvement of upper limbs alone.

Pathology

Various forms of this disorder are recognised:

Hypertrophic type — Segmental demyelination and hypertrophy with 'onion bulb' formation.

Neuronal type — Anterior horn cell/motor axon damage. No segmental demyelination.

Spinal muscular atrophy type — Anterior horn cell/motor axon damage. Usually autosomal dominant but occasionally recessive.

Clinically, these types differ and separation is aided by nerve conduction studies which reveal velocities as low as 15 m/sec in the hypertrophic type.

Treatment

Correction of foot deformities may be helpful.

PROGRESSIVE HYPERTROPHIC NEUROPATHY.   DEJERINE-SOTTAS DISEASE.

Commences in early childhood and is slowly progressive. Sensory symptoms are more prominent, otherwise the picture resembles peroneal muscular atrophy.

Inheritance is autosomal recessive.

The nerves can be seen or palpated with ease e.g. sural nerve or ulnar nerve.

Enlarged spinal roots may even result in spinal compression.

Nerve conduction velocity may be greatly reduced (5–10 m/sec).

Pathology

Enlargement seems due to connective tissue as well as Schwann cell whorling – 'onion bulb' formation.

Associated clinical features: Kyphosis is often found; myosis rarely.

ROUSSY-LEVY Syndrome

The features of distal limb wasting/weakness are associated with sensory ataxia, pes cavus.

The condition is separated from Friedreich's ataxia by the slow progression and lack of cerebellar signs, and slow conduction velocities.

Plexus Syndromes and Mononeuropathies.

Disease of a single peripheral or cranial nerve is termed *mononeuropathy*. When many single nerves are damaged one by one, this is described as *mononeuritis multiplex*. Damage to the brachial or lumbosacral plexus may produce widespread limb weakness which does not conform to the distribution of any one peripheral nerve. A knowledge of the anatomy and muscle innervation of the plexuses and peripheral nerves is essential to localise the site of lesion and thus deduce the possible causes.

Certain systemic illnesses are associated with the development of mononeuropathy or mononeuritis multiplex:

- diabetes mellitus.
- sarcoidosis.
- rheumatoid arthritis.
- polyarteritis nodosa.

Entrapment mononeuropathies result from damage to a nerve where it passes through a tight space such as the median nerve under the flexor retinaculum of the wrist. These are often related to conditions such as acromegaly, myxoedema and pregnancy, in which soft tissue swelling occurs. A familial tendency to entrapment neuropathy occasionally exists.

Cranial nerve mononeuropathies are dealt with separately.

The BRACHIAL PLEXUS

The plexus lies in the posterior triangle of the neck between scalenius anterior and scalenius medius muscles.

At the root of the neck the plexus lies behind the clavicle.

The plexus itself gives off several important motor branches:
1. Nerve to rhomboids.
2. Long thoracic nerve
   – to serratus ant.
3. Pectoral nerves
   – to pectoralis major.
4. Suprascapular nerve
   – to supraspinatus and infraspinatus.

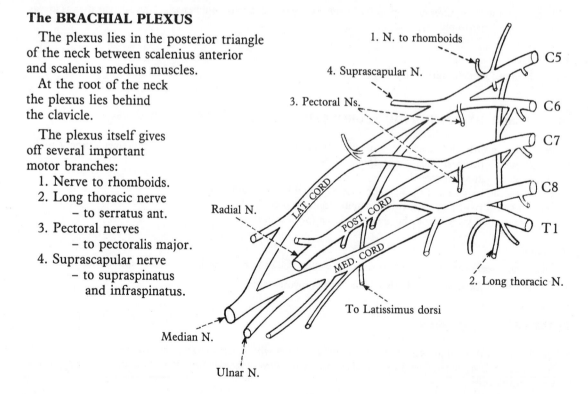

Brachial Plexus Syndromes

UPPER PLEXUS LESION
Erb-Duchenne Paralysis ($C_5 C_6$)

Traction on the arm at birth or falling on the shoulder may damage the upper part ($C_5 C_6$) of the plexus.

Deltoid ⎫
Supraspinatus ⎬ paralysed.
Infraspinatus ⎭

Biceps ⎫
Brachialis ⎬ elbow flexors – also paralysed.

Adductors of shoulder – mildly affected.

When damage to $C_5 C_6$ is more proximal – nerve to rhomboid and long thoracic nerve may be affected.

POSTERIOR CORD LESION ($C_5 C_6 C_7 C_8$)

Deltoid ⎫
Extensors of elbow (triceps) ⎪
Extensors of wrist (extensor carpi radialis longus and brevis, ⎬ paralysed
                extensor carpi ulnaris) ⎪
Extensors of fingers (extensor digitorum) ⎭

LOWER PLEXUS LESION ($C_8 T_1$)

Paralysis of all the intrinsic muscles of hand (small muscles) with paralysis also of the finger flexors.

N.B. A combined ulnar and median nerve lesion will produce a similar picture in the hand but with involvement also of flexor carpi ulnaris and pronator teres.

Klumpke's Paralysis

Injury to $C_8 T_1$ roots following forced abduction of the shoulder. Results in a claw hand with $C_8 T_1$ sensory loss and often a sympathetic palsy – a Horner's syndrome (see page 132).

TOTAL BRACHIAL LESION

This results in complete flaccid paralysis and anaesthesia of the arm. The presence of a Horner's syndrome suggests that the lesion is proximal and following trauma suggests root avulsion.

N.B. When trauma is the cause of brachial paralysis, early referral to a specialist unit with experience in the surgical repair of plexus injuries is advised.

Brachial Plexus Syndromes

The THORACIC OUTLET SYNDROME

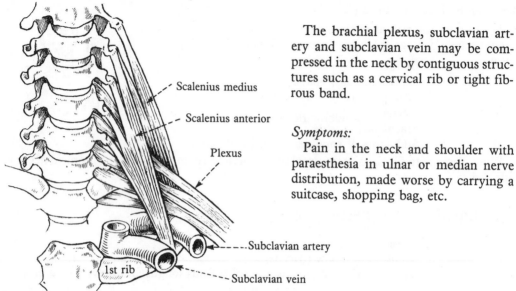

The brachial plexus, subclavian artery and subclavian vein may be compressed in the neck by contiguous structures such as a cervical rib or tight fibrous band.

Symptoms:

Pain in the neck and shoulder with paraesthesia in ulnar or median nerve distribution, made worse by carrying a suitcase, shopping bag, etc.

Signs:

Sensory loss detected in $\frac{1}{3}$ of patients.
Motor weakness and wasting ($C_8 T_1$) in $\frac{1}{2}$ of patients.
Signs of vascular compression:

> Unilateral Reynaud's phenomenon.
> Pallor of limb on elevation.
> Brittle trophic finger nails.
> Loss of radial pulse in arm on abduction and external rotation at the shoulder or on bracing the shoulders – ADSON's sign.
> Subclavian venous thrombosis may occur, especially after excessive usage of arm.

Investigation:

Plain radiology of the thoracic outlet may reveal a cervical rib or prolonged transverse process. Nerve conduction/electromyography may show a decrease in sensory potentials and evidence of denervation in the hand. Arteriography or venography is occasionally necessary if there are obvious vascular problems.

Treatment:

In middle aged people with poor posture and no evidence of abnormality on plain radiology, neck and postural exercises are helpful.

In young people with a cervical rib or abnormally long transverse process, exploration and removal or section of a fibrous band may afford relief.

Brachial Plexus Syndromes

BRACHIAL NEURITIS (Neuralgic amyotrophy)

Brachial neuritis is a relatively common disorder sometimes associated with:

Infection.
Injection of serum vaccine (3–10 days after typhoid, tetanus, etc.)
Strenuous exercise.
Following intravenous heroin abuse (mainlining)

Clinical features:

Acute onset with preceding shoulder pain.
Weakness is usually proximal, though the whole arm may be affected.
Occasionally both arms are affected simultaneously.
Sensory findings are negligible (loss over the outer aspect of the shoulder).
Reflex loss occurs.
Wasting is apparent after 3–6 weeks.
Recovery may be gradual over weeks or months and is not always complete.
Recurrent episodes can occur.

Differential diagnosis:

A painful weak arm.
Consider:
Cervical spondylosis.
Cervical disc lesion.
Brachialgia due to local bursitis.
Polymyalgia rheumatica.

Investigation:

Viral titres may be positive e.g. Coxsackie.

CSF may show a mild protein rise and a pleocytosis.

Nerve conduction studies will show slowing in affected nerves after 7–10 days.

When episodes are recurrent there is often a family history.
Familial Brachial Neuritis is associated with abnormalities of peripheral nerves (thickened myelin sheath) and electrical evidence on nerve conduction studies of a diffuse neuropathy.

PANCOAST's TUMOUR

Involvement of the plexus by an apical lung tumour (usually squamous cell carcinoma). The lower cervical and upper thoracic roots are involved.

Clinical features:

– severe pain.
– weak wasted hand muscles.
– sensory loss ($C_8 T_1$).
– Horner's syndrome.

BRACHIAL NEUROPATHY FOLLOWING RADIOTHERAPY

Irradiation of the axilla for breast carcinoma may damage the brachial plexus.
Onset may be delayed for some months.
Entrapment of the plexus by resultant fibrosis seems the probable cause.

Upper Limb Mononeuropathies

The LONG THORACIC NERVE (C$_5$C$_6$C$_7$)

Supplies: Serratus anterior muscle

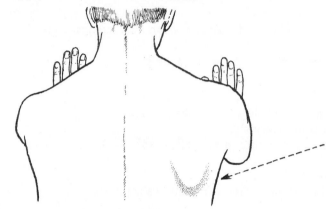

Damaged by:
Carrying heavy objects.
Strapping the shoulder.
Limited brachial neuritis.
Diabetes mellitus.

Results in:
Winging of the scapula
when arms are
stretched in front.

The SUPRASCAPULAR NERVE (C$_5$C$_6$)

Supplies: Supraspinatus and
Infraspinatus muscles.

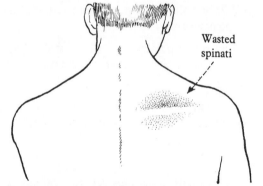

Wasted
spinati

Damaged by:
[as for Long Thoracic Nerve (above)]

Results in:
Weakness of abduction of arm
(supraspinatus).
Weakness of external rotation of arm
(infraspinatus).

The AXILLARY NERVE (posterior cord) (C$_5$C$_6$)

Supplies: Deltoid and Teres minor muscles.

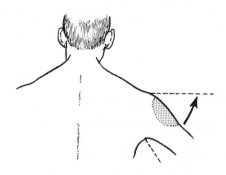

Damaged by:
Shoulder dislocation.
Limited brachial neuritis.

Results in:
Weakness of abduction of shoulder
between 15°–90°, and sensory loss
over the outer aspect of the shoulder.

Upper Limb Mononeuropathies

The MUSCULOCUTANEOUS NERVE (Lateral cord) $C_5 C_6$

Sensory supply: Lateral border of the arm.

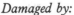

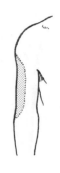

Damaged by:
Fracture of the humerus.
Systemic causes.

Results in:
Weakness of elbow flexion and forearm supination with characteristic sensory loss and absent biceps reflex.

Labels on diagram: Coracobrachialis, Biceps, Brachialis

The RADIAL NERVE (Posterior cord) $C_5 C_6 C_7 C_8$

Sensory supply: Dorsum of hand.

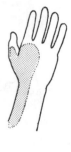

The nerve descends from the axilla, winding posteriorly around the humerus. The deep branch – the posterior interosseous nerve – lies in the posterior compartment of the forearm behind the interosseous membrane.

Damaged by:

Fractures of the humerus.
Prolonged tourniquet application.
Intramuscular injection.
Lipoma, fibroma or neuroma.
Systemic causes.

Results in:

Weakness and wasting of muscles supplied, characterised by wrist drop with flexed fingers (weak extensors). Sensory loss on dorsum of hand and forearm. Loss of triceps reflex (when lesion lies in the axilla) and supinator reflex.

Labels on diagram: Triceps, Brachioradialis, Extensor carpi radialis longus, Extensor carpi radialis brevis, Supinator, Anconeus, Extensor digitorum, Extensor digiti minimi, Extensor carpi ulnaris, Radius, Ulna, Abductor pollicis longus, Extensor pollicis longus, Extensor pollicis brevis, Extensor indicis

The *posterior interosseous branch* of the radial nerve can be compressed at its point of entry into the supinator muscle. The clinical picture is similar to a radial nerve palsy, only brachioradialis and wrist extensors are spared. Examination shows weakness of finger extension with little or no wrist drop.

Upper Limb Mononeuropathies

The MEDIAN NERVE (Lateral and medial cords) $C_7 C_8 T_1$

Sensory supply:

Palmar surfaces of the radial border of the hand.

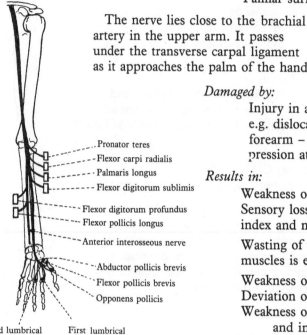

The nerve lies close to the brachial artery in the upper arm. It passes under the transverse carpal ligament as it approaches the palm of the hand.

- Pronator teres
- Flexor carpi radialis
- Palmaris longus
- Flexor digitorum sublimis
- Flexor digitorum profundus
- Flexor pollicis longus
- Anterior interosseous nerve
- Abductor pollicis brevis
- Flexor pollicis brevis
- Opponens pollicis
- Second lumbrical
- First lumbrical

Damaged by:

Injury in axilla
e.g. dislocation of shoulder, compression in the forearm – anterior interosseous branch, compression at the wrist (carpal tunnel syndrome).

Results in:

Weakness of abduction and apposition of thumb. Sensory loss is variable but most marked on index and middle fingers.

Wasting of thenar muscles is evident.

Weakness of pronation of the forearm. Deviation of wrist to ulnar side on wrist flexion. Weakness of flexion of distal phalanx of thumb and index finger.

The Carpal Tunnel Syndrome

Transverse carpal ligament

Median nerve

Flexor tendons

The median nerve is 'entrapped' under the transverse carpal ligament at the wrist.

Causes: Connective tissue thickening e.g.
Rheumatoid arthritis.
Acromegaly.
Hypothyroidism.
Infiltration of ligament e.g. Amyloid disease.
Fluid retention e.g. in pregnancy.
Weight gain.

Symptoms:

Pain, especially at night, and paraesthesia.

Objective findings may follow with cutaneous sensory loss and wasting and weakness of thenar muscles (abductor and opponens pollicis).

Nerve conduction studies are helpful in confirming diagnosis by showing slowing of conduction over the wrist.

Treatment: of the cause and local injection of hydrocortisone. Diuretics and surgical division of the transverse ligament may be necessary.

436

Upper Limb Mononeuropathies

The ULNAR NERVE (Medial cord) C_7C_8

Sensory supply:

Both palmar and dorsal surfaces of the ulnar border of the hand.

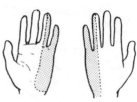

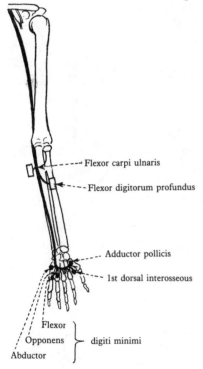

Flexor carpi ulnaris

Flexor digitorum profundus

Adductor pollicis

1st dorsal interosseous

Flexor
Opponens
Abductor
} digiti minimi

In the upper arm the nerve is closely related to the brachial artery and the median nerve, and passes behind the medial epicondyle of the humerus into the forearm,

In the hand, close to the hamate bone, it divides into deep and superficial branches.

Damaged by:

Injury at elbow either 'acute' e.g. dislocation, or 'delayed'.

Distal to the medial epicondyle, the ulnar nerve may be damaged by compression. Pressure on the nerve in the palm of the hand damages the deep branch resulting in wasting and weakness without sensory loss.

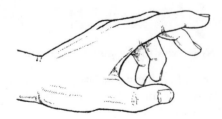

Results in:

Weakness and wasting of muscles supplied, with a characteristic posture of the hand – *Ulnar Claw Hand* – as well as sensory loss. The level of the lesion dictates the extent of the motor paralysis. Nerve conduction studies are helpful in confirming entrapment at the elbow.

Surgical transposition may be necessary in such cases.

Lumbosacral Plexus

The LUMBAR PLEXUS

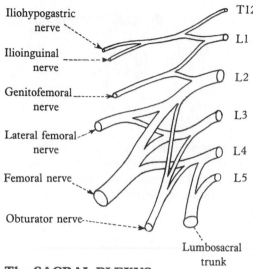

Iliohypogastric nerve

Ilioinguinal nerve

Genitofemoral nerve

Lateral femoral nerve

Femoral nerve

Obturator nerve

T12
L1
L2
L3
L4
L5

Lumbosacral trunk

The plexus is located in the psoas muscle. The important branches are the femoral and obturator nerves.

The femoral nerve $(L_2 L_3 L_4)$ emerges from the lateral border of the psoas muscle and leaves the abdomen laterally below the inguinal ligament with the femoral artery.

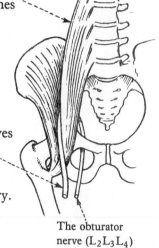

The obturator nerve $(L_2 L_3 L_4)$

The SACRAL PLEXUS

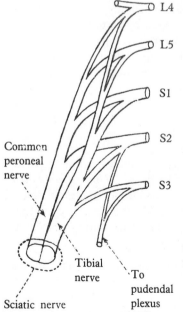

L4
L5
S1
S2
S3

Common peroneal nerve

Tibial nerve

To pudendal plexus

Sciatic nerve

The plexus is located on the posterior wall of the pelvis. The five roots of the plexus divide into anterior and posterior divisions. The $L_4 L_5 S_1 S_2$ divisions form the common peroneal nerve. The $L_4 L_5 S_1 S_2 S_3$ anterior divisions form the tibial nerve. Both these nerves fuse to form the sciatic nerve.

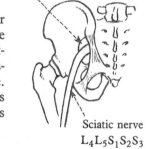

Greater sciatic foramen

Sciatic nerve $L_4 L_5 S_1 S_2 S_3$

The posterior divisions $S_2 S_3$ pass to the pudendal plexus.

The common peroneal and tibial nerves (sciatic nerve) leave the pelvis by the greater sciatic foramen. In the popliteal fossa the sciatic nerve splits into its constituent nerves.

438

Lumbosacral Plexus Syndromes

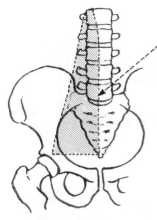

The proximity of the plexus to important abdominal and pelvic structures renders it liable to damage from diseases of these structures.

Trauma following abdominal or pelvic surgery e.g. hysterectomy, lumbar sympathectomy. Compression from an abdominal mass e.g. aortic aneurysm. Infiltration from tumour e.g. cervical carcinoma.

Symptoms may be unilateral or bilateral, depending upon causation. Weakness, sensory loss and reflex changes are dictated by the location and extent of plexus damage. Pain of a severe burning quality may be present; it may be worsened by coughing, sneezing, etc.

In general:

Lower plexus lesions produce:
Weakness of posterior thigh (hamstring) and foot muscles with posterior leg sensory loss.

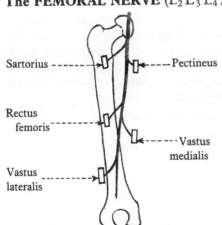

Upper plexus lesions produce:
Weakness of hip flexion and adduction with anterior leg sensory loss.

The lumbosacral plexus may be affected in the same way as the brachial plexus in brachial neuritis – lumbosacral neuritis – the association with infection etc., being similar. Recovery is usually good. Recurrent episodes may occur. Plexus lesions also occur in *diabetes mellitus* and *polyarteritis nodosa*. In both, the symptoms and signs may be bilateral.

Lower Limb Mononeuropathies

The FEMORAL NERVE ($L_2 L_3 L_4$)

Sartorius

Pectineus

Rectus femoris

Vastus medialis

Vastus lateralis

Damaged by:
Fractures of the upper femur.
Congenital dislocation of the hip.
Neoplastic infiltration.
Psoas muscle abscess.
Systemic ⟶ causes of mononeuropathy e.g. diabetes.

Results in:
Weakness of knee extension with wasting of thigh muscles.
Sensory loss over the anterior and medial aspects of the thigh.
The knee jerk is lost.

439

Lower Limb Mononeuropathies

The OBTURATOR NERVE ($L_2 L_3 L_4$)

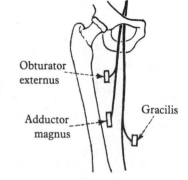

Damaged by: Same process as the femoral nerve.
During labour and occasionally as a consequence of compression by hernia in the obturator canal.

Results in: Weakness of hip external rotation and adduction.
The patient may complain of inability to cross the affected leg on the other.
Sensory loss is confined to the innermost aspect of the thigh.
The obturator reflex is absent (adductor response to striking the medial epicondyle).

The SCIATIC NERVE ($L_4 L_5 S_1 S_2 S_3$)

The nerve descends between the ischial tuberosity and the greater trochanter of the femur.

In the thigh it innervates the hamstring muscles (semitendinosus, semimembranosus and biceps).

Damaged by: Congenital or traumatic hip dislocation.
Penetrating injuries.
Accidental damage from 'misplaced' intramuscular injection.
Systemic $\longrightarrow$ causes of mononeuropathy

Results in: Weakness of hamstring muscles with loss of knee distal foot and leg muscles are also affected.
Sensory loss involves the outer aspect of the leg.
The ankle reflex is absent.
Plantar flexion of the big toe (Babinski reflex) is also lost.

The COMMON PERONEAL NERVE ($L_4 L_5 S_1 S_2$)

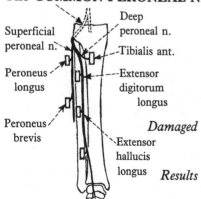

The nerve arises from the division of the sciatic nerve in the popliteal fossa. It bears a close relationship with the head of the fibula as it winds anteriorly. It divides into superficial and deep branches as well as giving off a purely sensory branch which, with sensory twigs from the tibial nerve, forms the *sural nerve*, mediating sensation from the dorsum and lateral aspect of the foot.

Damaged by: Trauma to the head of the fibula; pressure here from kneeling, crossing legs.
Systemic $\longrightarrow$ causes of mononeuropathy e.g. diabetes.

Results in: Weakness of dorsiflexion and eversion of the foot. The patient walks with a 'foot drop'. Sensory loss involves the dorsum and outer aspect of the foot. Partial common peroneal nerve palsies are common with very selective muscle weakness.

Lower Limb Mononeuropathies

The TIBIAL NERVE $(L_4 L_5 S_1 S_2 S_3)$

This nerve also arises from the division of the sciatic nerve in the popliteal fossa and descends behind the tibia, terminating in the medial and lateral plantar nerves which innervate the small muscles of the foot.

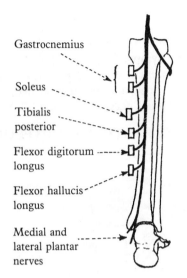

Gastrocnemius

Soleus

Tibialis posterior

Flexor digitorum longus

Flexor hallucis longus

Medial and lateral plantar nerves

The sensory branch forms the *sural nerve*.

Damaged by:
  Trauma in the popliteal fossa.
  Fracture of the tibia.
  Systemic   causes of mononeuropathy.

Results in:
  Weakness of plantar flexion and inversion of the foot.
  The patient cannot stand on toes.
  Sensory loss involves the sole of the foot.
  The ankle reflex is lost.

The Tarsal Tunnel Syndrome

This syndrome results from compression of the medial plantar nerve under the flexor retinaculum. Analogous to the carpal tunnel syndrome in the upper limbs, it presents with pain in the medial aspect of the foot and responds to operative division of the retinaculum.

The Autonomic Nervous System

The autonomic nervous system maintains the visceral and homeostatic functions essential to life. It is divided into SYMPATHETIC and PARASYMPATHETIC components and contains both motor (efferent) and sensory (afferent) pathways.

Both Sympathetic and Parasympathetic systems are regulated by the *limbic system, hypothalamus* and *reticular formation*. Fibres from these structures descend to synapse with preganglionic neurones in the intermediolateral column T1–L2 (sympathetic) and in the III, VII, IX and X cranial nerve nuclei and S2–S4 segments of the cord (parasympathetic).

PARASYMPATHETIC OUTFLOW

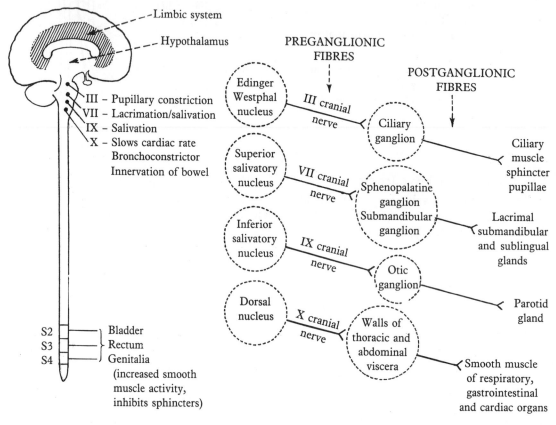

SACRAL OUTFLOW

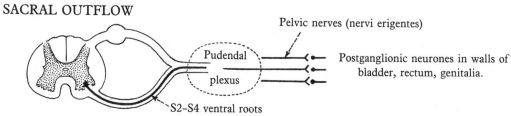

The Autonomic Nervous System

SYMPATHETIC OUTFLOW

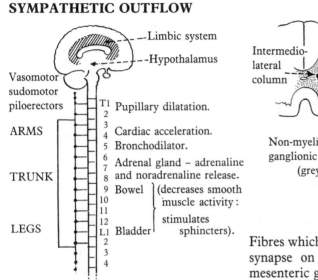

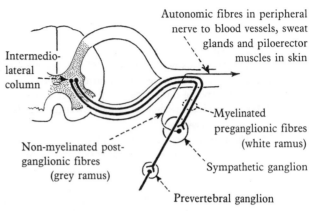

Autonomic fibres in peripheral nerve to blood vessels, sweat glands and piloerector muscles in skin

Intermedio-lateral column

Non-myelinated post-ganglionic fibres (grey ramus)

Myelinated preganglionic fibres (white ramus)

Sympathetic ganglion

Prevertebral ganglion

Vasomotor sudomotor piloerectors

ARMS

TRUNK

LEGS

T1 Pupillary dilatation.
Cardiac acceleration.
Bronchodilator.
Adrenal gland – adrenaline and noradrenaline release.
Bowel (decreases smooth muscle activity: stimulates sphincters).
Bladder

Fibres which pass through the sympathetic ganglion to synapse on a prevertebral ganglion e.g. coeliac or mesenteric ganglia constitute the *splanchnic nerves* and innervate the viscera.

The AFFERENT AUTONOMIC NERVOUS SYSTEM

Sympathetic

Terminate in spinal cord in intermediate zone of grey matter – in relation to preganglionic neurones.

Function: Important in the appreciation of visceral pain.

Parasympathetic

Afferent fibres from the mouth and pharynx, and respiratory, cardiac and gastrointestinal systems, travelling in the VII, IX and X cranial nerves, terminate in the nucleus of tractus solitarius.

Function: Important in maintaining visceral reflexes.

The sacral afferents end in the S2–S4 region in relation to preganglionic neurones.

Neuro-Transmitter substances

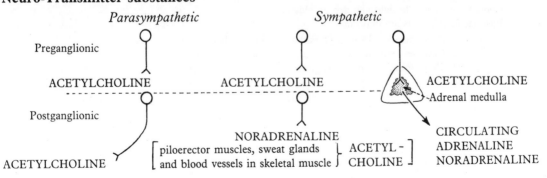

Parasympathetic   *Sympathetic*

Preganglionic

ACETYLCHOLINE   ACETYLCHOLINE   ACETYLCHOLINE
                                                      Adrenal medulla

Postganglionic

NORADRENALINE
[piloerector muscles, sweat glands and blood vessels in skeletal muscle] [ACETYL-CHOLINE]

ACETYLCHOLINE

CIRCULATING ADRENALINE NORADRENALINE

443

Tests of Autonomic Function

These tests help confirm suspected autonomic dysfunction.

BLOOD PRESSURE CONTROL

1. Maintenance of blood pressure with alteration in posture – dependent upon baroreceptor reflex function. A fall in BP occurs with efferent or afferent lesions – postural hypotension.

2. Exposure to cold induces vasoconstriction and a rise in BP – cold pressor test. Stress will produce a similar pressor response e.g. ask patient to do mental arithmetic.
Both central and peripheral lesions affect these tests.

3. Valsalva manoeuvre:
The patient exhales against a closed glottis, increases intrathoracic pressure and thus reduces venous return and systemic BP. The heart rate accelerates to maintain BP. On opening the glottis, venous return increases and an overshoot of BP with cardiac slowing occurs. An impaired response occurs with afferent or efferent autonomic lesions.

4. Noradrenaline infusion test:
A postganglionic sympathetic lesion results in 'supersensitivity' of denervated smooth muscle to adrenaline, with a marked rise in BP following infusion.

HEART RATE

1. Massage of the carotid sinus should stimulate the baroreceptors, increase vagal parasympathetic discharge and slow the heart rate. Either efferent or afferent lesions abolish this response.

2. Atropine test:
Intravenous atropine 'blocks' vagal action and with intact sympathetic innervation results in an increase in heart rate.

SWEATING

A rise in body temperature causes increased sweating, detectable on the skin surface with starch-iodide paper. Any lesion from the central to the postganglionic sympathetic system impairs sweating.

SKIN TEMPERATURE

Skin temperature is a function of the sympathetic supply to blood vessels. With pre- or postganglionic lesions the skin becomes warm and red. With chronic postganglionic lesions the skin may become cold and blue (denervation hypersensitivity). Compare the temperature of various regions.

PUPILLARY FUNCTION

Check the response to light and accommodation.
Pharmacological tests are important:

1. Atropine – blocks parasympathetic system – dilates pupil.
2. Cocaine – stimulates adrenergic receptors – dilates pupil.
3. Pilocarpine – normally innervated pupil – no response.
 – with preganglionic ——— constricts pupil
   parasympathetic lesion   (denervation hypersensitivity).

The Autonomic Nervous System — Specific Diseases

IDIOPATHIC ORTHOSTATIC HYPOTENSION
Two types of this condition are recognised:

(a) Due to degeneration of sympathetic postganglionic neurones.

(b) Due to degeneration of sympathetic preganglionic neurones of the intermediolateral column T1–L2 – the SHY-DRAGER SYNDROME.

In the latter disorder, features of extrapyramidal system involvement are also found.

Both disorders are characterised by: Postural hypotension: Anhidrosis (absent sweating):   Impotence: Sphincter disturbance: Pupillary abnormalities.

The disorders may be separated pharmacologically; the postganglionic disorder shows hypersensitivity (denervation hypersensitivity) to noradrenaline infusion.

Treatment:

Drugs such as fludrocortisone increase blood volume and may prevent postural hypotension.

DIABETIC AUTONOMIC NEUROPATHY
Symptoms of autonomic dysfunction are common in long standing insulin dependent diabetics:

Impotence/retrograde ejaculation.

Bladder dysfunction – decreased detrusor muscle action – resulting in increased residual volume.

Nocturnal diarrhoea.

Despite impairment of the cardiovascular reflexes (e.g. Valsalva manoeuvre), postural hypotension is never significant.

These problems arise from damage to both sympathetic and parasympathetic postganglionic neurones.

Treatment:

There is no specific treatment although improved diabetic control may help.

POST-INFECTIOUS POLYNEUROPATHY – Guillain-Barré syndrome (see previous chapter).

Autonomic involvement occurs commonly in this disorder and may present major problems in patient management. The lesion may involve the afferent or efferent limbs of the cardiovascular reflexes (baroreceptor reflexes) resulting in postural hypotension, episodes of hypertension and cardiac dysrhythmias.

Occasionally the post-infectious neuropathy is purely autonomic.

FAMILIAL DYSAUTONOMIA – RILEY-DAY syndrome.
This autosomal recessive disorder occurs in persons of Jewish descent.

Features of autonomic dysfunction: postural hypotension, pain insensitivity, hyperpyrexia – present from birth.

Pathology:

There is an absence of small unmyelinated sensory and sympathetic (postganglionic) axons.

PRIMARY AMYLOIDOSIS
Autonomic involvement with orthostatic hypotension, impotence, diarrhoea, bladder involvement, is striking in the hereditary type of primary amyloidosis.

TOXIC DISORDERS
Drugs may damage the autonomic nervous system e.g. cytotoxic agents, alcohol.

HORNER's SYNDROME
Pupil constriction, ptosis, enophthalmos and the absence of sweating on one side of the face, result from an interruption of sympathetic fibres to the pupil, lid and face (see page 132).

AUTONOMIC DYSFUNCTION IN QUADRIPLEGIA
A high cervical lesion which completely severs the spinal cord e.g. traumatic cervical fracture/dislocation will isolate all but the cranial parasymathetic outflow. As a result, disturbed autonomic function is inevitable but variable.

Autonomic reflexes are retained –   Passive movement or tactile stimulation of limbs may result in blood pressure rise, bradycardia, sweating, reflex penile erection (priapism).

The Autonomic Nervous System — Bladder Innervation

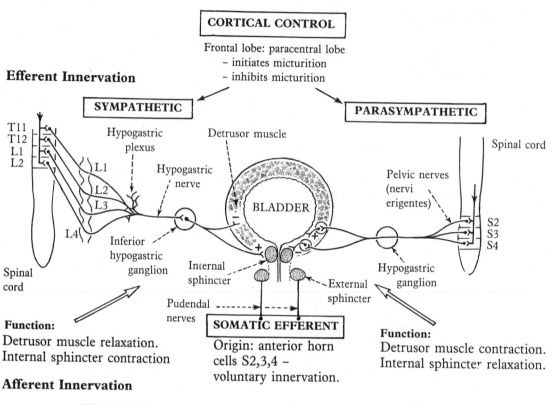

CORTICAL CONTROL

Frontal lobe: paracentral lobe
– initiates micturition
– inhibits micturition

Efferent Innervation

SYMPATHETIC

PARASYMPATHETIC

Hypogastric plexus

Detrusor muscle

Spinal cord

T11
T12
L1
L2

L1
L2
L3

L4

Hypogastric nerve

Pelvic nerves (nervi erigentes)

BLADDER

S2
S3
S4

Inferior hypogastric ganglion

Internal sphincter

External sphincter

Hypogastric ganglion

Spinal cord

Pudendal nerves

SOMATIC EFFERENT

Function:
Detrusor muscle relaxation.
Internal sphincter contraction

Origin: anterior horn cells S2,3,4 – voluntary innervation.

Function:
Detrusor muscle contraction.
Internal sphincter relaxation.

Afferent Innervation

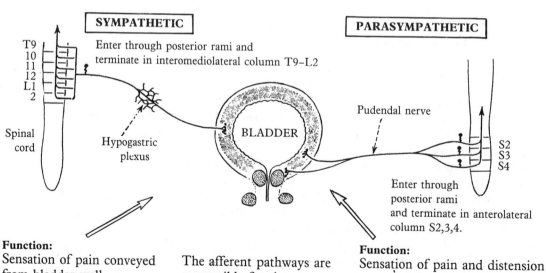

SYMPATHETIC

PARASYMPATHETIC

T9
10
11
12
L1
2

Enter through posterior rami and terminate in interomediolateral column T9–L2

Pudendal nerve

Spinal cord

Hypogastric plexus

BLADDER

S2
S3
S4

Enter through posterior rami and terminate in anterolateral column S2,3,4.

Function:
Sensation of pain conveyed from bladder wall.

The afferent pathways are responsible for the sensation of bladder filling.

Function:
Sensation of pain and distension conveyed from bladder wall and internal sphincter.

Micturition

The PROCESS of MICTURITION

1. Cortical centre – removal of conscious inhibition of micturition.
2. Voiding – wave-like detrusor muscle contractions with relaxation of internal and external sphincters.
3. Voiding completed – detrusor muscle relaxation,
   contraction of internal sphincter,
   contraction of external sphincter.
4. Voiding may be voluntarily interrupted before complete bladder emptying by forced voluntary contraction of the external sphincter.

DISORDERS of MICTURITION

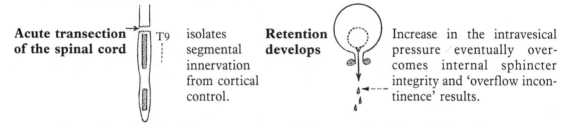

Acute transection of the spinal cord T9 isolates segmental innervation from cortical control.

Retention develops Increase in the intravesical pressure eventually overcomes internal sphincter integrity and 'overflow incontinence' results.

After some days or weeks a REFLEX BLADDER develops – automatic emptying may be induced by abdominal compression.

Lesions of the cauda equina 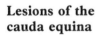 result in a parasympathetic denervated bladder which enlarges – flaccid neurogenic bladder – again with 'overflow incontinence'

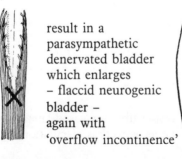

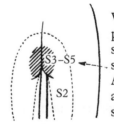

With impaired parasympathetic (S2–S4) action sensation is lost in the sacral dermatomes. Anal tone is diminished and the anal reflex absent.

Tabes dorsalis results in damage to the afferent sympathetic and parasympathetic fibres resulting in a painless bladder enlargement.

Bowel and Sexual Function

Sympathetic and parasympathetic supply to the rectum and internal anal sphincter resemble bladder innervation. The external anal sphincter is under voluntary control.

Sympathetic function is inhibitory – relaxation of the rectal musculature and contraction of the internal anal sphincter.

Parasympathetic function is concerned with emptying – contraction of the rectal musculature and relaxation of the internal anal sphincter.

The paracentral lobule of the frontal lobe also controls voluntary initiation or inhibition of defaecation.

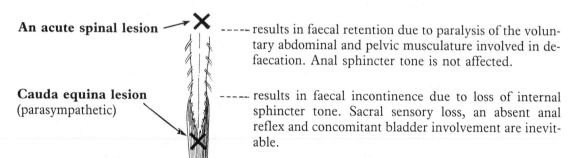

An acute spinal lesion ----- results in faecal retention due to paralysis of the voluntary abdominal and pelvic musculature involved in defaecation. Anal sphincter tone is not affected.

Cauda equina lesion (parasympathetic) ----- results in faecal incontinence due to loss of internal sphincter tone. Sacral sensory loss, an absent anal reflex and concomitant bladder involvement are inevitable.

In the childhood disorder – Hirschsprung's disease – the absence of parasympathetic innervation to the colon and rectum results in impaired bowel emptying, and colonic dilatation – megacolon – ensues.

SEXUAL FUNCTION

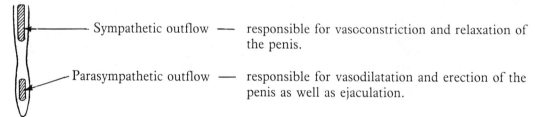

Sympathetic outflow — responsible for vasoconstriction and relaxation of the penis.

Parasympathetic outflow — responsible for vasodilatation and erection of the penis as well as ejaculation.

Spinal lesions may result in spontaneous reflex painful erection – priapism.

Cauda equina lesions result in failure of erection and ejaculation in addition to bladder/bowel and sensory problems.

Diseases of Skeletal (Voluntary) Muscle

Normal skeletal muscle morphology

A skeletal muscle is composed of a large number of muscle fibres separated by connective tissue (endomysium) and arranged in bundles (fasciculi) in which the individual fibres are parallel to each other. Each fasciculus has a connective tissue sheath (perimysium) and the muscle itself is composed of a number of fasciculi bound together and surrounded by a connective tissue sheath (epimysium).

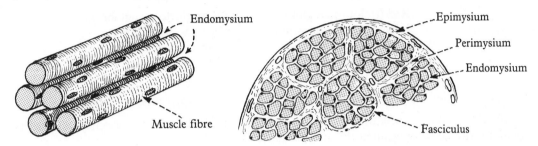

The three envelopes (sheaths) are made up of connective tissue richly endowed with blood vessels and fat cells (lipocytes).

The muscle fibre

This is a large multinucleated cell with an outer membrane – SARCOLEMMA and a cytoplasm – SARCOPLASM within which lie the MYOFIBRILS.

Each muscle fibre has its own end-plate approximately half way along its length.

The cell also contains mitochondria, endoplasmic reticulum and microsomes – the usual cellular constituents.

Fats, glycogen, enzymes and myoglobin lie within the sarcoplasm and related structures.

The MYOFIBRILS are the contractile components of muscle.

Each myofibril is 1μ in diameter and contains filaments of *myosin* and *actin* interdigitating with each other between each Z line. When muscle contracts or relaxes these filaments slide over each other producing shortening and lengthening of the muscle fibre. The striated appearance of skeletal muscle is a consequence of differing concentrations of actin and myosin. These resultant bands are designated as shown.

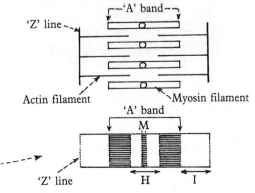

449

Muscle Morphology

Fibre Type:

Muscle fibres vary with function.   Two main types are recognised:

> Type I: Slow continuous contractions – TONIC.
> Type II: Sudden strong contractions – PHASIC.

Characteristics:

Type I	Type II
Red (rich in myoglobin),	White (little myoglobin),
Lower O_2 consumption,	High O_2 consumption,
Lower metabolism,	High metabolism,
Rich in sarcoplasm,	Little sarcoplasm,
AEROBIC.	May function ANAEROBICALLY.

Type I – small alpha motor neurone.   Type II – large alpha motor neurone.

Muscles contain a mixture of Type I and Type II fibres with a tendency for one type to predominate depending upon the specific muscle.

The Neuromuscular Junction

Muscle contraction is achieved by a nerve impulse. Each muscle fibre receives a nerve branch from the motor cell body in the anterior horn of the spinal cord or cranial nerve motor nuclei.

When a nerve fibre reaches the muscle it loses its myelin sheath and its neurilemma then merges with the sarcolemma under which the axon spreads out to form the motor end-plate.

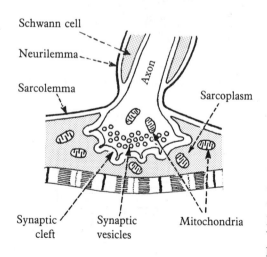

Schwann cell
Neurilemma
Sarcolemma
Axon
Sarcoplasm
Synaptic cleft
Synaptic vesicles
Mitochondria

The axon fibre with its endings and muscle fibres it supplies is called the MOTOR UNIT. The number of muscle fibres in a motor unit varies: in the eye muscles it is small (5–10), whereas in the limb muscles the number is large (in the gastrocnemius about 1800). Each motor unit contains only one type of muscle fibre i.e. Type I or Type II. The neuromuscular junction is the point at which neuromuscular transmission is effected. The motor end-plate is separated from the sarcoplasm by the synaptic cleft. Acetylcholine is found in the synaptic vesicles and released into the synaptic cleft when an electrical impulse passes down the axon. The end-plate potential is produced by such a release and when a certain threshold is reached a muscle action potential results which causes contraction.

The enzyme cholinesterase, found in high concentration at motor end-plates, destroys acetylcholine so that normally a single nerve impulse only gives rise to a single muscle contraction.

450

Clinical Examination

No muscle disease affects all muscle groups.
Topography (distribution) of weakness and wasting aids diagnosis and classification.

Certain points should be elicited from history:

1. Whether muscles fatigue with exercise and recover with rest –
   non-specific in muscle disease but may suggest defective
   neuromuscular transmission.

2. Tasks which are specifically difficult:
   proximal weakness – difficult in climbing stairs,
   lifting hands above head,
   combing hair.
   distal weakness – 'scuffing' toes when walking,
   weak hands e.g. cannot turn door handle, change gear in car.

3. Speed of onset of weakness (whether acute, subacute, chronic).

4. Muscle pains present at rest.

5. Muscle pains and cramps during or after exercise.

6. Whether contraction e.g. hand grip, is slow to relax (myotonia).

7. The presence of a family history of muscle disease or related disorders.

Examination should:

1. Note the distribution of wasting and weakness, and grade weakness according to the M.R.C. (Medical Research Council) scale:
   5 – Full strength.
   4 – Below normal.
   3 – Lift against gravity.
   2 – Movement with gravity eliminated.
   1 – Muscle twitch with no movement about the joint.
   0 – No muscle contraction.

2. Palpate muscles for tenderness.

3. Percussion to determine presence or absence of myotonia (see later).

4. Reflex examination, initially normal, may change with marked wasting and weakness – hyporeflexia becoming apparent.

5. General examination is essential. Muscle disease may be a reflection of an underlying metabolic, endocrine, neoplastic or connective tissue disorder, e.g. increased pigmentation in Addison's disease, malar rash in systemic lupus erythematosus, hepatosplenectomy in alcoholic liver disease.

The Muscular Dystrophies

Muscular dystrophies are genetically determined myopathies in which progressive degeneration and wasting of muscles occur.

The pathogenesis of the dystrophies is unknown.

Classification is based upon the clinical picture:

Type	*Usual mode of inheritance*
Duchenne dystrophy (Pseudohypertrophic muscular dystrophy)	Sex linked recessive or Autosomal recessive.
Benign X-linked muscular dystrophy (Becker's dystrophy)	Sex linked recessive.
Facioscapulohumeral dystrophy (Dejerine's dystrophy)	Autosomal dominant.
Scapuloperoneal	Autosomal dominant.
Limb girdle dystrophy (Erb's dystrophy)	Autosomal recessive.
Myotonic dystrophy	Autosomal dominant.
Oculopharyngeal dystrophy	Autosomal dominant.

The classification is based on topography of muscle involvement.

DUCHENNE DYSTROPHY

Duchenne dystrophy is the commonest form of muscular dystrophy. The disorder is generally X-linked recessive in mode of inheritance. This means that 50% of females are carriers (XX) and 50% of the male offspring may be affected (XY). In Turner's syndrome (XO) females may develop Duchenne dystrophy and infrequent female involvement can also be explained by rare autosomal recessive (non sex linked) inheritance.

Occurrence: 1 per 50,000 male births.

Spontaneous mutation (absence of family history) accounts for $\frac{1}{3}$ of cases.

Clinical features: Onset before 5 years of age.

Proximal muscle involvement initially:
- glutei/quadriceps $\longrightarrow$ WADDLING GAIT.
- shoulder girdle and upper forearm.
- axial muscles $\longrightarrow$ SWAY BACK POSTURE.

Muscular Dystrophies

Clinical features *(continued)*.

The child, at the initial stage of the illness, cannot climb stairs or rise from a low chair, and when attempting to rise from the ground will 'climb up himself' – Gower's sign (not diagnostic of the condition but indicative of pelvic muscle weakness).

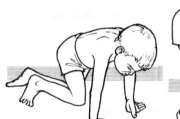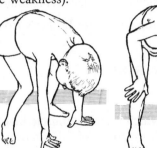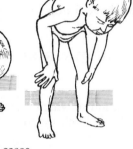

Pseudohypertrophy occurs in 80 per cent of cases.

The gastrocnemius commonly is enlarged and rubbery hard. Quadriceps/deltoid and tongue likewise may be affected.

Progression: Onset

Aged 12 years – child is no longer able to walk and weakness spreads distally in the limbs.

Kyphoscoliosis with respiratory distress and cardiac muscle involvement.

Aged 20 years – chest infection, cardiac failure and arrhythmias occur with severe muscle contractures. The patient by now is bed bound.

Survival is rare beyond mid-20's.

Investigation:

Muscle enzyme – creatine phosphokinase – is substantially elevated especially in early stages. The enzyme is raised at birth and is significantly elevated in the female carrier aiding detection of this state and genetic counselling.

Fetal blood sampling by fetoscopy requires further evaluation.

Electromyographic (EMG) studies will support the diagnosis and may be important in doubtful early cases with no family history i.e. spontaneous mutation. EMG studies do not detect carrier states.

Muscle biopsy will not always be necessary but will stablish the diagnosis beyond doubt.

Treatment: There is no effective treatment. Orthopaedic procedures such as tenotomy may prolong mobility. Steroids are of no value. Detection of the carrier state and advice are essential as preventive treatment.

Muscular Dystrophies

BECKER's DYSTROPHY

Becker's dystrophy is a rare X-linked recessive disorder.
The clinical features are similar to Duchenne but –

> Onset is later – aged 10 years and
>
> Progression is slower – patient remaining ambulant to mid 30's.

Muscle biopsies as well as above features separate Becker's from Duchenne's dystrophy.

FACIOSCAPULOHUMERAL DYSTROPHY

This is inherited as an autosomal dominant trait. Described by Dejerine (1885) it is referred to as Dejerine's dystrophy.

Abortive forms of this condition in which selective muscle involvement occurs (e.g. unilateral shoulder muscle) may 'mask' the dominant mode of inheritance.

Incidence: 0.4 per 100,000.

Clinical features:

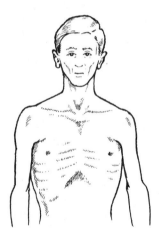

Onset in first or second decade.
Initially the lower half of the face is involved – cannot purse lips or whistle – then spread into trapezius and pectorals occurs.
Lumbar lordosis develops from spinal muscle weakness.
Pelvic musculature and quadriceps may eventually become involved. DROMEDARY or CAMEL BACKED gait with protrusion of the buttocks is characteristic.

Unlike Duchenne dystrophy the clinical course is slow and arrest of progression may occur.

In some cases weakness of facial muscles is noted in childhood without spread to other muscles until middle age. Cardiac muscle is not involved.

Life expectancy in this condition is normal.

Investigation:

EMG studies show myopathic changes.
Muscle enzymes are not elevated.
Muscle biopsy confirms diagnosis – fibre diameter is increased and a cellular response, lymphocytes and plasma cells between muscle fascicles, may be present.

Treatment: There is no specific treatment other than supportive with genetic guidance.

Muscular Dystrophies

SCAPULOPERONEAL MUSCULAR DYSTROPHY

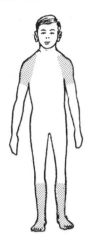

This is an autosomal dominant disorder with involvement of proximal upper limb and distal lower limb muscles. Onset is in early childhood and progression extremely slow. Cardiac muscle involvement may occur in later life. A more aggressive X-linked form of this dystrophy has been described.

The *creatine phosphokinase (CPK)* enzyme is elevated.

The *electrocardiogram* may be abnormal with atrial arrhythmias.

EMG studies show myopathic changes.

Muscle biopsy will show myopathic changes without inflammatory infiltrates.

Differentiation from spinal muscular atrophy with the same distribution of muscle involvement may require EMG and biopsy.

LIMB-GIRDLE MUSCULAR DYSTROPHY

This is an autosomal recessive disorder with onset in second or third decade which may be delayed to middle age.

Often muscle involvement is asymmetrical and onset is usually in the pelvic girdle muscles. Progression is slow. The disease may arrest in some patients. Muscle enlargement (calves) occurs in a proportion of cases.

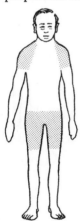

Attempts have been made to subdivide on the basis of pelvic or shoulder girdle onset – this has not been convincing.

The *creatine phosphokinase (CPK)* is elevated often 10 x normal.

Cardiac involvement does not occur (ECG normal).

EMG studies show non-specific myopathic features.

Muscle biopsy confirms myopathy with certain characteristic features.

Differentiation: This distribution of weakness in proximal muscles may be a feature of chronic spinal muscular atrophy, certain metabolic myopathies and polymyositis.

Investigation is essential to classify correctly as EMG and muscle biopsy will distinguish these disorders.

Treatment:

Treatment is symptomatic. Genetic counselling is difficult because of the high frequency of sporadic cases and absence of CPK elevation in the carrier state.

Muscular Dystrophies

MYOTONIC DYSTROPHY

Myotonic dystrophy is a disorder characterised by the presence of MYOTONIA – failure of immediate muscle relaxation after voluntary contraction has stopped.

It can be demonstrated by:

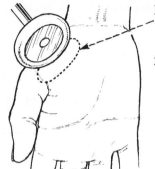

1. Striking a muscle with the tendon hammer and watching the resultant 'dimple' persist for a while before filling up.

2. Asking the patient to grip an object then suddenly release it. The slow relaxation and opening of the hand grip will make the object appear 'stuck' to the fingers.

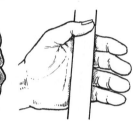

Physiologically, myotonia is due to instability of the muscle membrane with repetitive discharges following a short period of contraction.

Clinical features:

Myotonic dystrophy is an autosomal dominant inherited disorder with onset between 15 and 40 years.

The facial appearance is typical:

--Frontal baldness.
Myopathic face
- with ptosis.
Jaw hanging and
 wasting of muscles
 of mastication
 resulting in hollowing
 of temporal fossae and cheeks.
Wasting of neck and shoulder girdle
 muscles also is evident.

In the limbs –

weakness and wasting are distal though the hands are spared until late.

As the disease progresses, myotonia becomes less apparent and may disappear.

The disorder is progressive over 15–25 years.
Cataracts occur in 80 per cent of cases.
Testicular atrophy occurs in males.
Infertility, habitual abortion and menstrual abnormalities in females.
Cardiac dysrhythmias occur – occasionally resulting in sudden death.
Abnormalities of glucose/insulin metabolism with diabetes mellitus is present in some patients.
Mental deficiency is noted in a small proportion of patients.
Non-neurological manifestation – cataracts, frontal baldness, infertility – may predate the development of muscle weakness and myotonia.

Muscular Dystrophies

Myotonic dystrophy *(continued)*

Investigation:

The *creatine phosphokinase (CPK)* is elevated slightly.
The *ECG* may show conduction abnormalities.
The *EMG* shows classic features of myotonia, with waxing and waning in the amplitude and frequency of motor unit potentials.
Muscle biopsy may be normal or show a variety of changes.

Other investigations:

- Slit lamp examination of the eyes is essential to exclude cataract.
- Plain radiology may show certain bony abnormalities e.g. hyperostosis frontalis interna, small pituitary fossa.
- Elevated blood insulin levels may be found as may a diabetic glucose tolerance curve.

Myotonic dystrophy must be distinguished from other disorders in which myotonia occurs.

Treatment:

Drugs which act as membrane stabilisers e.g. procainamide, phenytoin, quinine, quinidine, acetazolamide, may reduce myotonia.
Identification and treatment of diabetes mellitus and cataract is important.
Genetic counselling should be given.
Sedative drugs are to be avoided as patients show an excessive sensitivity.
General anaesthesia when necessary should be given cautiously – there is risk of malignant hyperthermia.

Note that although a Mendelian disorder, in some generations cataract or diabetes mellitus may be sole manifestations.

OCULOPHARYNGEAL DYSTROPHY

This is an autosomal dominant disorder presenting in early middle age. Ptosis is the initial finding with progressive involvement of extraocular muscles until paralysis of all eye movements results. The pupillary reactions are spared. Dysphagia, facial weakness and proximal limb weakness develop later.
Laboratory findings demonstrate a high CPK (5 x normal). Muscle biopsy is characteristic. Treatment is supportive, with death eventually from intercurrent infection. Swallowing difficulties may necessitate nasogastric feeding.
Distinction must be made from myasthenia gravis and mitochondrial myopathy (see later) in which ptosis is a distinctive feature.

Inflammatory Myopathy

Inflammatory myopathy is a disorder of muscle in which there is clinical and laboratory evidence of an inflammatory process:

It is an acquired muscle disorder as opposed to the *inherited* dystrophies and may be classified into 4 types:

1. **Polymyositis**

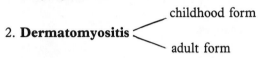

2. **Dermatomyositis** childhood form / adult form

3. **Inflammatory myopathy associated with neoplasia** (polymyositis or dermatomyositis forms).

4. **Inflammatory myopathy associated with collagen disorders** e.g. lupus erythematosus, systemic sclerosis, rheumatoid arthritis (polymyositis or dermatomyositis forms).

There are therefore two forms of inflammatory myopathy – polymyositis and dermatomyositis which are separated clinically by the dermatological findings in the latter – and classification into the four types depends on associated clinical features and the results of certain investigations.

Etiology:
Probably an autoimmune disorder.
This is supported by:
- response to immunosuppressive therapy.
- association with other known immunological disorders e.g. connective tissue disorders.
- elevated IgG in blood and presence of circulating autoantibodies e.g. antinuclear antibody in some cases.
- the reproduction of a similar disorder in laboratory animals by injection of muscle extract with Freund's adjuvant.

Inflammatory Myopathy

Clinical presentation:

Onset is acute or subacute over a period of several weeks and may follow systemic infect—ion, immunisation or even drug reaction.

(? Representing sensitisation to own muscle.)

Systemic symptoms prevail at onset, e.g. lassitude, and are then followed by muscle weakness.

1. Polymyositis

2. Dermatomyositis *usually more serious form and more acute in onset.*

Muscles may be painful and tender in 60% of cases though onset is usually painless.

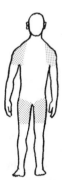 Proximal muscles are first involved and initially weakness may be asymmetrical e.g. one quadriceps only.

Weakness of posterior neck muscles will result in the head 'lolling' forwards.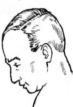

Occasionally weakness may spread into distal limb muscle groups.

Pharyngeal and laryngeal involvement results in dysphagia and dysphonia. Cardiac muscle may also be involved.

The eye muscles are *not* involved unless there is coexistent myasthenia gravis.

Reflexes are retained (if absent, consider underlying carcinoma with added neuropathy).

Characterised by skin rash.
Violet discoloration of light exposed skin.

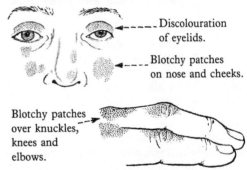

Discolouration of eyelids.

Blotchy patches on nose and cheeks.

Blotchy patches over knuckles, knees and elbows.

Telangiectasia and tightening of skin also occurs.

Childhood form   Adult form

Not associated with malignancy.
Multisystem involvement.
Calcification develops in skin and muscle with extrusion through skin.
Muscle contractures develop – tip-toe gait.
Gastro-intestinal ulceration occurs.

The muscle weakness is as in polymyositis but in childhood dermatomyositis may be very severe, involving chewing, swallowing and breathing.

Inflammatory Myopathy

3. Polymyositis and Dermatomyositis associated with neoplasia.

Approximately 15% of adults with inflammatory myopathy have underlying neoplasia. In dermatomyositis, of those over 40 years of age as many as 60% harbour neoplasia. Neoplasms in almost every organ have been associated and up to 2 years may elapse from onset of myopathy to the detection of such a neoplasm.

4. Polymyositis and Dermatomyositis associated with collagen disorder.

Approximately 25% of adults with inflammatory myopathy have symptoms and signs of an associated connective tissue disorder.

Diagnosis: The clinical picture is suggestive and diagnosis is supported by the following investigations:

Muscle enzymes
Creatine phosphokinase elevated in most patients along with other muscle enzymes.

Circulating antibodies
E.g. rheumatoid factor, antinuclear factor. Present in 40%.

Electromyogram
Shows a typical myopathic pattern with fibrillations.

Erythrocyte sedimentation rate (ESR)
Elevated in most patients.

Muscle biopsy shows necrosis of muscle fibres with inflammatory cells – lymphocytes, plasma cells, leucocytes – in the endomysium.

Prior to the availability of treatment the outcome in inflammatory myopathy was variable and obviously influenced by the presence of associated neoplasia or collagenosis. Periods of relative improvement could occur but generally progression prevailed. Death occurred as a result of chest infection, gastrointestinal haemorrhage, perforation and cardiac arrest in 20 – 30% of all patients.

Treatment:

Steroids — Prednisolone 60mg daily in divided doses with gradual reduction to maintenance dose once improved. If stopped too early, relapse may occur.

Cimetidine protects against the risk of gastrointestinal haemorrhage or perforation.

In refractory cases immunosuppressive drugs – methotrexate, azothiaprine or cyclo-phosphamide – may be used.

Outcome: Mortality is now low though only 10% recover completely. In the rest, the disease becomes inactive after 2 years and patients are left with varying degrees of disability. When associated with collagen disease, eventual outcome will depend on the nature of that disease. When associated with neoplasm, steroids may cause temporary improvement. Removal of the tumour, if feasible, may result in complete remission.

Endocrine/Metabolic Myopathies

Unlike inflammatory myopathy the weakness in these conditions is more chronic and is unassociated pathologically with inflammation. Correction of the underlying endocrine disturbance results in recovery. Usually the other features of endocrine dysfunction are more problematical and myopathy is of secondary importance.

Pituitary

Acromegaly
Proximal weakness with fatigue. Entrapment neuropathies, e.g. carpal tunnel syndrome may complicate the clinical picture of myopathy.

Parathyroid

Hyperparathyroidism and osteomalacia.
Weakness of a proximal distribution with muscle tenderness occurs in 50% of patients with osteomalacia but is less common in primary hyperparathyroidism. The legs are mainly affected and a waddling gait results.

Adrenal

Hyperadrenalism and Hypoadrenalism
These may both be associated with proximal myopathy. In patients treated with steroids, a similar picture may develop rapidly when drug induced. Reduction of steroid dosage may result in improvement.

Thyroid

Hyperthyroidism
Weakness occurs in 20% of thyrotoxic patients. Shoulder girdle weakness is more marked than pelvic. Reflexes are brisk, fasciculation may be present and bulbar muscles can become involved. *Distinction must be made from motor neurone disease.* There is always clinical evidence of thyrotoxicosis in these patients. Diagnosis is confirmed by thyroid function studies.

Hypothyroidism
Proximal weakness involves pelvic girdle more than shoulder. Painful cramps are present and reflexes are diminished with slow relaxation phase. There is always clinical evidence of hypothyroidism in these patients. Diagnosis is confirmed by thyroid function tests.

In chronic proximal weakness, careful clinical history taking, examination and appropriate investigation will separate the various endocrine causes.

Metabolic Myopathies: The Periodic Paralyses

Acute episodes of weakness may result from alterations in serum potassium levels. Three separate forms exist:

Hypokalaemic Periodic Paralysis

Autosomal dominant.
Onset in second decade.
Precipitated by: exercise, carbohydrate load.
Commences in proximal lower limb muscles and rapidly becomes generalised. Onset usually in morning on wakening.
Bulbar muscles/respiration unaffected.
K^+ falls as low as 1.5meq/l.

Treatment:
  Acute – oral KCl.
  Prophylactic – acetazolamide;
    low carbohydrate,
    high K^+ diet.
  With age, attacks become progressively less frequent.
Non familial hypokalaemic periodic paralysis may occur in patients suffering from hyperthyroidism.

Hyperkalaemic Periodic Paralysis

Autosomal dominant or recessive.
Onset in infancy/childhood.
Precipitated by: rest after activity or by cold.
Commences in the lower limbs and evolves rapidly.
Attacks are of short duration (less than 60 min).
Myotonia is evident in some patients.
K^+ rises only slightly.

Treatment:
  Acute – intravenous calcium gluconate or sodium chloride.
  Prophylactic – acetazolamide.

Paramyotonia Congenita
  A rare related disorder.
  Periodic paralysis + myotonia – induced by exercise/cold.

Normokalaemic Periodic Paralysis

Autosomal dominant.
Onset variable.
Precipitated by: ingestion of K^+ containing substances.
Attacks appear more severe and prolonged.
Myotonia is absent.

Treatment:
  Acute – supportive.
  Prophylactic – acetazolamide or
    9α fluorohydrocortisone.

NON-PROGRESSIVE CONGENITAL POLYMYOPATHIES

These are disorders which result from an abnormality in basic muscle morphology and usually have a familial incidence No treatment exists, but they do not lead to progressive disability. Muscle biopsy with histochemical staining and electron microscopy should achieve the diagnosis.

Central Core Disease

Pathology: Hyaline changes in myofibrils lying centrally within the muscle fibres.
Clinically: Variable age of onset.
Proximal muscle involvement (may resemble limb girdle dystrophy).
Dominant inheritance.

Nemaline Myopathy

Pathology: Presence of rod-like structures below the muscle sarcolemma.
Clinically: Onset in infancy.
Bulbar muscles may be involved.
Dominant or recessive inheritance.

Mitochondrial Myopathy

Pathology: Large and excessive mitochondria within the muscle fibres.
Clinically: Onset in infancy/childhood.
Initial hypotonia and delayed motor development.
Several variations are recognised with variable inheritance.

Metabolic Myopathies

Disorders of glycogen or lipid metabolism may result in muscle weakness and diminished exercise tolerance.

McARDLE's DISEASE – due to phosphorylase deficiency.

Clinically: Exercise ⟶ Pain and hardening of muscles ⟶ Muscles fail to relax and contractions occur.

Biochemically: Glycogen ⟶ Glucose 6-phosphate

Absence of phosphorylase enzyme blocks conversion

Myoglobin appears in the urine

Diagnosis: Failure of serum lactate to rise following exercise.
Muscle biopsy – absence of phosphorylase activity with appropriate histochemical staining.

McArdles's disease should be suspected in a patient who develops painful contracted muscles following exercise. Treatment with oral fructose may help, but persistent weakness often results.

ACID MALTASE DEFICIENCY

The development in adult life of limb girdle weakness characterises this disorder. In some, selective involvement of the respiratory muscles causes respiratory failure.

Acid maltase deficiency occasionally presents in infancy with a floppy hypotonic weakness associated with an enlarged tongue.

Diagnosis: Confirmed by muscle biopsy.

CARNITINE DEFICIENCY

This results in disordered fatty acid transport.

Clinically, muscle weakness and contractures occur with exercise in children or adults. A failure to produce ketones following prolonged fast and a normal elevation in serum lactate following exercise differentiates this condition from McArdle's disease.

Myasthenia Gravis

Myasthenia gravis is a disorder of neuromuscular transmission characterised by:

    1. Abnormal weakness and fatiguing of some or all muscle groups.

    2. Weakness worsening on sustained or repeated exertion, or towards the end of the day and relieved by rest.

This condition is a consequence of an autoimmune destruction of the NICOTINIC POSTSYNAPTIC RECEPTORS FOR ACETYLCHOLINE.

Myasthenia gravis is rare, with a prevalence of 40 per million. The tendency for patients to carry certain histocompatibility (HLA) antigens and the increased incidence of autoimmune disorders in first degree relatives suggests an IMMUNOLOGICAL BASIS.

AETIOLOGY

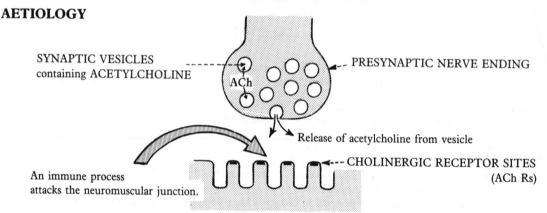

SYNAPTIC VESICLES containing ACETYLCHOLINE

PRESYNAPTIC NERVE ENDING

Release of acetylcholine from vesicle

An immune process attacks the neuromuscular junction.

CHOLINERGIC RECEPTOR SITES (ACh Rs)

Antibodies bind to the receptor sites resulting in their destruction (complement mediated). These antibodies are referred to as ACETYLCHOLINE RECEPTOR ANTIBODIES (ACh R antibodies) and are found in the patient's serum.

An experimental form – experimental autoimmune myasthenia gravis (EAMG) – can be produced in animals by injecting acetylcholine receptor (ACh R) protein which has been extracted from the electric eel. EAMG is similar to human myasthenia gravis. Serum from such an animal contains ACh R antibodies.

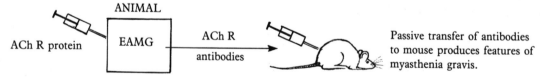

ANIMAL

ACh R protein

EAMG

ACh R antibodies

Passive transfer of antibodies to mouse produces features of myasthenia gravis.

In human myasthenia gravis a reduction of acetylcholine receptor sites has been demonstrated in the postsynaptic folds. Reduced receptor synthesis and increased receptor resorption, as well as the blocking of receptor response to acetylcholine, all seem responsible for the disorder. All are a consequence of immunological attack.

The rôle of the Thymus: Thymic abnormalities occur in 80% of patients. The main function of the thymus is to effect the production of T-cell lymphocytes, which participate in immune responses. Thymus dysfunction is noted in a large number of disorders which may be associated with myasthenia gravis e.g. systemic lupus erythematosus.

Myasthenia Gravis — Pathology

Changes are found in THYMUS gland and in muscle.

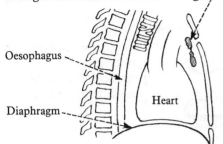

Oesophagus

Heart

Diaphragm

The gland is most active in the induction of normal immune responses in the neonatal period and attains its largest size at puberty after which it will involute.

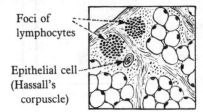

Foci of lymphocytes

Normal structure

Epithelial cell (Hassall's corpuscle)

In myasthenia gravis :

20%: involuted gland;

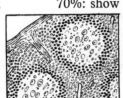

70%: show hyperplasia with lymphoid follicles demonstrating germinal centres;

10%: thymoma, a tumour of lymphoid and epithelial cells which rarely metastasises but may be locally invasive.

Muscle biopsy may show abnormalities:
1. Lymphocytic infiltration associated with small necrotic foci of muscle fibre damage.
2. Muscle fibre atrophy (Type I and II or Type III alone).
3. Diffuse muscle necrosis with inflammatory infiltration. This is associated with thymoma producing anti striated muscle antibody.

Motor point biopsy may show abnormal motor end-plates. Supravital methylene blue staining will show abnormally long and irregular terminal branching.

Light and electron microscopy show destruction of ACh receptors with simplification of the secondary folds of the postsynaptic surface.

Clinical Features

90 per cent of cases are adult.

The disorder may be selective, involving specific groups of muscles.

Several clinical subdivisions are recognised:

Group I   – Ocular muscles only ——————— 20%
Group IIA – Mild generalised weakness ——— 30%
Group IIB – Moderate generalised weakness – 30%
Group III – Acute fulminating
Group IV – Severe upon mild or moderate at onset } – 20%

Approximately 40 per cent of Group I will eventually become Group II. The rest remain purely ocular throughout the illness.

Groups IIB, III and IV develop respiratory muscle involvement.

Peak age of onset is between 20 – 40 years.

Under 40 years is more common in females. Over 40 years, sex incidence is equal.

Myasthenia Gravis — Clinical Features *(continued)*

Bulbar signs and symptoms

Ocular involvement produces ptosis and muscle paresis.

Weakness of jaw muscles allows the mouth to hang open.

Weakness of facial muscles results in expressionless appearance.

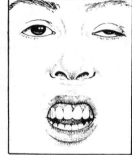

On smiling, buccinator weakness produces a characteristic smile (myasthenic snarl).

Bulbar involvement may result in:
Dysarthric speech. Dysphonic speech. Dysphagia.
Nasal regurgitation of fluids. Nasal quality to speech.

Weakness of eye opening.... 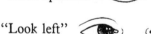 (ptosis) ....and closing....   ....in the same patient is characteristic. (failure to 'bury' eyelashes)

The demonstration of *fatiguing* is important in reaching diagnosis and in monitoring the response to treatment.

"Look upwards" SECONDS ----> SECONDS ----> Ptosis becomes apparent and the eye drifts to neutral position.

"Look left" SECS ----> SECS ---->

Ptosis becomes apparent and there is asymmetrical drift of eyes to the neutral position.

Fatiguing of other bulbar muscles may be demonstrated by:
Blowing out cheeks against pressure.
Counting as far as possible in one breath, etc.

The tongue occasionally shows the characteristic triple grooved appearance with two lateral and one central furrow.

Limb and trunk signs and symptoms.

Weakness of neck muscles may result in lolling of the head. Limb muscles tend to be involved proximally. Fatigue may be demonstrated by movement against a constant resistance.

Limb reflexes are often hyperactive and fatigue on repeated testing.

Muscle wasting occurs in 15 per cent of cases.

Natural history:
(Before treatment became available)
10% of cases went into a period of remission of long duration.
20% experienced short periods of remission (one – several months).
30% progressed to death.
The remainder showed varying degrees of disability accentuated by exercise.

466

Myasthenia Gravis — Differential Diagnosis

Distinguish from:
1. The patient who complains of fatiguing easily – neurotic, hysterical or depressed individual.
2. The patient with progressive ophthalmoplegia e.g. ocular myopathy.
3. The patient with multiple sclerosis – diplopia, dysarthria and fatigue with a relapsing and remitting course.
4. The patient with the Lambert-Eaton myasthenic syndrome (see page 528).

Investigation

PHARMACOLOGICAL

Anticholinesterase drugs are used to confirm diagnosis.

Tensilon (edrophonium) – short action, 2-4 minutes, given i.v. 2-10mg *slowly*, with atropine available to counter muscarinic side effects. This is positive when noticeable improvement in weakness occurs on objective testing.

SEROLOGICAL

Acetylcholine receptor antibodies are detected in 90% of patients and are specific to this disease.

Other antibodies – microsomal, colloid, rheumatoid factor gastric parietal cell antibody – are occasionally found. These reflect the overlap between myasthenia gravis and other auto-immune disorders.

In thymoma, anti striated muscle antibodies are found.

ELECTROPHYSIOLOGICAL

Reduction of the amplitude of the compound muscle action potential evoked by repetitive supramaximal nerve stimulation – 'the decrementing response'.

Various rates of stimulation may be used; even at rates as low as 3/sec a decrementing response may be seen.

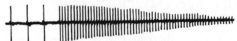

Measure of 'JITTER' – the time interval variability of action potentials from two single muscle fibres of the same motor unit – is a more sensitive index of neuromuscular function and is increased.

PROVOCATIVE

These investigations need only be performed in a small group of patients, serological and advanced neurophysiological investigations rendering them largely obsolete.

Drugs which compete or block at the receptor site may be used to aid diagnosis e.g. curare – patients with myasthenia gravis respond to only 10% of the normal curarising dose, weakness being reversed by edrophonium or neostigmine.

Regional curarisation – injecting into a forearm vein with an applied sphygmomanometer cuff and combining with electrical tests – aids diagnosis.

ADDITIONAL

When thymoma is suspect, especially when the disease presents later than usual in life, conventional and computerised tomography of the anterior mediastinum and an isotope (Gallium) scan should be carried out.

Myasthenia Gravis — Treatment

In the severely ill patients, the first priority is to protect respiration by intubation if necessary, and ventilation.

Anticholinesterase drugs

This is the longest established form of treatment (1934).

Anticholinesterase drugs interfere with CHOLINESTERASE, the enzyme responsible for the breakdown of acetylcholine allowing enhanced receptor stimulation.

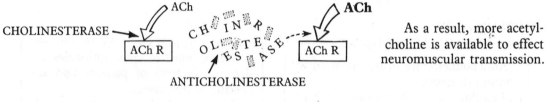

CHOLINESTERASE

ANTICHOLINESTERASE

As a result, more acetylcholine is available to effect neuromuscular transmission.

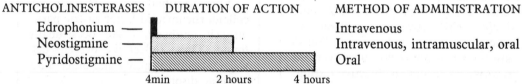

ANTICHOLINESTERASES	DURATION OF ACTION	METHOD OF ADMINISTRATION
Edrophonium —		Intravenous
Neostigmine —		Intravenous, intramuscular, oral
Pyridostigmine —		Oral
	4min 2 hours 4 hours	

A muscarinic inhibitor, Atropine, may be required to counter side effects.

Anticholinesterases rarely give complete symptomatic relief.

The balance between myasthenic and cholinergic (overdose) symptoms is very fine. The same patient may show myasthenic weakness and cholinergic weakness simultaneously in different muscle groups.

CHOLINERGIC OVERDOSAGE:

Muscle fasciculation.
Increased secretions – sweating,
                 – bronchorrhoea.
Respiratory difficulty.
Pupillary signs – miosis.

} All these warnings of overdosage may be masked if atropine is being taken.

Ultimately cholinergic overdosage will result in generalised weakness – *cholinergic crisis*.

Steroids

Prednisolone may be used in patients who do not satisfactorily respond to anticholinesterase therapy. Thirty per cent remain in remission for up to 5 years following steroid treatment. Care should be taken as an exacerbation of symptoms is common 5–10 days after commencement. Alternate day dosage is used to reduce the incidence of drug induced complications.

Immunosuppressants other than steroids

Azathioprine. This drug appears useful in stabilising the disease and reducing the requirements for anticholinesterases. It is especially useful in patients who have proved refractory to steroids. The influence of azathioprine therapy may take some time to be noticeable, beneficial response being noted between 6 – 12 months after commencement. Complications of infection and bone marrow suppression must be weighed against advantages.

Cyclophosphamide has been used to a limited extent.

468

Myasthenia Gravis — Treatment *(continued)*

Thymectomy

When thymoma is not suspected, the benefits of thymectomy (20–30% remission, 50% improvement) must be weighed against the risk of sternotomy in myasthenics – post operative respiratory difficulties.

Thymectomy seems to be of most benefit to young patients with generalised symptoms and a history of less than 5 years duration.

The transcervical operative approach is recommended by many; this procedure avoids splitting the sternum and has a lower associated morbidity, but many groups have shown that this does not always achieve total thymectomy, residual tissue being regularly found.

Thymectomy is contraindicated in congenital myasthenia as this is not an autoimmune disorder.

Plasmapheresis

This is a procedure in which the patient's plasma is 'exchanged' for albumin or another plasma expander. In this way IgG is removed with a fall in acetylcholine receptor antibody levels.

Several 'exchanges' are initially required and because of the 'rebound' of antibody levels after 2 – 3 weeks, either chronic intermittent exchange or simultaneous immunosuppressive therapy, e.g. steroids, azathioprine, is essential to maintain remission.

Plasmapheresis is probably most effective in producing short term improvement and can be used in: 1. myasthenic crisis. 2. to improve clinical state before thymectomy.

3. to control exacerbation evoked by initiation of steroid therapy.

4. repeatedly in severely ill patients who might otherwise require prolonged hospitalisation.

SUMMARY OF TREATMENT

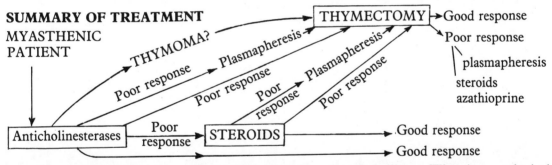

Anticholinesterases should not be required throughout the whole illness. When immunological control of the disease is obtained, these drugs may be stopped.

NEONATAL form of myasthenia gravis.   This develops in a number of infants of myasthenic mothers.
- Suggested by poor crying/sucking and floppy limbs.
- Presents within 48 hours of birth and may persist until the end of 3rd month.
- Caused by passive transplacental passage of IgG (acetylcholine receptor antibodies).
- Treatment with anticholinesterases is required.

This disorder may occur in infants even when their mother has been in remission for many years.

CONGENITAL form of myasthenia gravis.

This usually commences in infancy and persists through adult life. Receptor antibodies are not found and the disease may result from structural abnormalities of the receptors themselves. (A number of such disorders have been identified.)

SECTION V

Multifocal Neurological Disease
and its Management

Bacterial Infections — Meningitis

ACUTE BACTERIAL MENINGITIS

Meningitis is an inflammation of arachnoid, pia mater and the intervening subarachnoid space. When such inflammation results from bacterial infection the onset is acute. Bacteria invade the subarachnoid space *directly* by spread from contiguous structures e.g. sinuses, or *indirectly* from the blood stream.

Causative organisms:

In neonates – Gram -ve bacilli e.g. E.coli, Klebsiella.
Haemophilus influenzae.

In children – H.influenzae.   Streptococcus pneumoniae.
Neisseria meningitidis.

In adults – Strep. pneumoniae.   N.meningitidis.

Other bacteria – Listeria monocytogenes, streptococcus pyogenes and staphylococcus aureus – are less commonly responsible.

Infections of 'mixed' etiology (two or more bacteria) may occur following head injury, mastoiditis or iatrogenically after lumbar puncture.

Pathology:

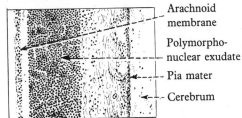

Arachnoid membrane
Polymorpho-nuclear exudate
Pia mater
Cerebrum

A purulent exudate most evident in the basal cisterns extends throughout the subarachnoid space.

The underlying brain, although not invaded by bacteria, becomes congested and oedematous.

The integrity of the pia mater protects against brain abscess formation.

The inflammatory exudate may affect vascular structures crossing the subarachnoid space producing an *arteritis* or *venous thrombophlebitis* with resultant *cerebral infarction*. Similarly, cranial nerves may suffer direct damage.

Hydrocephalus can result from obstruction to CSF flow in the ventricles and subarachnoid space.

Clinical:

Prodromal features	Meningitic features
A respiratory infection, otitis media or pneumonia, associated with muscle pain, backache and lethargy.	High fever. Severe frontal/occipital headache. Stiff neck. Photophobia. Drowsiness.

Acute Bacterial Meningitis

Clinical *(continued)*

Meningitic signs:

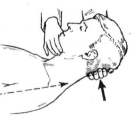

Neck stiffness –
gentle flexion of
the neck is met
with boardlike
stiffness

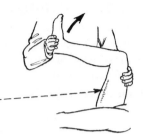

Kernig's sign –
stretching the
lumbar roots
produces pain

Associated neurological signs

Focal or generalised seizures are common.
Cranial nerve signs occur in 15 per cent of patients.
Sensorineural deafness, not due to concurrent otitis media but to direct cochlear involvement –
20%.
Focal neurological signs – hemiparesis, dysphasia, hemianopia – occur in 10% of patients.

Non-neurological complications

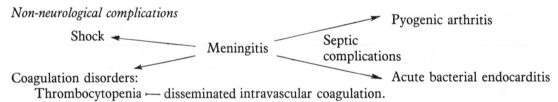

Shock ←— Meningitis —→ Pyogenic arthritis / Septic complications —→ Acute bacterial endocarditis

Coagulation disorders:
Thrombocytopenia ⊢— disseminated intravascular coagulation.

Features specific to causative bacteria

H. influenzae *Haemophilus meningitis*	*N. meningitidis* *Meningococcal meningitis*	*Strep. pneumoniae* *Pneumococcal meningitis*
Generally occurs in children. Preceding upper respiratory tract infection. Onset abrupt with a brief prodrome. Infection in adults associated with CSF rhinorrhoea, otorrhoea, diabetes or alcoholism.	Often occurs in epidemics where the organism is carried in the nasopharynx. Septicaemia can occur with arthralgia, purpuric skin rash. When overwhelming confluent haemorrhages appear in the skin due to disseminated intravascular coagulation as circulatory shock develops.	Predominantly an adult disorder. Often associated with debilitation e.g. alcoholism. May result from pneumonia or middle ear sinus infection or follow splenectomy. Onset may be explosive, progressing to death within a few hours.
Outcome:		
Generally good. Less than 5% mortality.	Gradual onset – good prognosis. Sudden onset with septicaemia – poor outcome. Overall mortality – 10%	Mortality – 20%. Poor prognostic signs – coma, seizures, low cell count in CSF.

Acute Bacterial Meningitis

Investigations:
1. If patient is in coma or has papilloedema or focal neurological signs ⟶ exclude an intracranial mass with a *CT scan.*
2. If above signs are absent or CT scan excludes a mass lesion ⟶ *confirm diagnosis with a lumbar puncture and identify the organism.*

          CSF examination – moderate increase in pressure < 300 mm CSF.
                     – Gram stain of spun down sediment.

Gram +ve paired cocci = pneumococcus	Gram -ve bacilli = haemophilus	Gram -ve intra and extracellular cocci = meningococcus

     – cell count is elevated, 100–10,000 cells/mm³ (80–90% polymorphonuclear leucocytes).
     – glucose is depressed.   – enzyme lactic dehydrogenase is elevated.

Serological/immunological tests:
     – countercurrent immunoelectrophoresis detects capsular antigen in CSF; leads to rapid diagnosis if CSF microscopy is unhelpful.

Blood cultures:
     – Haemophilus isolated in 80% of cases of Haemophilus meningitis.
     – Pneumococcus and meningococcus in less than 50% of patients.

3. Check Serum electrolytes.
     – important in view of the frequency of inappropriate antidiuretic hormone excretion in meningitis.

4. Detect the source of infection.
         Chest X-ray – ? pneumonia.   Skull X-ray – ? fracture.
         Sinus X-ray – ? sinusitis.   Petrous views – ? mastoiditis.

Treatment:
Once meningitis is suspected, treatment must commence immediately, before identification of the causative organism. Such identification may be rapid if gram stain is helpful (70–80%), but may depend on cultures or countercurrent immunoelectrophoresis.

Initial therapy (before organism identification):
     Neonates (above 1 month) — Ampicillin, 300 mg/kg/day i.v.
     Children (under 5 years) — Ampicillin, 300 mg/kg/day +
                               Chloramphenicol, 50–100 mg/kg/day i.v.
            Adults — Penicillin G, 24 million units/day i.v.
                   Chloramphenicol, 4–8 g/day.

Therapy after organism identification :	*Adults*	*Children*	*Alternative*
Pneumococcus or Meningococcus	Penicillin G, 24 million units/day i.v.	300,000 units/ kg/day i.v.	(penicillin allergy) Chloramphenicol
Haemophilus	Ampicillin, 12–14 g/day i.v. Chloramphenicol, 4 g/day i.v.	300 mg/kg/day i.v. 50–100 mg/kg/day i.v.	Chloramphenicol
Listeria	Penicillin G, 24 million units/day i.v.	300,000 units/ kg/day i.v.	Tetracycline

Acute Bacterial Meningitis

Treatment *(continued)*

Duration:

Meningococcus ⎫
Haemophilus ⎬———— continue for at least 1 week after afebrile.
Pneumococcus ———— continue for 10–14 days after afebrile.

Remove any source of infection e.g. mastoidectomy or sinus clearance.
Offer contacts of patients with meningococcal infection chemoprophylaxis – rifampicin 600 mg twice daily for 48 hours.

Meningitis/CSF shunts

Meningitic infection may follow CSF drainage operations for hydrocephalus. This may occur in the immediate post-operative period or be delayed for weeks or months. Clinical features of raised intracranial pressure may coexist due to shunt blockage. Bacteraemia is inevitable and blood cultures identify the responsible organism – usually staphylococcus albus. The infection seldom resolves with antibiotic therapy alone and shunt removal is usually required.

Bacterial Infections — Tuberculous Meningitis

Meningitis is the commonest clinical manifestation of tuberculous infection of the nervous system. In children, it results from bacteraemia following the initial phase of primary pulmonary tuberculosis. In adults, it may occur many years after the primary infection.

Following bacteraemia, metastatic foci of infection lodge in:

1. Meninges.
2. Cerebral or spinal tissue.
3. Choroid plexus.

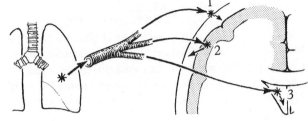

Rupture of these encapsulated foci results in spread of infection into the subarachnoid space. In adults, reactivity of metastatic foci may occur spontaneously or result from impaired immunity (e.g. recent measles, alcohol abuse, administration of steroids).

The clinical features of tuberculous meningitis (TBM) result from:

1. Infection.
2. Exudation – which may obstruct the basal cisterns and result in hydrocephalus.
3. Arteritis – secondary to inflammation around vessels, resulting in infarction of brain and spinal cord.

The meninges around the brain stem are generally most severely affected.

Clinical features:

The majority of patients are adults; childhood TBM is now rare.

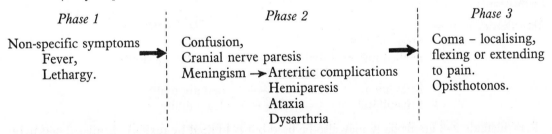

Phase 1	*Phase 2*	*Phase 3*
Non-specific symptoms Fever, Lethargy.	Confusion, Cranial nerve paresis Meningism → Arteritic complications Hemiparesis Ataxia Dysarthria	Coma – localising, flexing or extending to pain. Opisthotonos.

Seizures may occur at the onset.

Untreated, the illness may progress from phase 1 to death over a 3 week period. The rate of progression varies considerably, at times being as rapid as an acute bacterial meningitis.

Organisation of the inflammatory exudate may result in *hydrocephalus/dementia/blindness*.

Tuberculous Meningitis

Investigations:

Cerebrospinal fluid:
    A lymphocytic pleocytosis is usually present, though in acute cases polymorphonuclear cells may predominate – 500/mm³
    The protein is elevated – 100–400 mg/100 ml.
    The glucose level falls (check blood glucose simultaneously to exclude hypoglycaemia).
    Microscopy (Ziehl Neelsen stain) reveals acid fast bacilli in 20% of patients.
    CSF culture (6 weeks in Lowenstein-Jensen medium) should confirm the diagnosis.
Chest X-ray: Reveals changes of old or recent tuberculosis in 50–70%
PPD skin test (tuberculin): Positive to intermediate strength in 90%. Patients developing TBM while on steroids or with recently acquired primary tuberculosis may give a negative response.
CT scan: Shows meningeal enhancement on basal views and occasional ventricular enlargement.

Diagnosis:

Diagnosis is based on the clinical presentation with characteristic CSF findings. Even if Ziehl Neelsen staining is negative in view of the progressive disease course do not await the results of cultures – *if suspect, commence antituberculous treatment.*

Differential diagnosis of subacute/chronic meningitis (see page 496).

{ Viral meningoencephalitis (with *normal* CSF sugar)
Carcinomatous meningitis (with *high* CSF protein, *low* CSF sugar).
Partially treated bacterial meningitis.
Fungal meningitis. Sarcoidosis.

Treatment:

Antituberculous drugs: *Daily dose*
        – Streptomycin ——————— 1 g i.m.
        – Isonicotinic acid dydrazide —— 300–600 mg orally.
               (isoniazid)
        – Rifampicin ——————— 600 mg orally.
        – Ethambutol ——————— 1.5 g orally.

    Pyrazinamide 2–3 grams daily may also be used but is limited by toxicity. Isoniazid and pyrazinamide penetrate meninges well; other drugs penetrate less well especially when the inflammation begins to settle. Continue streptomycin for 3 months. Once sensitivities are known, reduce the number of drugs but continue therapy for 18–24 months.

Side effects:
    Streptomycin may cause 8th cranial nerve damage.
    Ethambutol may produce optic atrophy – check colour vision.
    Isoniazid may produce peripheral neuropathy – protect with *pyridoxine* 50 mg daily.
    Nausea, vomiting, abnormal liver function and skin rashes may occur with all antituberculous drugs.

Tuberculous Meningitis

Treatment *(continued)*

Intrathecal therapy:

Since CSF penetration, especially with streptomycin, is poor, some recommend intrathecal treatment. Streptomycin 50 mg may be given daily or more frequently in seriously ill patients.

When an obstructive hydrocephalus occurs, combined intraventricular (through the shunt reservoir or drainage catheter) and lumbar intrathecal injections may be administered.

Steroid therapy:

Many clinicians combine antituberculous therapy with steroids in the hope that these will minimise the risk of obliterative endarteritis and arachnoid adhesions, but benefits are uncertain.

Hydrocephalus

Progressive dilatation of the ventricles impairing conscious level requires CSF drainage – either temporarily with a ventricular catheter (permitting intraventricular drug administration) or permanently with a ventriculo-peritoneal/atrial shunt.

The Course of treated tuberculous meningitis:

Even with modern treatment, mortality remains at 20%. Of those who survive, neurological sequelae persist in 30% – hydrocephalus, blindness, deafness, dementia and epilepsy.

With treatment, CSF sugar quickly returns to normal; the cellular reaction gradually diminishes over 3–4 months; the protein level may take a similar time to return to normal.

Other Forms of CNS Tuberculous Infection

TUBERCULOMA:
Tuberculomata may occur in cerebral hemispheres, cerebellum or brain stem, and may produce a space occupying effect. Most resolve with antituberculous therapy. See page 338.

POTT's DISEASE
Chronic epidural infection follows tuberculous osteomyelitis of the vertebral bodies. This arises in the lower thoracic region, can extend over several segments and may spread through the intervertebral foramen into pleura, peritoneum or psoas muscle (psoas abscess) – see page 389.

SPINAL ARACHNOIDITIS

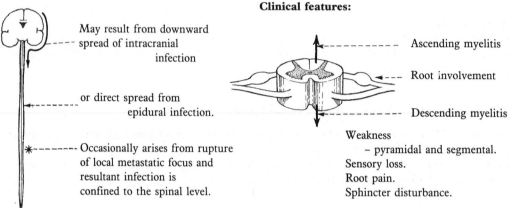

Clinical features:

May result from downward spread of intracranial infection

or direct spread from epidural infection.

✱ Occasionally arises from rupture of local metastatic focus and resultant infection is confined to the spinal level.

Ascending myelitis

Root involvement

Descending myelitis

Weakness
 – pyramidal and segmental.
Sensory loss.
Root pain.
Sphincter disturbance.

Dignosis: Plain radiology, myelography and CSF examination.
Treatment: As for Pott's paraplegia
 – Surgical decompression if indicated and antituberculous treatment.

TUBERCULOUS ENCEPHALOPATHY
An autoimmune encephalopathy with features of acute allergic encephalomyelitis or haemorrhagic leukoencephalopathy (pages 509,510). This may complicate the course of tuberculous infection and may significantly contribute to the degree of neurological dysfunction resulting from tuberculous meningitis. Clinically, convulsions and deepening coma with extensor posturing characterise this complication.

TRANSVERSE MYELITIS
Transverse myelitis may occur during the successful treatment of tuberculosis and is not related to the usage of intrathecal therapy. It probably represents a delayed endarteritis.

Non-viral Infections of the CNS — Syphilis

Syphilis is an infectious disease caused by the organism *Treponema pallidum*. Entry is by:
   (a) inoculation through skin or mucous membrane (sexually transmitted) – acquired syphilis.
   (b) transmission in utero – congenital syphilis.
The natural history of infection is divided into:

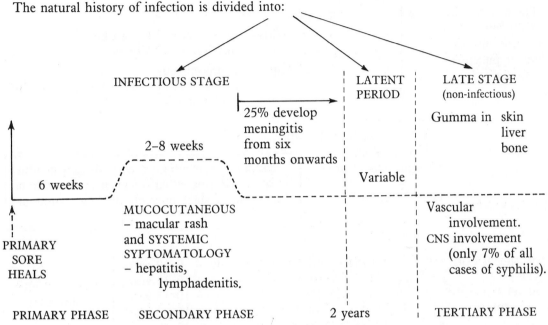

The *chancre* or *primary sore* on skin or mucous membrane represents the local tissue response to inoculation and is the first clinical event in acquired syphilis.

The organism, although present in all lesions, is more easily demonstrated in the primary and secondary phases.

In congenital syphilis fetal involvement can occur even though many years may elapse between conception and the mother's primary infection.

Widespread recognition and efficient treatment of the primary infection have greatly reduced the late or tertiary consequences.

Not all patients who avoid treatment develop the tertiary phase.

Investigations

Serological diagnosis depends on detection of antibodies.
   1. Non-specific (Reagin) antibodies.
      Reagin tests involve complement fixation.
      The Venereal Disease Research Laboratory (VDRL) test is the commonest and when positive in CSF is diagnostic of neurosyphilis. If negative, test for:
   2. Specific treponemal antibodies.
      Fluorescent Treponemal Antibody Absorption (FTA) test and
      Treponema Immobilisation (TPI) test.
      These tests are positive in every case of neurosyphilis.

Neurosyphilis

The initial event in neurosyphilis is meningitis. Of all untreated patients 25 per cent develop an acute symptomatic syphilitic meningitis within 2 years of the primary infection.

ACUTE SYPHILITIC MENINGITIS: 3 clinical forms are recognised:

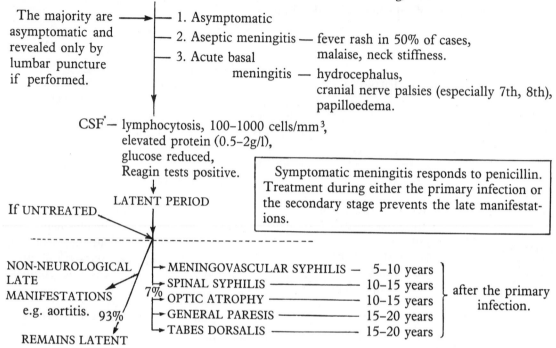

The majority are asymptomatic and revealed only by lumbar puncture if performed.

1. Asymptomatic
2. Aseptic meningitis — fever rash in 50% of cases, malaise, neck stiffness.
3. Acute basal meningitis — hydrocephalus, cranial nerve palsies (especially 7th, 8th), papilloedema.

CSF — lymphocytosis, 100–1000 cells/mm³,
elevated protein (0.5–2g/l),
glucose reduced,
Reagin tests positive.

LATENT PERIOD

If UNTREATED

Symptomatic meningitis responds to penicillin. Treatment during either the primary infection or the secondary stage prevents the late manifestations.

NON-NEUROLOGICAL LATE MANIFESTATIONS e.g. aortitis.

REMAINS LATENT

7%

93%

MENINGOVASCULAR SYPHILIS — 5–10 years
SPINAL SYPHILIS ———————— 10–15 years
OPTIC ATROPHY ——————————— 10–15 years
GENERAL PARESIS ——————— 15–20 years
TABES DORSALIS ——————— 15–20 years

after the primary infection.

Late neurological complications occur in only 7 per cent of UNTREATED cases.

These forms are exceptionally rare and the clinical syndromes mentioned above seldom occur in a 'pure' form.

MENINGOVASCULAR SYPHILIS

'Early' late manifestation resulting in an obliterative endarteritis and periarteritis.

Presents as a 'stroke' in a young person – hemisphere, brain stem or spinal. Granulations around the base of the brain may produce cranial nerve palsies or even hydrocephalus.

CSF – lymphocytes 100/mm³, protein↑, gammaglobulin↑, positive serology.   Penicillin arrests progression.

SPINAL SYPHILIS

Chronic meningitis with sub-pial damage to the spinal cord.

Presents as a progressive paraplegia, occasionally with radicular pain and wasting in upper limbs – ERB's PARAPLEGIA.   CSF – as meningovascular syphilis.   Penicillin arrests progression.

OPTIC ATROPHY

Meningitis around optic nerve with sub-pial necrosis may be the only manifestation of late syphilis.

Presents as a constriction of the visual fields with a progressive pallor of the optic disc:
    if both eyes are affected, the vision is rarely saved.
    if only one eye is involved, treatment with penicillin will save the other.

Neurosyphilis

GENERAL PARESIS

Characterised by dementia – with memory impairment, disordered judgement and disturbed affect – manic behaviour, delusions of grandeur (rare).

There are two phases: 1. Pre-paralytic – with progressive dementia.

2. Paralytic – when corticospinal and extrapyramidal symptoms and signs develop associated with involuntary movements (myoclonus).

Argyll Robertson pupils may be present (see page 133).

At autopsy, meningeal thickening, brain atrophy and perivascular infiltration with plasma cells and lymphocytes are evident; culture from the cortex may reveal an occasional treponema.

CSF – lymphocytes 50/mm³, protein ↑ 0.5–2g/l, gammaglobulin↑.

Reagin tests in CSF positive in the majority.

Treatment in the pre-paralytic phase will halt progression in 40 per cent.

TABES DORSALIS

Posterior spinal root and posterior column dysfunction - - - - - - - - →
account for symptoms.

Pupillary abnormality (Argyll Robertson) and optic atrophy occur. Peripheral reflexes are lost and joint position and vibration sensation is impaired. A positive Romberg's test (page 178) indicates a sensory ataxia.

Pain loss results in trophic lesions and occasionally a Charcot joint may develop. - - - - - - - - - - →

Urinary incontinence, impotence and constipation also occur.

'Lightning pains', visceral crises (abdominal pain/diarrhoea) and rectal crises (tenesmus) are frequent.

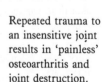

Repeated trauma to an insensitive joint results in 'painless' osteoarthritis and joint destruction.

The CSF is more normal than in general paresis. The Reagin test may be negative in 30 per cent. Treatment may produce some improvement; it will not reverse joint destruction.

SYPHILITIC GUMMA presenting as an intracranial mass is extremely rare.

TREATMENT of Neurosyphilis

Penicillin G. ——— 2–4 megaunits i.v.
    or   4 hourly for 10 days.
Procaine Penicillin —— 600,000 units i.m.
    or   daily for 15 days.
Benzathine Penicillin— 2–4 megaunits i.m. weekly x 3.

(When patient sensitive to penicillin
↓
Erythromycin or
Tetracycline may be given
orally over 30 days.)

The Jarisch-Herxheimer reaction – tachycardia/fever – occurs in one-third of patients within a few hours of commencing treatment but is of no neurological consequence.

CSF follow up: CSF is checked initially and at 6 monthly intervals until normal.

Cell count is the best indicator of persistent infection.

In the presence of a normal CSF cell count and protein, a weakly positive VDRL does not indicate the need for further treatment.

Non-viral Infections of CNS — Protozoal

TOXOPLASMOSIS

Toxoplasmosis is an infection of man contracted from animals – cattle, sheep, pigs, dogs and cats.

Organism: An anaerobic intracellular protozoan, *Toxoplasma Gondii.*

The majority of infections in man are asymptomatic (30% of the population have specific antibodies indicating previous exposure).

In the host

Organism ----- enters R.E. cell → Multiplies and cell ruptures → Blood stream → To involve organs e.g. liver, spleen, CNS, eye.

Lymphatics →

Transmission: Eating uncooked meat or contact with faeces of an infected dog or cat.

There are two forms of toxoplasmosis:

Congenital – when a non-immune woman contracts infection during pregnancy (subclinical infection); transplacental spread results in fetal infection.

↓

Premature delivery occurs in 25%.

Contributes to 20% of neonatal mortalities.

Causes: – hydrocephalus,
– aqueduct stenosis,
– microcephaly.

Non-neurological features:
– skin rash, jaundice,
hepatosplenomegaly, choroidoretinitis.

Skull X-ray shows:
– curvilinear calcification (basal ganglion and peri-ventricular).

Varying degrees of organ involvement may occur. The only manifestation may be choroidoretinitis in an otherwise healthy child.

Of all patients with choroidoretinitis, 25% result from toxoplasmosis.

Acquired – Infection of children and young adults is uncommon and may be associated with underlying systemic disease or immunosuppressive therapy.

↓

Fever and fatigue with muscle weakness and lymphadenopathy result. Abnormal lymphocytes in peripheral blood leads to confusion with infectious mononucleosis. The neurological features are those of a meningoencephalitis with seizures, myoclonus and deepening coma. CSF examination shows a pleo-cytosis.

Rarely pneumonitis, hepatitis, myocarditis and choroidoretinitis occur.

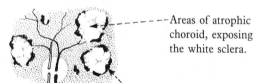

Areas of atrophic choroid, exposing the white sclera.

Retinal pigment epithelium becomes hyperplastic – densely pigmented areas result.

Infection with *T.Gondii* results in an allergic state. Although encysted protozoon are found within various organs, damage results from delayed hypersensitivity rather than direct attack.

Diagnosis:

Organisms are seldom identified.

Mouse inoculation aids isolation of the encysted zoite form.

Sabin Feldman Dye Test may demonstrate a rising titre.

Complement fixation antibody test may provide a positive result.

N.B. Rubella, cytomegalovirus and herpes simplex can also spread transplacentally and cause jaundice and hepato-splenomegaly. Cytomegalovirus may also produce choroidoretinitis and intracranial calcification.

Treatment:

Sulphonamide and pyrimethamine (Dapaprim) for at least 28 days. Give steroids when choroidoretinitis is present.

Viral Infections

GENERAL PRINCIPLES

Invasion of the nervous system may occur as part of a generalised viral infection. Occasionally nervous system involvement is disproportionately severe and symptoms of generalised infection are slight.

Viruses enter the body through the: *Respiratory tract,*
Gastro-intestinal tract,
Genito-urinary tract or by
Inoculation through the skin.

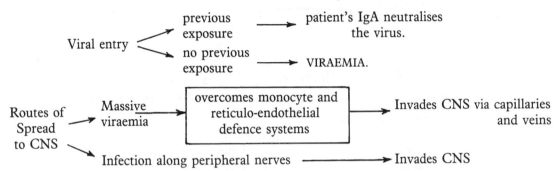

Viral entry → previous exposure → patient's IgA neutralises the virus.

Viral entry → no previous exposure → VIRAEMIA.

Routes of Spread to CNS → Massive viraemia → overcomes monocyte and reticulo-endothelial defence systems → Invades CNS via capillaries and veins

Routes of Spread to CNS → Infection along peripheral nerves → Invades CNS

After CNS penetration, the clinical picture depends upon the particular virus and the cells of the nervous system which show a specific susceptibility.

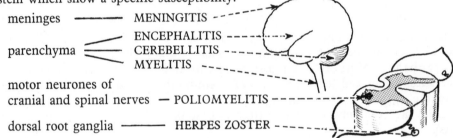

meninges ———— MENINGITIS

parenchyma ⟨ ENCEPHALITIS
CEREBELLITIS
MYELITIS

motor neurones of cranial and spinal nerves — POLIOMYELITIS

dorsal root ganglia ——— HERPES ZOSTER

Some viruses appear to remain latent for many years within the nervous system before producing symptoms - SLOW VIRAL INFECTIONS.

MENINGITIS

Aseptic meningitis (fever/meningism and lymphocytic or monocytic CSF response) is usually viral especially when the onset is acute, although this is not always the case.

Attempts at identification of the causal organisms may fail, or may reveal the following (in order of frequency):

ENTEROVIRUSES ⟨ echovirus
coxsackievirus

MUMPS VIRUS
HERPES SIMPLEX (sub-type 2)
EPSTEIN-BARR VIRUS
HERPES ZOSTER
LYMPHOCYTIC CHORIOMENINGITIS VIRUS

485

Viral Infections — Meningitis

Incidence

Enterovirus infection — affects children/young adults and occurs seasonally in late summer. Spread is by the faecal/oral route.

Mumps — affects children/young adults. Winter/spring incidence.

Lymphocytic choriomeningitis — affects any age and is a consequence of airborne spread from rodent droppings.

Clinical features of acute aseptic meningitis

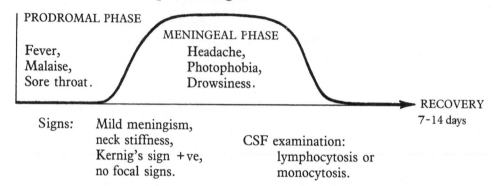

Echovirus	Coxsackie virus	Mumps	Lymphocytic choriomeningitis
Maculopapular skin rash with or without petechiae. Muscle weakness of an isolated muscle group some weeks later (poliomyelitis).	A paralytic disorder resembling poliomyelitis and associated with outbreaks of 'epidemic myalgia' (BORNHOLM's DISEASE).	Prolonged clinical course with deafness.	Clinical resemblance to infectious mononucleosis. Choroidal involvement and an encephalitic component are not uncommon.

Specific features *may* occur:

Differential Diagnosis:

From other causes of an aseptic meningitis which are usually subacute or chronic in onset –

Tuberculous or *Fungal* meningitis.

Leptospirosis.   *Carcinomatous* meningitis.

Sarcoidosis.   Partially treated *bacterial* meningitis.

Parameningeal chronic infection which evokes a meningeal response e.g. mastoiditis.

The self-limiting and mild nature of viral meningitis should not lead to confusion with these more serious causes   – see page 496).

Viral Isolation: Confirmation of diagnosis depends upon successful isolation of the causative virus. E.g. echovirus and coxsackievirus from the CSF, throat or stool.

In lymphocytic choriomeningitis, a rise in antibody titre may be demonstrated.

Prognosis is excellent and **Treatment** symptomatic.

486

Viral Infections — Parenchymal

Viruses may act:

> *directly* —→ acute viral encephalitis or meningoencephalitis,
>
> *after a latent period* —→ 'slow' virus encephalitis,
>
> or *indirectly via the immune system* —→ allergic or post infectious encephalomyelitis, post vaccinial encephalomyelitis.

Finally, an encephalopathy may develop during the course of a viral illness in which inflammation is not a pathological feature – REYE's SYNDROME.

ACUTE VIRAL ENCEPHALITIS

In acute encephalitis attempts to identify the causative virus often fail.

Encephalitis following childhood infections – measles, mumps, varicella, rubella – is presumed *post-infectious* and not due to direct viral invasion, though, in both mumps and measles, viruses have occasionally been isolated from the brain.

Herpes simplex is the commonest cause of severe sporadic encephalitis.

Clinical features:

3 sets of features are present

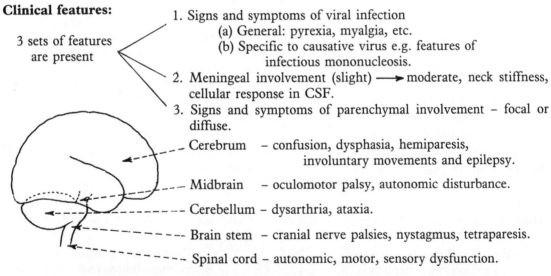

1. Signs and symptoms of viral infection
   (a) General: pyrexia, myalgia, etc.
   (b) Specific to causative virus e.g. features of infectious mononucleosis.
2. Meningeal involvement (slight) —→ moderate, neck stiffness, cellular response in CSF.
3. Signs and symptoms of parenchymal involvement – focal or diffuse.

Cerebrum – confusion, dysphasia, hemiparesis, involuntary movements and epilepsy.

Midbrain – oculomotor palsy, autonomic disturbance.

Cerebellum – dysarthria, ataxia.

Brain stem – cranial nerve palsies, nystagmus, tetraparesis.

Spinal cord – autonomic, motor, sensory dysfunction.

All or some of these features may be present. The terminology may vary depending on the predominant site involved i.e.

BRAIN STEM ENCEPHALITIS,
CEREBELLITIS,
MYELITIS.

In general, the illness lasts for some weeks.

Prognosis is uncertain and depends on the specific virus –

> Herpes simplex – high mortality.
> Mumps – excellent outcome.

487

Viral Infections — Parenchymal

HERPES SIMPLEX ENCEPHALITIS
Two sub-groups of Herpes Simplex Virus (HSV) are recognised:
  (a) Type I, responsible for oral and labial rashes as well as ENCEPHALITIS.
  (b) Type II, responsible for genital and neonatal infection as well as ASEPTIC MENINGITIS.

Most cases of encephalitis probably result from reactivation of the latent virus rather than from primary infection.

Clinical features:
General symptoms at onset – headache, fever – with evolution over several days to seizures and impaired conscious level.

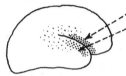

Inferior frontal and temporal lobes are specifically involved and signs and symptoms reflect this – olfactory or gustatory hallucinations, behavioural disturbance, complex partial seizures, dysphasia (dominant hemisphere) and hemiparesis.

Cerebral oedema may follow resulting in tentorial herniation.

In those who recover, a profound memory disturbance may persist.

Investigations:
CT scan shows low attenuation in the inferior frontal and temporal lobes unless haemorrhage has occurred into necrotic regions. In early stages, the CT scan may be normal; in those patients an isotope brain scan may detect an area of increased uptake.

CSF examination reveals 5–500 lymphocytes but the protein is only mildly elevated and the glucose is normal. CSF pressure may be raised.

EEG examination shows generalised slowing with bursts of 'periodic' high voltage slow wave complexes over the involved temporal lobe.

N.B. In some patients only serial investigations may demonstrate the characteristic changes.

Differential diagnosis: Consider: – other forms of viral encephalitis.
  – other causes of lymphocytosis in CSF e.g. tuberculosis, cryptococcus, toxoplasma,
  – brain tumour.   cerebral abscess.

Diagnosis is confirmed by biopsy, guided by CT scan, isotope brain scan and EEG evidence of a lateralised lesion.

Biopsy will show evidence of a necrotising encephalitis with intranuclear eosinophilic inclusion bodies.

Demonstrate antigen by immunofluorescence

Isolate virus by culture

Serological tests and CSF immunofluorescence tests are less reliable.

Treatment:
Antiviral drugs. Previous studies convincingly demonstrate a reduction in mortality from 70% in an untreated control group to 30% in patients treated with *adenine arabinoside*. A recent study compares adenine arabinoside with *acyclovir* and shows a further reduction in mortality to 19% in patients on acyclovir. If the above results are confirmed, since side effects are minimal, acyclovir may prove invaluable in the treatment of herpes simplex encephalitis.

488

Viral Infections — Reye's Syndrome

REYE's SYNDROME

This is a 'toxic encephalopathy' which occurs in young children. It is associated with fatty changes in the liver and occurs after viral or bacterial infections or, rarely, after immunisation.

Pathologically there is acute cerebral oedema without inflammation.

Incidence: 1 per 100,000 children per year.   Commonest in rural communities.
Outbreaks described with certain virus infections.

Pathology:

Neurones and glial cells are swollen; the liver and heart show fatty infiltration.
Associated virus infections: Influenza A,   Influenza B,   Varicella.

Pathogenesis:

Viral synergism with an environmental factor e.g. salicylates, may be responsible.

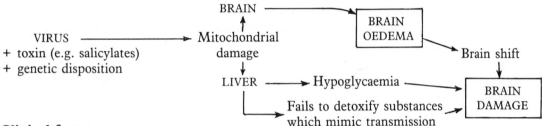

Clinical features:

<u>Initial stage</u>

Virus infection → which begins to improve

Vomiting, Delirium,
Depressed conscious level → coma
with a flexion or extension response.
to stimulation. Focal signs are absent.
Hepatomegaly occurs in 50% of patients.

Death may result from raised intracranial pressure.

Investigations:

Raised liver enzymes, elevated serum ammonia and hypoglycaemia (in infants) are characteristic.

Differential diagnosis:

Consider other causes of raised intracranial pressure in childhood especially.

— lead encephalopathy,
— lateral sinus thrombosis e.g. following mastoiditis,
— steroids,
— vitamin A overdosage.

Treatment:

Treatment aims at lowering intracranial pressure with the aid of intracranial pressure monitoring (see page 489). In addition, blood glucose must be maintained and any associated coagulopathy treated.

Prognosis: The overall mortality is 20%.

When raised intracranial pressure is present, mortality increases to 40% and a high proportion of survivors have cognitive disorders.

Viral Infections — Parenchymal

'SLOW' VIRUS DISORDERS

'Slow' virus disorders are diseases in which virus infection results in a chronic progressive neurological condition.

The evidence of a viral etiology is: *direct* — finding of inclusion bodies, demonstration of viral particles, isolation of virus,

and *indirect* — relationship of onset of symptoms to a preceding viral illness, transmission of illness from one host to the next.

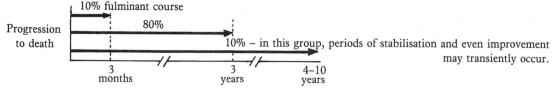

Not all these features are present in any one illness.
'Slow' infection refers to the long incubation period.

SUBACUTE SCLEROSING PANENCEPHALITIS (SSPE)

Caused by measles-like *paramyxovirus* – isolated from brain biopsy.

Clinical features: A world-wide disorder. Incidence: 1 per million per year. Onset: between ages 7–10 years.

Stage 1	*Stage 2*	*Stage 3*
Behavioural problem,	Development of myoclonic jerks,	Lapses into rigid
Declining school performance,	Seizures,	stuporous state
Progression ⟶ dementia.	Cerebellar ataxia, Dystonia.	

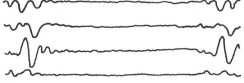

Progression to death

10% fulminant course

80%

10% – in this group, periods of stabilisation and even improvement may transiently occur.

3 months   3 years   4–10 years

The illness may occur after measles vaccination or following clinical infection at an early age (under 2 years).
Accompanying features of infection i.e. pyrexia, leucocytosis, are *absent*.

Investigations:

CSF examination shows elevated γglobulin with IgG oligoclonal bands; elevated measles antibodies (75% of total CSF IgG).

Blood examination shows elevated serum measles antibodies.

EEG – shows periodic high voltage slow wave complexes on a low voltage background trace.

Pathology:

Changes involve both white and grey matter, especially in the posterior hemispheres. Brain stem, cerebellum and spinal cord are also affected.

Oligodendrocytes contain eosinophilic inclusion bodies. Marked gliosis occurs with perivascular lymphocyte and plasma cell cuffing.

Treatment: There is no specific treatment.

Subacute measles encephalitis may follow measles infection in children on *immunosuppressive drug treatment* or with *hypogammaglobulinaemia*. The clinical course is different however from SSPE.

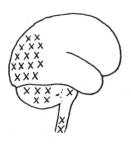

490

Viral Infections — Parenchymal

PROGRESSIVE RUBELLA PANENCEPHALITIS

Similar to SSPE with a fatal outcome, caused by Rubella virus.

Presents at a later age (10–15 years).

Progressive dementia.

Ataxia.   Spasticity.   Myoclonus.

CSF shows high γglobulin.

EEG does *not* show periodic complexes of SSPE.

Antibodies elevated in serum and CSF to rubella.

Biopsy does *not* show inclusion bodies.

Treatment: No specific treatment.

CREUTZFELDT-JAKOB DISEASE

Spongiform encephalopathic changes characterise this disorder, which presents as a presenile dementia.

Incidence: 1 per million per year.   10–15% of cases are familial.   **Onset:** 5th to 6th decade.

Clinical course: 3 phases are recognised:

1. *Prodromal*
   Vague onset,
   Unsteadiness,
   Memory disturbance,
   Visual symptoms.

2. *Progressive*
   Progressing dementia,
   Ataxia, Corticospinal signs,
   Visual loss (cortical),
   Myoclonus, Chorea,
   Muscle wasting (amyotrophy).

3. *Terminal*
   Mute, Profoundly demented,
   80% die within 12 months
   of onset.

Investigation:

CSF – usually normal.

EEG – bilateral high voltage sharp waves on a
   background of slow wave activity.

The clinical picture and electroencephalogram suggest the
diagnosis which is ultimately confirmed pathologically.

Pathology:

Moderate to severe atrophy occurs.

Frontal lobes are most affected

then parietal and occipital lobes

then cerebellum

and anterior horn

cells in spinal cord.

Vacuolation

Microscopically – Neuronal degeneration occurs with marked astrocytic proliferation.
   Vacuolation of glial cells results in a characteristic spongiform appearance.

Aetiology:

The realisation that other disorders characterised by spongiform changes – KURU (a degenerative disorder found in New Guinea associated with cannibalism) and SCRAPIE (a disorder in sheep) – were transmissible, led to the demonstration of transmission in Creutzfeldt-Jakob disease.

Following primate inoculation, an illness characterised by confusion ataxia and amyotrophy developed in 12–18 months.

The mode of transmission in humans is unclear; it has been documented following corneal grafting and following the use of depth electrodes in neurosurgery but does not appear communicable in that conjugal cases are unknown.

Care should be taken in handling material from patients.

Treatment: There is no treatment.
   Antiviral drugs are of no benefit.

491

Viral Infections — Poliomyelitis

Poliomyelitis is an acute viral infection in which the anterior horn cells of the spinal cord and motor nuclei of the brain stem are selectively involved.

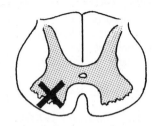

Causative viruses:

The poliovirus is an enterovirus (RNA virus).

Three immunologically distinct strains have been isolated. Immunity to one does *not* result in immunity to the other two.

Coxsackie and echoviruses may produce a clinically indistinct disorder.

Pathology:

Initially – inflammatory meningeal changes, followed by – inflammatory cell infiltrates (polymorphs and lymphocytes) around the brain stem nuclei and anterior horn cells. Neurones may undergo necrosis or central chromatolysis.

Microglial proliferation follows.

Mode of Spread:

Spread by faecal/oral route. Once ingested the virus multiplies in the nasopharynx and gastrointestinal tract penetration of GI tract results in viraemia but CNS involvement occurs in only a very small proportion. Most infected patients are asymptomatic. Virus excretion continues in the faeces for as long as three months after the initial infection – carrier state.

Epidemiology:

A highly communicable disease which may result in epidemics.

Seasonal incidence – late summer/autumn.

World-wide distribution, although more frequent in northern temperate climates.

Prophylactic inoculation has produced a dramatic reduction in incidence in the last 25 years.

Clinical features:

Infection may result in:

- Subclinical course + resultant immunity (majority).
- Mild non-specific symptoms of viraemia + resultant immunity.
- Meningism without paralysis
    (PRE-PARALYTIC) + resultant immunity.
- Meningism followed by paralysis
    (PARALYTIC) + resultant immunity.

Viral Infections — Poliomyelitis

Preparalytic stage:

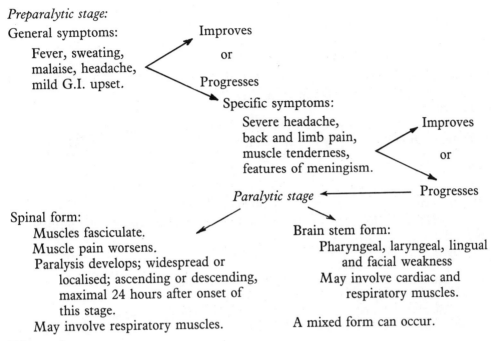

General symptoms:

    Fever, sweating,
malaise, headache,
mild G.I. upset.

Improves

or

Progresses

    Specific symptoms:

        Severe headache,
back and limb pain,
muscle tenderness,
features of meningism.

Improves

or

Progresses

Paralytic stage

Spinal form:
    Muscles fasciculate.
    Muscle pain worsens.
    Paralysis develops; widespread or
        localised; ascending or descending,
        maximal 24 hours after onset of
        this stage.
    May involve respiratory muscles.

Brain stem form:
    Pharyngeal, laryngeal, lingual
        and facial weakness
    May involve cardiac and
        respiratory muscles.

    A mixed form can occur.

Diagnosis:
    During the meningeal phase, consider other causes of acute meningitis.
    Once the paralytic phase ensues, distinguish from the Guillain Barré syndrome and transverse myelitis.
    The clinical picture + CSF examination (polymorphs and lymphocytes increased; protein elevated with normal glucose) are sufficient to reach the diagnosis.
    Serological tests + virus isolation will confirm later.

Prognosis:
    In epidemics, a mortality of 25% results from respiratory paralysis. Improvement in muscle power usually commences one week after the onset of paralysis and continues for up to a year.
    Only a proportion of muscles remain permanently paralysed; in these, fasciculation may persist. In affected limbs, bone growth becomes retarded with shortening as well as thinning.

Treatment:
    The patient is kept on bed rest and fluid balance carefully maintained.
    Respiratory failure may require ventilation.
    Avoid the development of deformities in affected limbs with physiotherapy and splinting.

Prophylaxis:

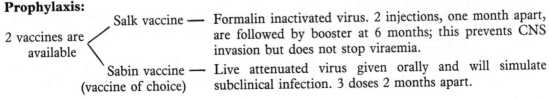

2 vaccines are available

Salk vaccine — Formalin inactivated virus. 2 injections, one month apart, are followed by booster at 6 months; this prevents CNS invasion but does not stop viraemia.

Sabin vaccine — Live attenuated virus given orally and will simulate (vaccine of choice) subclinical infection. 3 doses 2 months apart.

Viral Infections — Herpes Zoster

Varicella (chickenpox) and Herpes Zoster (shingles) are different clinical manifestations of infection by the same virus – a DNA virus, varicella zoster (VZ).

Varicella may cause: – an acute encephalitis,   – post-infectious encephalomyelitis,
                          – viral meningitis,   – post-infectious polyneuropathy.

Herpes Zoster appears to be due to reactivation of an earlier varicella exposure or infection; such reactivation may result from steroid/immunosuppressive treatment.

Pathology: The virus invol-

ves the *dorsal root* (sensory) ganglion of the spinal cord or the *cranial nerve* sensory ganglion – trigeminal or geniculate.

The inflammatory process may spread into the spinal cord and involve posterior and anterior horns. Similarly inflammatory changes may occur in the brain stem.

Haemorrhage occurs with neural loss and intense lymphocytic infiltration.

Clinical features:

Incidence increases with age. Both sexes are affected equally.
Recurrent attacks occur but are rare.

Occurs more frequently in association with disorders in which immunity is disturbed e.g. lymphoma, Hodgkin's disease.

Initial feature: A vesicular skin rash associated with burning, painful sensation. Vesicles contain clear fluid and conform to a *dermatome distribution.*

After 1–3 weeks, the vesicles crust over and leave irregular pigmentation of the skin with scarring. The distribution of lesions reflects the particular nerve involved.

Motor weakness occurs in 20% due to spread of inflammation into the anterior horn cell When cranial nerve ganglia are involved: territory.

Trigeminal: usually ophthalmic division with vesicles above the eye and associated corneal ulceration – HERPES ZOSTER OPHTHALMICUS.

Geniculate: vesicles within the external auditory meatus and ear drum with a lower motor neurone VII nerve palsy – RAMSAY HUNT SYNDROME.

Diagnosis:

Based on clinical features. CSF examination reveals lymphocytic response.

Treatment:

When herpes zoster is uncomplicated, treatment is symptomatic. In patients with defective cellular immunity with spread from a dermatomal presentation to a generalised vesicular eruption, adenine arabinoside (ARA-A) will accelerate healing.

POST-HERPETIC NEURALGIA

This is a condition which occurs in 50% of elderly patients after herpes zoster. A chronic, uncomfortable, burning pain presents in the territory of the involved dermatome. Touching the skin may evoke severe, lancinating pains.

Treatment with antidepressants, anticonvulsants e.g. carbamazepine, transcutaneous stimulation (TCS) or sympathetic ganglion block may help, but results are unpredictable.

494

Opportunistic Infections

An opportunistic infection is produced by an organism not normally pathogenic in a person with a disturbed immune response. Such impaired immunity may result from disease or from drug treatment with steroids or cytotoxic agents. Invasion of the CNS may be the sole manifestation of such infection or represent a part of more widespread dissemination.

Conditions which predispose to opportunistic infection:

Leukaemia.   Acquired immune   Cytotoxic drugs.   Multiple antibiotic treatment.
Lymphoma.   deficiency syndrome (AIDS)   Steroid drugs.   Following splenectomy.

Organisms involved:

Bacteria– m. tuberculosis.   staph. aureus.   *Fungi*–cryptococcus.   *Viruses*–herpes zoster.
      gram -ve bacilli.   anaerobic bacilli.   candida.   cytomegalovirus.
      listeria.   aspergillus.   papovavirus.

Protozoa – toxoplasmosis (see page 484).

1. Bacteria

These present with signs and symptoms of *meningitis* or *brain abscess* and are diagnosed by gram stain and culture. Treatment (see pages 337 and 338).

Listeria meningitis deserves separate mention.

Onset is sudden and an encephalitic component with altered consciousness may be associated with meningeal symptoms. Pneumonia and evidence of bacteraemia are found. The CSF may show polymorphs, or monocytic cell excess with elevated protein/low sugar. The organism is intracellular and difficult to culture.   Treatment: i.v. ampicillin.

2. Fungi

Cryptococcus neoformans: A meningitic illness in which the patient presents with headache, drowsiness, cranial nerve palsies and disturbed vision. Culture from CSF is difficult. Indian ink staining of centrifuged CSF *may* demonstrate cryptococcus. Antigen in CSF/serum or anticryptococcal antibody in serum aid diagnosis.

This condition is *fatal without treatment*. Intravenous amphotericin B is sometimes used in conjunction with 5-fluorocytosine. These drugs are toxic. Relapse following treatment is frequent and drug resistance not uncommon.

Candida:
Aspergillus: } Produce meningitis, multiple abscess or granuloma formation.

Diagnosis depends on serological tests or isolation from biopsy material.

Treatment is with amphotericin B and/or 5-fluorocytosine.

3. Viruses

Herpes Zoster: See page 494.

Cytomegalovirus: Produces an encephalitic illness or a peripheral neuropathy

Papovavirus: Produces a distinct neurological syndrome – progressive multifocal leuko-encephalopathy (see page 510), a progressive disorder over months or weeks in which dementia, seizures and focal neurological deficits occur.

Diagnosis is dependent on brain biopsy.   Treatment: Antiviral drugs – cytosine arabinoside has been used with limited success.   Remissions rarely occur.

The opportunistic infections are not in themselves characteristic. Diagnosis depends on the recognition of infection in the immunocompromised host and then applying appropriate serological investigations.

Subacute/Chronic Meningitis

This entity is characterised by symptoms and signs of meningeal irritation which persists for 3 to 4 weeks without improvement. Unlike acute meningitis, the onset is insidious; cranial nerve signs and focal deficits such as hemiparesis, dementia and gradual deterioration of conscious level may dominate the clinical picture. The outcome depends upon etiology and the instigation of appropriate treatment.

Chronic meningitis is associated with certain CSF findings.

- Lymphocytosis + low glucose.
- Lymphocytosis + normal glucose.

Diagnosis depends upon CSF examination.

Lumbar puncture should be performed in suspicious cases as soon as CT scan has ruled out a mass lesion.

Subacute/Chronic meningitis with low CSF glucose

Causes	Diagnosis	Specific features	Treatment
M. tuberculosis	See page 478		
Fungi Cryptococcus neoformans Coccidiodes Candida Histoplasma	CSF Identification of organism with India ink stain. Antigen detected (latex agglutination). Culture. Serum Anticryptococcal antibody tests.	— Hydrocephalus may develop with progressive dementia.	See page 495
Carcinomatous meningitis lung/breast/ gastro-intestinal tract. Leukaemia/ lymphoma. Glioma. Medulloblastoma.	Evidence of primary neoplasm. CSF Malignant cells seen in fresh centrifuged filtered sample.	Back pain/ radicular involvement common. Hydrocephalus in 30%	Consider irradiation followed by intrathecal methotrexate. Leukaemia/lymphoma requires specialist advice.

Subacute/Chronic Meningitis

Subacute/Chronic meningitis with normal CSF glucose.

Causes	Diagnosis	Specific features	Treatment
Parameningeal infections Cerebral abscess. Epidural abscess. Sinusitis. Mastoiditis.	Evidence of primary infected source. *X-rays* Sinuses, mastoids. *CT scan* cerebral or cerebellar abscess. *CSF* microscopy/ culture. *Blood* cultures.	Prodromal sinus or middle ear infection.	Appropriate antibiotic therapy and surgical drainage of loculated parameningeal infection.
Bacteria Treponema Brucella Leptospira	See page 481. *CSF* Isolate organism. Serological tests. *Serum* Serological tests.	*Brucella* —— Contact with infected cattle. *Leptospira* —— Contact with contaminated rat, dog or cattle urine. Jaundice, renal damage and cutaneous haemorrhages may be present.	Tetracycline, Streptomycin. Benzyl penicillin, Erythromycin.
Miscellaneous Parasites e.g. toxoplasma. Sarcoidosis. Behçet's disease. Systemic lupus erythematosus.			

Despite extensive investigation, a group of patients with chronic meningitis exists in whom no cause is found. This is referred to as – Chronic lymphocytic meningitis of unknown etiology.

The Demyelinating Diseases – Introduction

Demyelinating disorders of the central nervous system affect *myelin* and/or *oligodendroglia* with relative sparing of *axons*.

The central nervous system is composed of *neurones* with *neuroectodermal* and *mesodermal* supporting cells.

The neuroectodermal cells comprise:

> *astrocytes,*
> *ependymal cells,*
> *oligodendrocytes.*

The oligodendrocytes, like Schwann cells in the peripheral nervous system, are responsible for the formation of *myelin* around central nervous system *axons*.

One Schwann cell myelinates one axon but one oligodendrocyte may myelinate several contiguous axons, and the close proximity of cell to axon may not be obvious by light microscopy.

Oligodendrocytes are present in grey matter near neurones and in white matter near axons.

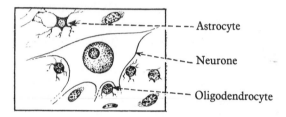

Myelin is composed of *protein* and *lipids*.
Protein accounts for 20 per cent of total content.
The lipid fraction may be divided into:

> cholesterol,
> glycophosphatides
> (lecithins),
> sphingolipids
> (sphingomyelins).

The laying down of myelin in the central nervous system commences at the fourth month of foetal life in the median longitudinal bundle, then in frontal and parietal lobes at birth and spreads. Most of the cerebrum is myelinated by the end of the 2nd year. Myelination continues until the 10th year of life.

Myelin disorders may be classified as diseases in which:

1. Myelin is inherently abnormal or was never properly formed – these disorders generally presenting in infancy and early childhood e.g. *leukodystrophy.*
2. Myelin which was normal when formed breaks down as a consequence of inflammation e.g. *multiple sclerosis.*

Multiple Sclerosis

Multiple sclerosis is a common demyelinating disease, characterised by focal disturbance of function and a relapsing and remitting course.

The disease occurs most commonly in temperate climates.

PREVALENCE RATES

	LATITUDE	RATE/100,000
Orkney and Shetland Islands ———	60° N	128
North Scotland ———————	58° N	55
San Francisco ————————	38° N	30
Queensland, Australia —————	20° S	7

The disease usually occurs in young adults with a peak age incidence of 20–40 years. Slightly more females than males are affected.

PATHOLOGY

Scattered lesions with a greyish colour, 1mm to several cm in size, are present in the white matter of the brain and spinal cord and are referred to as *plaques*.

The lesions lie in close relationship to veins (post-capillary venules) – perivenous distribution.

RECENT LESIONS ⟶ LATER ⟶ OLD LESIONS

RECENT LESIONS	LATER	OLD LESIONS
Myelin destruction. Relative axon sparing. Perivenous infiltration with mononuclear cells and lymphocytes. Oedema is evident in acute lesions.	Astrocyte proliferation.	Relatively acellular. Occasional perivenous macrophages and lymphocytes. Axon degeneration may occur.

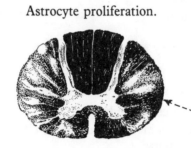

Dorsal spinal cord showing established plaques of demyelination.

PATHOGENESIS

Immune deficiency has been suggested. This might explain the possible persistence of a latent virus and variations in immune status could be the basis of 'relapses and remissions'. Studies of humoral and cellular immunity both *in vivo* and *in vitro* have been conflicting.

Hereditary/genetic factors appear significant. There is an increased familial incidence of multiple sclerosis. This has led to the study of *Histocompatibility Antigens* (HL-A). An association between A3, B7, B18 and DW2/DRW2 and multiple sclerosis has been demonstrated.

Viruses may be important in the development of multiple sclerosis, possibly viral infection in a genetically/immunologically susceptible host.

Elevated serum and CSF antibody titres have been found to:

varicella zoster, measles, rubella and herpes simplex during relapse.

It has been suggested that these antiviral antibodies are produced within the CSF.

Oligoclonal bands present in M.S. in the CSF contain antibodies to several viruses.

Biochemical: No biochemical effect has been demonstrated – myelin appears normal before breakdown and proposed excess of dietary fats or malabsorption of unsaturated fatty acids unproven.

Multiple Sclerosis

Pathogenesis *(continued)*

In summary – the causation is probably multifactorial.

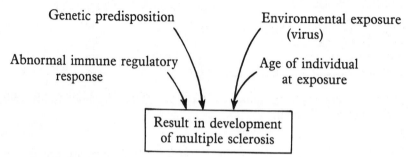

CLINICAL FEATURES

Precipitating factors:

> Infection.
> Trauma.
> Surgery.
> Pregnancy and puerperium.

These may result in the initial presentation or in a relapse.

Following trauma, symptoms and signs may relate to the site of injury.

Multiple sclerosis is characterised clinically by:
1. Signs and symptoms of dissemination (widespread CNS involvement).
2. A relapsing and remitting course.

Symptoms at onset

1. *Vague symptoms* – lack of energy, headache, depression, aches in limbs – may result in diagnosis of psychoneurosis. These symptoms are eventually associated with:

2. *Precise symptoms:*
   (Initial symptom of multiple sclerosis expressed as a %)

Limb weakness	40%
Sensory disturbance	20%
Visual loss	25%
Disturbance of ocular movements	
Vertigo	
Ataxia	15%
Sphincter disturbance	

Trigeminal neuralgia may be an early symptom of multiple sclerosis, and this disorder should always be considered in the young patient with paroxysmal facial pain.

Multiple Sclerosis

Motor Symptoms

Monoparesis and paraparesis are the common presentations of motor weakness. Hemiparesis and quadriparesis occur less commonly.

Paraparesis is the result of spinal demyelination, usually in the cervical region.

Signs are those of increased tone:

> hyperactive deep tendon reflexes,
> extensor plantar response and
> often absent abdominal reflexes.

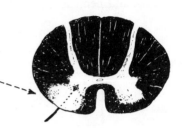

A plaque at the anterior root exit zone will result in lower motor neurone signs (reflex loss and segmental wasting)

Sensory Symptoms

Fleeting sensory numbness and paraesthesia are common and often so transient as to be forgotten.

Paraesthesia is more often due to posterior column demyelination than to spinothalamic tract involvement.

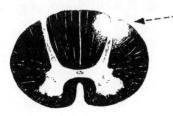

Posterior column lesions result in impaired vibration sensation and joint position sensation.

In such cases a limb may be rendered 'useless' by the absence of position sensation.

On flexion of the neck with cervical posterior column involvement, Lhermitte's sign is elicited – sudden shock-like sensation down the back to arms/legs.

Spinothalamic lesions result in thermal dysaesthesia, a painful feeling of burning, coldness or warmth, with associated sensory loss to pain and temperature contralateral to the lesion.

A plaque at the posterior root entry zone will result in loss of all sensory modalities in that particular root distribution.

Multiple Sclerosis

Disturbance of Vision

Retrobulbar neuritis (R.B.N.) – Rapid partial or total loss of vision in one eye evolving over seconds, hours or days.

A central visual field defect – scotoma – is often present due to selective involvement of macular fibres.

Altitudinal and hemianopic field defects may occur.

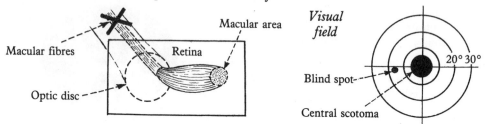

As colour vision (cones) is a function of the macular area some disturbance in colour perception will occur.

Pain may be present, especially on movement of the eye, and occurs if the dural membrane covering the nerve is involved.

Fundal examination may reveal swelling – *papillitis* in 50 per cent of cases.

The development of papillitis in R.B.N. depends upon the proximity of the plaque to the optic nerve head.

Reduced acuity distinguishes from papilloedema.

> Usually only one eye is affected.
> Occasionally both eyes, simultaneously or consecutively, are affected.
> 30% recover completely.
> 40% show almost complete return of vision.
> 30% show none to only moderate improvement.

Retrobulbar neuritis can be categorised as follows:

1. No evidence of multiple sclerosis occurs in patient's life time.
2. Acute bilateral R.B.N. is followed by a transverse myelitis (Neuromyelitis optica).
3. Signs and symptoms of further demyelination elsewhere in the nervous system follow – multiple sclerosis. Over a 15 year period from presentation with R.B.N. 35–40% of patients fall into this group.

Following recovery from R.B.N. the optic disc may develop an atrophic appearance with a pale temporal margin – Temporal pallor. (The temporal side of the optic disc receives the macular fibres.)

It is important to appreciate that plaque formation in the optic nerve may be asymptomatic and pallor may be found on fundoscopy in a patient with pure motor or sensory symptomatology.

Rarely visual loss results from chiasmal or optic radiation plaques.

Multiple Sclerosis

Disturbance of Ocular Movement

Diplopia may result from demyelination affecting the intramedullary course of the III, IV or VI cranial nerves. Abnormality of eye movements without diplopia occurs when supranuclear or internuclear connections are involved. The latter results from a lesion in the medial longitudinal bundle (MLB) – *Internuclear ophthalmoplegia* – and in young persons is pathognemonic of MS.

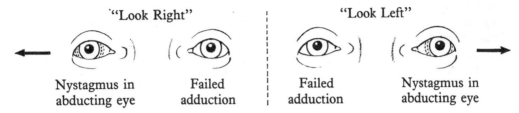

"Look Right"   "Look Left"

Nystagmus in abducting eye   Failed adduction   Failed adduction   Nystagmus in abducting eye

Nystagmus may be an incidental finding on neurological examination. Its presence should be sought as evidence of a second lesion. It is unusual in multiple sclerosis when the eyes are in the primary position, and is commonly seen on lateral gaze.

Pupillary abnormalities may occur from:

- sympathetic involvement in the brain stem (Horner's syndrome),
- III nerve involvement

or – II nerve involvement.

The swinging light test is a sensitive test of impaired afferent conduction in the II nerve. Alternating the light from one eye to the other results eventually in 'pupillary escape' – the pupil dilates despite the presence of direct light.

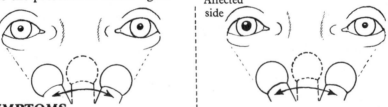

Affected side

OTHER SYMPTOMS

Vestibular symptoms: Vertigo of central type may be a presenting problem or develop during the course of the illness. Hearing loss is rare.

Ataxia of gait and limb incoordination are frequently present. The gait ataxia may be cerebellar or sensory type (see Romberg's test). Limb incoordination, intention tremor and dysarthria indicate cerebellar involvement. The most gross intention tremor encountered in clinical practice occurs in MS, the limbs being widely flung about when attempting the simplest of tasks.

Sphincter disturbance with urgency or precipitancy of micturition and eventual incontinence occurs. Conversely urinary retention in a young person may be the first symptom of disease. On direct questioning, impotence is frequently found.

Mental changes: Mood change – euphoria or depression occur. Pseudobulbar palsy gives rise to emotional lability (uncontrolled outbursts of crying or laughing). Dementia may occur in advanced cases.

Multiple Sclerosis

CLINICAL COURSE

Relapses occur within 1 year in 30% of patients and after 10 years in 10%. Initial remissions may be complete with a return of normal function. Diversity is a characteristic of the disease and the following clinical patterns may be defined:

1. Acute MS:

    Explosive onset.
    Death may occur in months.
    Dramatic recovery and prolonged remission may occur.
    Separation from acute disseminated encephalomyelitis is difficult.

2. Slowly progressive course with no relapse/remission. Often spinal form (see below).

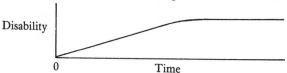

3. Relapsing course with accumulating disability.

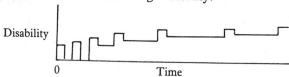

4. Benign form:

    Abrupt onset – good remission – long latent period.

    Within this group could be included those in whom plaques appear as an incidental finding at autopsy.
    25 years after onset as many as two thirds of surviving patients are ambulant and of those one third remain in employment.

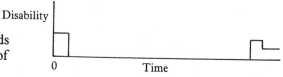

Of all patients diagnosed with MS, 75% survive for 25 years.

Classification can be made depending on pattern of CNS involvement.
The majority have a *generalised* form with optic nerve, cerebellum/brain stem and spinal lesions.
One third develop an almost exclusively *spinal* form with spastic/ataxic gait and sphincter disturbance. Asymptomatic optic nerve involvement is frequent (abnormal VERs).
A *cerebellar* form occurs in a minority.

Multiple Sclerosis

INVESTIGATIONS

There is no diagnostic test. Investigations only support the clinical suspicion.

Neurophysiological: Measurements of conduction within the central nervous system to detect a second symptomatic lesion (see page 50).

1. *Visual evoked potential (VEP).* In optic nerve involvement the latency of the large positive wave is delayed beyond 110 msec. The amplitude of the waves may also be reduced.

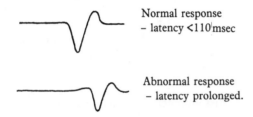

Normal response
– latency <110 msec

Abnormal response
– latency prolonged.

2. *Somatosensory evoked response (SSEP)* may detect central sensory pathway lesions.

3. *Brainstem auditory evoked potentials (BAEP)* may detect brainstem lesions.

Cerebrospinal fluid examination by lumbar puncture

A mild pleocytosis (25 cells/mm^3), mainly lymphocytes, is occasionally found.
The total protein may be elevated.
An increase in gammaglobulin with a normal albumin occurs in 50–60% of cases.
Electrophoresis of CSF using agar or acrylamide shows discrete bands which are not present in serum – rather than a diffuse increase in CSF immunoglobulins.

Oligoclonal bands

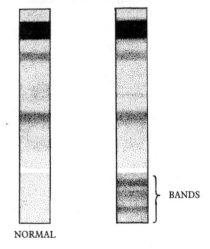

NORMAL

BANDS

These bands are found in up to 95% of established cases and 50–60% of cases after first attack of symptoms.
Oligoclonal bands are found in a few other neurological diseases e.g.
    chronic meningitis,
    neurosyphilis,
    subacute sclerosing panencephalitis.

CT-scanning may show small areas of reduced density corresponding to plaques and ventricular dilatation occurring secondary to periventricular plaques.
Nuclear magnetic resonance (NMR) scanning shows greater promise for the detection of small multiple lesions.

Multiple Sclerosis

DIFFERENTIAL DIAGNOSIS

Diagnosis is based on demonstrating clinical or neurophysiological lesions disseminated in time (relapses) and space (anatomical localisation).

In the established case diagnosis is obvious, with scattered signs and history of relapse.

Difficulty arises:

1. With the first attack   2. With non-remitting progressive form of disease   3. In differentiating from other neurological disorders in which dissemination is a feature

Full investigation of that part of neuroaxis involved:

   With *spinal presentation,*
      myelography is necessary.
   With *cerebellar presentation,*
      posterior fossa CT-scan is required.

e.g. lupus erythematosus

Check ESR
      Antinuclear antibodies,
      Anti-DNA binding.

Acute MS may be clinically inseparable from acute disseminated encephalomyelitis.

Solitary lesions strategically placed may give the impression of disseminated disease. This is especially so at the foramen magnum where a lesion may produce:

Nystagmus
Cranial nerve signs
Cerebellar signs   e.g. Neurofibroma
Brainstem signs   or
Corticospinal signs   Arnold Chiari malformation

Multiple Sclerosis – Treatment

SYMPTOMATIC/SUPPORTIVE

1. Spasticity. Spasms of flexor or extensor nature are painful and contractures will develop.

> Drugs – antispastic,
> e.g. Baclofen, Dantrolene,
> Diazepam.

Care must be taken not to make muscles too floppy and remove their 'splinting' effect. In severe contractures – tenotomy. When bladder/bowel function is lost – consider intrathecal alcohol or phenol.

2. Urinary symptoms. Probanthene may be useful in the uninhibited bladder. The patient with precipitancy of micturition may need to pay close attention to his fluid load. Mandelamine and ascorbic acid will acidify urine and protect against infection.
Urinary infection, when it occurs, should be promptly treated.

3. Bowel symptoms. Stool softeners and high roughage diet should be recommended when constipation is a problem.

4. Paroxysmal pain of a burning dysaesthetic type may respond well to the anticonvulsants carbamazepine and phenytoin.

5. Seizures of a tonic/clonic or occasionally tonic nature will require anticonvulsants.

6. Pain and sphincter disturbance may respond to dorsal column stimulation (DCS). The results of such electrical treatment are variable.

SPECIFIC AGAINST DISEASE PROCESS

1. Anti-inflammatory and Immunosuppressive therapy
ACTH (Adrenocorticotrophic Hormone) may shorten the duration of relapses but will not influence the outcome.
Regime: I.M. 80 i.u. ACTH daily x 7 followed by I.M. 40 i.u. ACTH daily x 7.
Immunosuppressives
– cyclophosphamide, azothiaprine –
no evidence of value and potentially dangerous; marrow toxicity, etc. Occasionally used in acute MS.

2. Enhancement of cell mediated immunity (depressed in MS?).
Transfer factor – disappointing.
Interferon (antiviral substance made by immunocompetent cells) has been suggested but not evaluated.

3. Physical treatment. Elevation of body temperature may aggravate symptoms – consequently body cooling has been applied in acute situations, also hyperbaric oxygen therapy, which appears to modify the animal model of MS (acute experimental allergic encephalomyelitis). This has not yet been conclusively proven of value in patients with MS.

4. Dietary measures e.g. low gluten or polyunsaturated fat supplemented diets again of no proven value.

IN SUMMARY – No available specific therapy of proven value.

507

Other Demyelinating Diseases

Neuromyelitis Optica (Devic's disease)

Neuromyelitis optica is characterised by a simultaneous or successive optic neuritis/transverse myelitis.

A history of upper respiratory infection may precede neurological symptoms.

Visual loss is rapid – either unilateral or bilateral with large central scotomata. Papillitis may be present or the optic disc may appear normal.

Spinal cord symptoms follow – hours, days or occasionally weeks later.

   Back pain and girdle pain. Paraesthesia in lower limbs.

   Urinary retention. Paralysis may ascend to involve respiratory muscles.

EXAMINATION

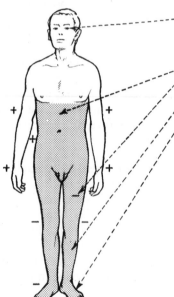

Papillitis with reduced visual acuity and central scotoma.

Sensory loss extending up to mid thorax.

Reduced lower limb reflexes initially.

Reduced power in lower limbs.

Extensor plantar responses.

The disorder may be:

1. A presentation of multiple sclerosis in adults. A relapsing and remitting course typical of MS ensues.

2. A monophasic illness occurring in childhood akin to acute disseminated encephalomyelitis. Cavitation within the spinal cord may occur, resulting in permanent deficit.

INVESTIGATION

Visual evoked responses are prolonged. The CSF shows an elevated protein with a lymphocytosis occasionally as high as 1000 cells per mm^3. Gammaglobulin may be elevated and oligoclonal bands present.

TREATMENT

Steroids may prove effective in 2 (above), the postinfectious form. Treatment otherwise is supportive.

Other Demyelinating Diseases

Acute Disseminated Encephalomyelitis (ADEM)

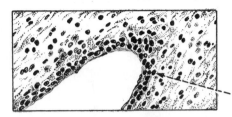

ADEM is an acute demyelinating disorder in which small foci of demyelination with a perivenous distribution are scattered throughout the brain and spinal cord. Lesions are 0.1 – 1.0mm in diameter.

Microglial, plasma cell and lymphocyte exudate around the vein.

This disorder may follow upper respiratory and gastro-intestinal infections (viral), viral exanthems (measles, chickenpox, rubella etc.) or immunisation.

The synonymous titles 'post-infectious' and 'post-vaccinal' encephalomyelitis can also be applied to this condition.

CLINICAL FEATURES: Within days or weeks of resolution of the viral infection, fever, headache, nausea and vomiting develop. Meningeal symptoms (neck stiffness, photophobia) are then followed by drowsiness and multifocal neurological signs and symptoms – hemisphere brain-stem/cerebellar/spinal cord and optic nerve involvement.

Predominantly *spinal* or *cerebral* forms occur though usually the picture is mixed. Optic nerve involvement takes the form of optic neuritis. Rarely the peripheral nervous system is involved.

OUTCOME: 20% mortality.

Recovery may be complete. The cerebral form often results in permanent intellectual and behavioural deficits.

Relapse occurs in a few – the clinical picture being indistinguishable from MS.

DIAGNOSIS: No diagnostic test.

CSF – 20–200 mononuclear cells.

Total protein elevated with γglobulin raised also.

Peripheral blood may be normal or show neutrophilia, lymphocytosis or lymphopenia.

The electroencephalogram (EEG) shows diffuse slow wave activity.

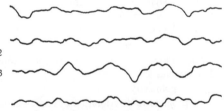

Generalised asynchronous delta activity

Diagnosis is straight forward when there is obvious preceding viral infection or immunisation. When viral infection immediately precedes, distinction from acute encephalitis is impossible.

Separation from acute MS may be difficult. Fever, meningeal signs with elevated CSF protein above 100 mg/ml with cell count greater than 50 per mm^3 suggest ADEM.

Pathologically, demyelination is limited to perivascular areas and lesions do not approach the same size as in MS.

TREATMENT: Steroids should be used and appear effective. Large dosage is recommended during the acute phase.

Other Demyelinating Diseases

Acute Haemorrhagic Leukoencephalitis

This is a rare demyelinating disease. It is regarded as a very acute form of post-infectious/acute disseminated encephalomyelitis.

The clinical picture is: Antecedent viral infection, depression of conscious level and multifocal signs and symptoms. Very focal features may suggest a mass lesion or even herpes simplex encephalitis.

The diagnosis is only really possible at biopsy or autopsy, but elevated CSF pressure, lymphocytosis and erythrocytes in CSF and xanthochromic appearance of fluid are all suggestive.

Pathology: Perivascular polymorph infiltration.
Microscopic and macroscopic haemorrhage.
Perivascular demyelination and necrotising changes in vessels.

Treatment: Steroids in high doseage should be used though evidence of value in this rare condition is scant.

Progressive Multifocal Leukoencephalopathy

This is a demyelinative disease occurring in association with systemic illness in which cell mediated and occasionally humoral mediated immunity is depressed e.g. lymphoma, sarcoidosis, systemic lupus erythematosus.

Clinical picture: Features of diffuse process – personality change, hemiparesis, cortical visual loss, seizures etc.

Duration of illness: 3–6 months. Non-remitting and fatal.

Pathology: Demyelination without inflammatory response.
Electron microscopy – papovavirus in oligodendroglia.
Antibodies may be detected in serum to papovavirus.

Treatment: No specific treatment.

Dysmyelinating Diseases

Inborn errors of metabolism involving myelin formation may result in abnormal or arrested myelination. Several groups of disorders may express themselves in this way.

The *Leukodystrophies* represent one such group and may be subdivided into:
1. Metachromatic leukodystrophy,   3. Adrenoleukodystrophy,
2. Globoid cell leukodystrophy,   4. Spongy sclerosis,
depending on pathological features.

Clinical features: Onset is in infancy or childhood. Metachromatic leukodystrophy may develop in early adult life.
The features are those of:
– hypotonicity,
– progressive deterioration of conscious level with eventual flexion or extension to pain,
– seizures will occur throughout the illness.
Cerebellar ataxia and optic atrophy can occur.

Metachromatic leukodystrophy affects not only the central but also the peripheral nervous system. This disorder, when presenting in adult life may be mistaken for psychotic illness before the dementia becomes evident.

In adrenoleukodystrophy, features of Addison's disease coexist.

All show recessive Mendelian inheritance except adrenoleukodystrophy which is an X-linked recessive disorder.

Diagnosis: CSF examination may show protein elevation.
In metachromatic leukodystrophy, metachromatic bodies may be present in urine and diagnosis is confirmed by sural nerve biopsy.

Brain biopsy may help in diagnosis.

Prognosis: These disorders are all progressive with death within months to 2–3 years.

510

Neurological Complications of Drugs and Toxins

INTRODUCTION

Drugs and toxins do not often produce well defined clinical syndromes but usually a diffuse neurological picture in which impairment of conscious level may occur.

Diagnosis is especially dependent upon history:
- Availability of drugs.
- Occupational/industrial exposure to toxins.

Drug toxicity may result from:
- The chronic abuse of drugs e.g. barbiturates, opioids.
- The side effects of drug therapy e.g. anticonvulsants, steroids.
- The willfull overdosage of drugs e.g. sedatives, antidepressants.

Toxin exposure may be:
- Accidental: Industrial or household poisons e.g. organophosphates, carbon monoxide, turpentine.
- Wilfull: Solvent abuse.

HISTORY and EXAMINATION

When drugs or toxins are suspected, the following clinical features are supportive.

Mental state
Confusion, delirium, coma occur with acute exposure.

Seizures
may occur with some drugs.

Pupillary findings
Generally unaffected by drugs.
Narcotics will produce small pupils.
Glutethamide ⟶ large pupils.

Multisystem Dysfunction
Cardiac, respiratory, hepatic and gastrointestinal systems may be involved.

Brain stem Reflexes
e.g. Dolls eye reflex – may be transiently lost.
Also: Note:
- Puncture marks in narcotic addicts.
- The presence of a snout area rash in solvent abusers.
- Rashes in barbiturate poisoning.
- Respiration rate in salicylate poisoning.
- Skin colour in carbon monoxide poisoning.

Clinical features:

While the neurological picture is generally diffuse, certain pronounced symptoms occur with one drug or toxin and not with another. The following table should act as a guide to diagnosis and direct the clinician in the appropriate usage of the 'drug screen'

For treatment, the reader is advised to consult an appropriate pharmacology text.

Neurological Syndromes of Drugs and Toxins

This table is not all inclusive but includes common drugs/toxins.

Syndrome of optic nerve damage

Chloramphenicol. Streptomycin.
Ethambutol. Vitamin A (papilloedema).
Chloroquine (retinopathy).

Syndrome of VIII nerve (vestibular) damage

Aminoglycoside antibiotics.
   Gentamicin. Neomycin. Streptomycin.
   Kanamycin (cochlear damage also).

Syndrome of progressive confusion/delirium

Amphetamines. Amantadine.
Barbiturates. Beta blockers.
Lithium. Phenytoin. Salicylates.

Heavy metals (lead).
Carbon monoxide. Caffeine.

Syndrome of seizures/myoclonus with hypo- or hyperreflexia

Amphetamines. Clonidine.
Lithium. Phenytoin. Theophylline.
Tricyclic antidepressants.

Organophasphates.
Lead. Caffeine.

Syndrome of involuntary movements – Parkinsonian, Dystonic etc.

Butyrophenones. Phenothiazines.
L.dopa. Na valproate.
Tricyclic antidepressants.

Heavy metals. Organophosphates.

Syndrome of progressive weakness and/or paraesthesia (muscle, neuro- muscular junction, peripheral nerve)

Antifungal drugs. Clofibrate. Dapsone.
Metronidazole. Isoniazid. Steroids.
Sulphonamides. Phenytoin. Vincristine.
Organophosphates. Solvents.

Syndrome of progressive ataxia

Anticonvulsants e.g. phenytoin. Metronidazole.
Solvents.

The DRUG SCREEN

Too often the clinician, when managing suspected drug or toxin overdosage requests a 'drug screen'.

The techniques used in detection e.g. gas chromatography, thin-layer chromatography and immunological tests, are sophisticated and time consuming and may require samples of serum, urine or both.

The clinician must 'narrow down the field' from the history and presenting symptoms/signs and discuss with the laboratory the class of drug or toxin he suspects. In this way detection will be more successful.

A knowledge of the blood level of some drugs, e.g. salicylates, barbiturates, is important in deciding the approach to treatment.

Specific Syndromes of Drugs and Toxins

The commonest toxic cause of central and peripheral nervous system damage is alcohol abuse, which is dealt with on page 525.

SOLVENT ABUSE

This is an increasing problem with inner city children. The purpose of inhalation is to achieve a state of euphoria. Habituation develops. The following substances are commonly used: Aerosols, cleaning fluids, nail varnish remover, lighter fluids, 'model' glue. The causative contents of these probably are aromatic e.g. toluene and chlorinated hydrocarbons, acetone and ketones.

Symptoms of acute intoxication: Euphoria.
Dysarthria, ataxia, diplopia.
Delusions and hallucinations may occur, followed by seizures if exposure has been prolonged.

Death may result – Aspiration/asphyxiation.
Cardiac arrhythmias.
Accidental while intoxicated.
Renal or hepatic damage.

Symptoms of chronic abuse: Behavioural disturbance.
Chronic ataxia.
Sensorimotor peripheral neuropathy.

LEAD EXPOSURE

Lead has no biological function. It is present in normal diet as well as in the atmosphere from automobile fumes and the water supply of old buildings containing lead tanks and piping. Occupation exposure occurs in plumbers, burners and smelters.

Lead excess interferes with *haem* synthesis. This results in the accumulation of 'blocked' metabolites such as aminolevulinic acid (ALA) in serum and urine.

Anaemia occurs with a characteristic finding in the blood film (basophilic stippling).

Both the peripheral and central nervous systems are affected.

ADULTS

A chronic motor neuropathy with some sensory symptomatology. Axonal damage predominates.

rarely

Acute encephalopathy

CHILDREN

Peripheral neuropathy is rare. Encephalopathy is characteristic.

Acute fulminating with confusion, impaired conscious level, coma, seizures, papilloedema.

Chronic with fatigue and irritability, headache, apathy.

In encephalopathy, diffuse neurological symptoms and signs may occur e.g. vertigo, ataxia, paraparesis, hemiplegia.

Treatment:

Chelating agents (e.g. calcium disodium edetate (EDTA) or D penicillamine) and i.v. mannitol in acute encephalopathy with papilloedema.

In acute fulminating encephalopathy the mortality has been reduced to 5% but neurological sequelae are common.

Specific Syndromes of Drugs and Toxins

NARCOTIC ADDICTION
The alkaloids derived from opium include morphine and codeine.

A large number of synthetic and semisynthetic agonists are available in the drug treatment of pain e.g. methadone.

Heroin is diacetylmorphine; because of the ease with which this crosses the blood/brain barrier it is 3 times more effective than morphine.

Clinical effects of administration

Alteration in mood – euphoria.   Analgesic effect.   Pupillary constrictor.

Depresses body temperature.   Slow gastrointestinal motility.

Induces orthostatic hypotension.

Tolerance develops with physical dependence and

Repeated exposure

$\longrightarrow$ withdrawal symptoms: – drug craving.

– sweating, anorexia/vomiting.

Death from – cardiac arrhythmia,   – seizures, abdominal pain.

pulmonary oedema or

massive overdosage may occur, especially when combined with alcohol.

Frequent medical complications in drug addicts include:

Thrombophlebitis, pulmonary embolism and sepsis – local infection at site of administration.

Endocarditis, pulmonary infection, tuberculosis or serum hepatitis (Type B).

The neurological complications of such infections (meningitis, abscess etc) may ensue.

Specific neurological complications in drug addicts:

Transverse myelitis – hypersensitivity response?

Peripheral neuropathy – Guillain Barré type.

Mononeuropathy – pressure palsy or 'misplaced' injection.

Brachial or lumbar sacral plexitis – hypersensitivity?

Cerebral infarction – arteritis?

Neurological sequelae on recovery from overdosage

Dementia, seizures, involuntary movements.

The treatment of narcotic addiction is complex and not dealt with here. To the neurologist and neurosurgeon, recognition is important lest an addict be missed. Antagonists e.g. naloxone, may be life saving in the emergency room when respiration is depressed; thereafter the patient should be referred to a specialist dealing with problems of drug addiction.

Metabolic Encephalopathies

Encephalopathy is a loose term implying a diffuse disorder of the cerebral hemispheres.
In general terms, the clinical features of metabolic or drug induced encephalopathy are relatively stereotyped.

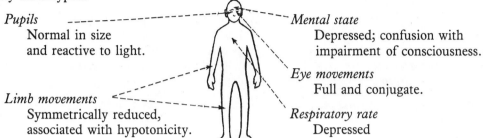

Pupils
Normal in size and reactive to light.

Mental state
Depressed; confusion with impairment of consciousness.

Eye movements
Full and conjugate.

Limb movements
Symmetrically reduced, associated with hypotonicity.

Respiratory rate
Depressed

These features are characteristic but exceptions occur in specific encephalopathies –

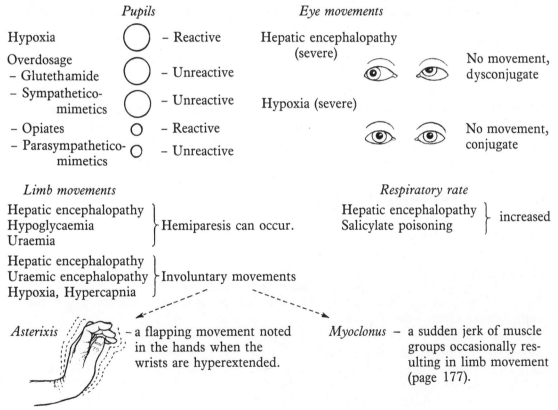

Pupils

Hypoxia – Reactive

Overdosage
– Glutethamide – Unreactive
– Sympathetico-mimetics – Unreactive
– Opiates – Reactive
– Parasympathetico-mimetics – Unreactive

Eye movements

Hepatic encephalopathy (severe) — No movement, dysconjugate

Hypoxia (severe) — No movement, conjugate

Limb movements

Hepatic encephalopathy
Hypoglycaemia
Uraemia
} Hemiparesis can occur.

Hepatic encephalopathy
Uraemic encephalopathy
Hypoxia, Hypercapnia
} Involuntary movements

Respiratory rate

Hepatic encephalopathy
Salicylate poisoning
} increased

Asterixis – a flapping movement noted in the hands when the wrists are hyperextended.

Myoclonus – a sudden jerk of muscle groups occasionally resulting in limb movement (page 177).

Beware the possibility of dual pathology e.g. an alcoholic patient with a chronic subdural haematoma may also be in liver failure as well as having thiamine deficiency.

Classification and Biochemical Evaluation

Many metabolic disturbances cause an *acquired* encephalopathy in adults.
The most frequently encountered are:

Hypoxic	– less commonly
Hypercapnoeic	Hyponatraemia. Hypernatraemia.
Hypoglycaemic	Hypokalaemia. Hyperkalaemia.
Hyperglycaemic	Hypocalcaemia. Hypercalcaemia.
Hepatic	Hypothyroidism. Lactic acidosis.
Uraemic	Addison's disease.

Drugs and toxins producing encephalopathy are dealt with separately (page 511).

Laboratory Assessment of suspected metabolic encephalopathy

All patients should have a basic biochemical screen:
– Serum urea and electrolytes.
– Liver function (albumin, globulin, bilirubin, alkaline phosphatase and enzymes) and random blood glucose.
– Blood gases (pH, PO_2 PCO_2).
– Electroencephalography – slow wave activity (theta or delta) supports the diagnosis of a diffuse dysfunction: hepatic encephalopathy shows a specific triphasic slow wave configuration.
– CT scan – if the above tests are normal or coexisting structural brain disease is suspected.

Calculation of the *anion gap* may be helpful in the diagnosis of encephalopathies, especially *lactic acidosis.* The sum of the anions (Cl^- and HCO_3^-) normally equals the sum of the cations (Na^+ and K^+). An increase in the gap in the absence of ketones, salicylates and uraemia suggests lactic acidosis.

Specific Encephalopathies

HYPOXIC ENCEPHALOPATHY

Impaired brain oxygenation results from:
– Reduced arterial oxygen pressure – lung disease.
– Reduced haemoglobin to carry oxygen – anaemia or blood loss.
– Reduced flow of blood containing oxygen (ischaemic hypoxia) – due to reduced cardiac output (with reduced cerebral blood flow).
– Biochemical block of cerebral utilisation of oxygen – rare (e.g. cyanide poisoning).

When cerebral arterial pO_2 falls below 35 mm Hg (4.5 kPa), anaerobic metabolism takes over; this is not efficient and a further drop in pO_2 will result in neurological dysfunction. The extent of hypoxic damage depends not only upon the duration of hypoxia but also on other factors e.g. body temperature – hypothermia protects against damage. The irreversibility of hypoxic damage is explained by the 'no flow phenomenon' – after 3–5 minutes the endothelial lining of small vessels swells – even with reversal of hypoxia, flow through these vessels is no longer possible.

Specific Encephalopathies

HYPOXIC ENCEPHALOPATHY *(continued)*

Pathology:

As a consequence of high metabolic demand, some areas are more susceptible than others.

Vulnerability to hypoxia:

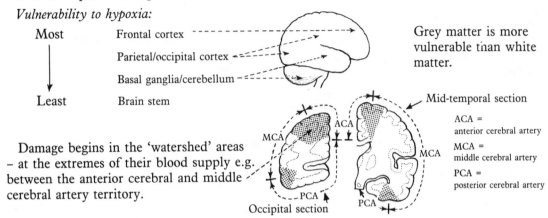

Most   Frontal cortex

Parietal/occipital cortex

Basal ganglia/cerebellum

Least   Brain stem

Grey matter is more vulnerable than white matter.

Damage begins in the 'watershed' areas – at the extremes of their blood supply e.g. between the anterior cerebral and middle cerebral artery territory.

Mid-temporal section

ACA = anterior cerebral artery

MCA = middle cerebral artery

PCA = posterior cerebral artery

Occipital section

Microscopic changes depend upon the delay between the onset of hypoxia and death.

Immediate:	*At 48 hours:*	*At several days/weeks:*
Scattered petechial haemorrhages.	Cerebral oedema associated with petechial haemorrhage.	Necrosis in cortical grey matter and globus pallidus with associated astrocytic proliferation. The cerebellum and brain stem may also be affected.

Clinical features: Severe hypoxia e.g. circulatory arrest.

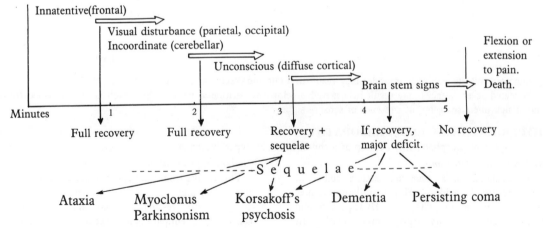

Innatentive(frontal)

Visual disturbance (parietal, occipital)

Incoordinate (cerebellar)

Unconscious (diffuse cortical)

Brain stem signs

Flexion or extension to pain. Death.

Minutes   1   2   3   4   5

Full recovery   Full recovery   Recovery + sequelae   If recovery, major deficit.   No recovery

– – – – – – – – – – Sequelae – – – – – – – – – –

Ataxia   Myoclonus Parkinsonism   Korsakoff's psychosis   Dementia   Persisting coma

Delayed hypoxic encephalopathy refers to the rare occurrence of a full clinical recovery followed after some weeks by a progressive picture ⟶ deterioration of conscious level ⟶ death. Widespread subcortical demyelination is found at autopsy.

517

Specific Encephalopathies

HYPERCAPNOEIC ENCEPHALOPATHY: the consequence of an elevated arterial carbon dioxide level.

Clinical features:

Headache, confusion, disorientation, involuntary movements.
Papilloedema, depressed limb reflexes, extensor plantar responses.

Diagnosis:

A pCO_2 greater than 50 mm Hg (6 kPa) with a reduced pO_2 is found on arterial blood sampling.

The presence of headache, confusion and papilloedema may suggest intracranial tumour. If hypercapnia has not been diagnosed, such patients inevitably are referred for CT brain scan.

HYPOGLYCAEMIC ENCEPHALOPATHY: the consequence of insufficient glucose reaching the brain and may result from:
- Overdosage of diabetic treatment.
- Insulin secreting tumour – insulinoma.
- Hepatic disease with reduction of liver glycogen.

Serum glucose levels of 1.5 mmol/l are associated with the onset of encephalopathy. Levels of 0.5 mmol/l are associated with coma.

Pathology:

Changes occur in the cerebral cortex – focal necrosis surrounded by neuronal degeneration. Subcortical grey matter (caudate nucleus) and cerebellum are vulnerable.

Clinical features:

These, like those of hypoxia, are dependent upon the duration and severity of hypoglycaemia.

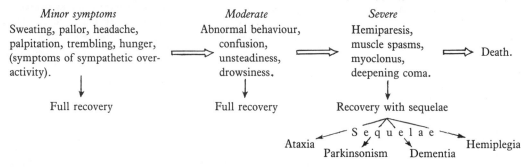

Repeated mild to moderate episodes may result in a chronic cerebellar ataxia.

Repeated severe attacks may result in a mixed myelopathy/peripheral neuropathy which is distinguished from motor neurone disease by the presence of sensory signs.

HYPERGLYCAEMIC ENCEPHALOPATHY

Two types of encephalopathy develop as a consequence of hyperglycaemia:

Diabetic ketoacidotic coma

Accumulation of acetone and ketone bodies in blood results in acidosis. Hyperventilation ensues with a reduction in pCO_2 and HCO_3^-. Osmotic diuresis due to hyperglycaemia results in dehydration.

The neurological presentation is that of confusion progressing to coma and, if untreated, death.

Diabetic hyperosmolar non-ketotic coma

This results from the hyperosmolar effect of severe hyperglycaemia. Reduction of the intracellular compartment results. Involuntary movements, seizures and hemiparesis may occur. Vascular thrombosis is not uncommon. Ketoacidosis is mild or does not occur.

Specific Encephalopathies

HEPATIC ENCEPHALOPATHY

Neurological signs and symptoms secondary to hepatic dysfunction may arise in:
- acute liver failure.
- chronic liver failure complicated by infection or gastrointestinal haemorrhage.
- chronic liver failure producing characteristic *hepatocerebral degeneration.*

Clinical features:

These may be divided into two groups:

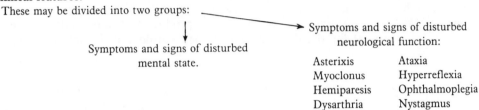

Symptoms and signs of disturbed
mental state.

Symptoms and signs of disturbed
neurological function:

Asterixis	Ataxia
Myoclonus	Hyperreflexia
Hemiparesis	Ophthalmoplegia
Dysarthria	Nystagmus

The encephalopathy is progressive.

Pathology:

Neuronal loss with gliosis is noted in the cerebral cortex as well as basal ganglia, cerebellum and brain stem. Astrocytes with irregular and enlarged nuclei are characteristic.

Hepatocerebral degeneration produces varying symptoms and signs. Dementia is associated with dysarthria and ataxia. Primitive reflexes, choreoathetosis, myoclonus, tremor and pyramidal signs may also be present. Consciousness is *not* impaired.

URAEMIC ENCEPHALOPATHY

Clinical features:

These may be divided into two groups:

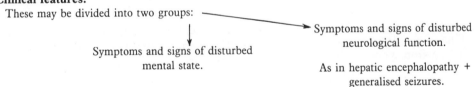

Symptoms and signs of disturbed
mental state.

Symptoms and signs of disturbed
neurological function.

As in hepatic encephalopathy +
generalised seizures.

Pathology:

Uraemia may produce non-specific pathological findings in the nervous system. Peripheral nervous system involvement occurs in chronic renal failure (page 422).

Dialysis encephalopathy is encountered in persons on renal dialysis exposed to high aluminium levels in the dialysate. The features are those of dementia, behavioural changes, seizures and myoclonus. Previously progressive, this condition may be halted or avoided by controlling aluminium levels.

Specific investigations and treatment of individual metabolic encephalopathies do not come within the scope of this book.

Nutritional Disorders

INTRODUCTION

Nutritional deficiency presents a major problem in the developing world. In Western countries, alcoholism is the major cause of the neurological syndromes resulting from dietary deficiency with faddism and malabsorption disorders accounting for only a small number.

Vitamins appear important nutrients and certain disorders such as Wernicke Korsakoff syndrome (thiamine) or subacute combined degeneration (vit B12) can be attributed to a single deficiency whereas others such as polyneuropathy result from multiple deficiency.

Vitamin deficiency alone (as in starvation) does not always produce symptoms; a dietary excess of carbohydrate seems essential for the development of the neurological features of thiamine deficiency.

The deficiency syndromes may occur in pure forms, especially subacute combined degeneration, but those with a common aetiological factor occur in combination with each other.

Wernicke Korsakoff Syndrome

This syndrome is comprised of two parts:

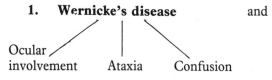

1.   Wernicke's disease   and   **2.   Korsakoff's psychosis**

Ocular involvement   Ataxia   Confusion

Selective impairment of short term (immediate) memory.

Cause:

Thiamine deficiency arising from poor nutrition. ——— Prevalent in alcoholics. Hyperemesis gravidarum and other causes of poor nutrition.

N.B.   Korsakoff's psychosis may also be caused by head injury, anoxia, epilepsy, encephalitis and vascular diseases.

WERNICKE's DISEASE

Pathology:

Lesions take the form of parenchymal necrosis with vacuolation of remaining tissue and haemorrhage.

Lesions are symmetrically present, adjacent to III and IV ventricles, around the aqueduct of Sylvius, mamillary bodies and the dorsal nucleus of the vagus.

Wernicke Korsakoff Syndrome

Wernicke's disease *(continued)*

Clinical features: Develops acutely.

Ocular involvement: - - - - - - - - - - - - - -
   Nystagmus is always present.
   Unilateral or bilateral VI nerve paresis present in $\frac{2}{3}$.
   Gaze palsies are less common.
   Pupillary involvement and complete ophthalmoplegia are rare.
   Retinal haemorrhages occasionally occur.

Confusion:
   Disorientated.
   Disinterested and innatentive.
   Withdrawal symptoms of alcohol:
   – agitation, delusions and hallucinations develop following admission to hospital.

Ataxia – is often the presenting symptom.
   Mild ataxia of gait or gross ataxia with inability to stand.
   Limb involvement is rare.
   No dysarthria.

Associated features:
   Polyneuropathy is present in 80% of cases.
   Vestibular disturbances will occur occasionally and accentuate the ataxia.
   Autonomic disturbances may be seen.

KORSAKOFF's PSYCHOSIS

Pathology:
   Bilateral lesions in the dorsomedial nuclei of the thalamus and the hippocampal formation.

Clinical features:
   There is a disturbance of memory in which new information cannot be stored. In addition the normal temporal sequence of established memories is disrupted, resulting in a semi-fictionalised account of the circumstances which the patient may find himself in – *confabulation.* This memory disturbance can only be tested for when the confusion of Wernicke's disease has cleared.

Investigation of Wernicke Korsakoff Syndrome:
   Haematological and biochemical evidence of alcohol/nutritional deficiency e.g. elevated MCV, abnormal LFT's, elevated γGT.
   The blood *transketolase* (enzyme in hexose monophosphate shunt) is an index of thiamine levels, and should be measured immediately before being modified by hospital diet.
   The blood *pyruvate* is less accurate.

Treatment of Wernicke Korsakoff Syndrome:
   Beware, when giving i.v. infusions to confused patients, as dextrose will use up the remaining thiamine and aggravate the condition.

   50 mg thiamine i.v.
   +   } daily until normal diet is commenced.
   50 mg thiamine i.m.

   Eyes improve – in days, though nystagmus may persist for months.
   Ataxia improves – in weeks.
   Memory disturbance once established will persist despite treatment in the majority (80%) of patients.
   Overall mortality: 15% ⟶ coma ⟶ death.

Subacute Combined Degeneration of the Spinal Cord

Cause:

B12 deficiency   – Impaired absorption due to lack of intrinsic factor (idiopathic).
                          – Following total or partial gastrectomy.
                          – Malabsorption syndrome.
                          – Dietary deficiency (rare).

Pathology:

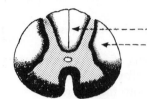

Spinal cord demyelination – affects:
Posterior columns and
Lateral columns (corticospinal and spinocerebellar tracts).
Corticospinal degeneration is most evident in the lower cord, posterior column degeneration in the upper cord.
Peripheral nerve large myelinated fibre degeneration also occurs.

B12 deficiency resulting in neurological damage is usually associated with a *megaloblastic anaemia* in most cases, though a normal peripheral blood film may be found.

The exact role of B12 in tissue metabolism, especially within the nervous system, has not been defined.

Clinical features:

Onset is subacute, not chronic.
Paraesthesia of extremities is the presenting symptom.
                   Numbness and distal weakness follow.
Walking becomes unsteady and spasticity is evident in the lower limbs with flexor or extensor spasms.

Examination:

– Gait is ataxic (sensory ataxia).
– Motor power is diminished distally.
– Plantar responses are extensor.
– Sensory loss: loss of vibration and joint position sensation in the lower limbs. Stocking/glove sensory loss is found when peripheral nerves are involved.
– Reflex findings are variable and depend on the predominance of peripheral nerve or corticospinal tract involvement.

Associated features:

Mental changes, due to anaemia or hemisphere demyelination, may progress from dullness to dementia.

Optic nerve involvement similar to tobacco/alcohol amblyopia may ocur.

Subacute Combined Degeneration of the Spinal Cord

Diagnosis:

Suspect in paraparesis with combined upper and lower motor neurone signs with 'stocking/glove' sensory loss.

Differentiate from other causes of acute myelopathy e.g. . cord compression, multiple sclerosis.

Investigation:

Peripheral blood film
- anaemia,
- elevated MCV,
- normal MCHC,
- mild leukopenia/thrombocytopenia.

Bone marrow – megaloblastic erythropoesis.

B12 (serum) low.

Investigation of underlying cause of B12 deficiency is essential:
- Schilling test,
- gastroscopy,
- barium meal,
- investigation of absorption.

Treatment:

Parenteral B12 (Hydroxocobalamin – 1mg/ml).

1mg daily for 1 week.

1mg 3 times per week until peripheral blood film is normal.

1mg monthly thereafter.

Course and Progression:

Untreated, the disorder is progressive, the patient eventually becoming bed bound.

If diagnosed and treated early (within 2 months of onset), complete recovery can be anticipated.

In established cases, only progression may be halted.

Caution:

When folic acid is prescribed for megaloblastic anaemia, it will improve the haematological picture of B12 deficiency with rapid and occasionally irreversible deterioration of the neurological symptoms and signs.

Polyneuropathy

The combination of polyneuropathy and cardiac involvement is referred to as BERI-BERI. When oedema is also present it is termed wet beri-beri and, when absent, dry beri-beri. Beri-beri occurs in rice eating countries.

In Western countries, alcoholism is the major cause of nutritional polyneuropathy with or without cardiac involvement.

Deficiency of vitamin B complex – THIAMINE, PYRIDOXINE, PANTOTHENIC ACID – results in peripheral nerve damage.

Pathology:

Nerve cell → Axon

Segmental demyelination and axonal degeneration occur simultaneously

Longest and largest diameter nerve fibres are affected first.

Anterior horn cells and dorsal root ganglion cells undergo chromatolysis.

Vagus nerve and sympathetic trunk involvement occurs in severe cases.

Clinical features:

Onset: Subacute

Symptoms Weakness. Distal paraesthesia – burning feet. Pain – lancinating quality.

Signs

1. Varying degrees of *areflexia* (only ankle reflexes are lost initially).
2. *Weakness* which is more marked distally than proximally and initially involves the lower limbs.
3. *Sensory loss* of a 'stocking/glove' type involving all modalities of sensation.
4. *Sympathetic* involvement results in sweating soles of feet and occasionally demonstrable orthostatic hypotension.
5. *Vagus nerve* involvement results in a hoarse voice and disturbance of swallowing.

Associated signs: Shiny skin on legs with poor distal hair growth. 'Hyperpathic' painful soles of feet.

Diagnosis:

Suggested by nutritional/alcohol history.

Supported by investigations such as peripheral blood film (MCV), LFT's and γGT.

Nerve conduction studies confirm the clinical picture and detect asymptomatic cases with minimal signs e.g. reduced ankle reflexes, diminished peripheral vibration sensation.

Differential diagnosis:

Other causes of acute/subacute neuropathy.

Treatment:

Balanced diet with vitamin B group supplementation.

Burning paraesthesia may respond to carbamazepine or to a lumbar sympathetic block.

Recovery may be very slow but with the withdrawal of alcohol and adequate vitamin supplementation some recovery will occur.

524

Optic Neuropathy

The development of chronic visual loss as a result of optic neuritis occurs in the malnourished patient with high tobacco consumption (Tobacco alcohol amblyopia). It is much less common than polyneuropathy.

Pathology:
Damage to myelinated fibres in the papillomacular bundle of the optic nerve. Retinal ganglion cells at the macular area are also damaged.

Clinical features:
The condition slowly develops over weeks.
Vision becomes hazy and blurred.
Colour vision (red green discrimination) is involved early.

Examination:
Bilateral involvement.
Reduced visual acuity.
Centrocaecal scotoma
   (a field defect of an
   eliptical shape spreading
   from blind spot to macula and most easily detected with a red target).

Blind spot   Macula

Fundal examination is normal, though optic atrophy will occur eventually.
Coexistent Wernicke Korsakoff syndrome or polyneuropathy are common.

Treatment:
Improvement in nutrition will halt progression and even result in gradual shrinkage of the scotoma.
Vitamin B supplementation, especially B12, should be administered.

Alcohol Related Disorders

ALCOHOLIC MYOPATHY
Muscle damage (elevated creatine phosphokinase) is not uncommon in alcoholics following acute ingestion. But rarely is this symptomatic.

Acute alcoholic myopathy occurs after 'binge' drinking.
Acute muscle necrosis ensues with pain/cramping and muscle tenderness/swelling.
Myoglobin is excreted in the urine (myoglobinuria) after release
   from damaged muscles.
Symptoms of alcohol withdrawal – delirium, etc – coexist.
Limb involvement may be markedly asymmetrical.
Sometimes both calf muscles are swollen and tender.
Improvement occurs with hospitalisation.
Marked myoglobinuria may result in *renal failure*.
Elevated serum K^+ may provoke cardiac arrhythmias.
Aetiology appears due to the direct toxic effect of alcohol on muscle.
Chronic proximal weakness has been described, but is rare.

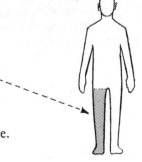

Alcohol Related Disorders

ALCOHOLIC CEREBELLAR DEGENERATION

Ataxia occurs as a component of Wernicke's disease or as a distinct clinical entity with a chronic progressive course.

A long history of alcohol abuse is obtained. Male alcoholics are predominantly affected. Onset is gradual and symptoms often stabilise.

Ataxia of gait with lower limb incoordination predominates. The upper limbs are spared.

Nystagmus is rarely present and cerebellar dysarthria very uncommon.

Coexistent signs of neuropathy are often found.

Investigations: – Abnormal liver function tests. Macrocytosis in peripheral blood film.
CSF examination normal.
CT scanning may reveal cerebellar atrophy with an enlarged IV ventricle.

Progression → may evolve rapidly and reverse with improved nutrition and alcohol withdrawal.
may evolve subacutely.
may evolve chronically and slowly progress over many years.

Pathology: —— Purkinje cell loss in cerebellar hemispheres and in superior cerebellar vermis.

Pathogenesis: – Cerebellar degeneration occurs in malnutrition as well as alcohol abuse and the response of acute ataxia in Wernicke's disease to thiamine would suggest that this is important in the genesis of cerebellar degeneration.

Differential diagnosis: — Distinguish from hereditary and other acquired ataxias e.g. hypothyroidism, remote effects of carcinoma.

Treatment: — Alcohol withdrawal, a well balanced diet and adequate vitamin supplementation.

CENTRAL PONTINE MYELINOLYSIS

A history of alcohol abuse or debilitating disease such as carcinoma is obtained.

The lesion is one of demyelination with cavitation. Microscopically, myelin is lost, oligodendrocytes degenerate but neurones and axons are spared.

Clinically, an acute or subacute pontine lesion is suspected, evolving over a few days, with bulbar weakness and tetraparesis.

The limbs are flaccid with extensor plantar responses.

With progression of the lesion, eye signs become evident and conscious level becomes depressed → coma → death.

Pons

Investigations:

Electrolytic disturbances (low sodium, low phosphate) are found.
Liver function is normal. CSF examination is normal.

Recognition of this condition before death is important in view of its reversibility, though it is usually diagnosed at autopsy. Vigorous supportive therapy with correction of metabolic abnormalities and vitamin supplementation is advised.

CORPUS CALLOSUM DEMYELINATION (Syn: Marchiafava-Bignami disease)

This is a rare disorder occurring in malnourished alcoholics. It is rarely diagnosed in life.

The clinical picture is that of personality change with signs of frontal lobe disease.

The condition occurs most commonly in persons of Italian origin.

Non-Metastatic Manifestations of Malignant Disease

Disturbance of neurological function can occur in association with neoplasm without evidence of metastases. Brain, spinal cord, peripheral nerve and muscle may be affected, either separately or in combination with one another. Other forms of malignancy such as the reticuloses may produce similar neurological syndromes.

Bronchial carcinoma is the commonest malignancy to be associated with the non-metastatic syndromes. However this develops in only 20% of patients with bronchial carcinoma.

The non-metastatic manifestations of malignancy are rare, and all types of neoplasia may be incriminated.

NON-METASTATIC NEUROLOGICAL SYNDROMES ⟶

- Encephalitis
- Cerebellar degeneration
- Myelopathy
- Neuropathy
- Myopathy
- Neuromuscular junction disturbance
  Myasthenic syndrome

The syndromes are not discreet e.g. neuropathy and myopathy may coexist – carcinomatous neuromyopathy; encephalitis and myelopathy may coexist – carcinomatous encephalomyelitis.

ENCEPHALITIS

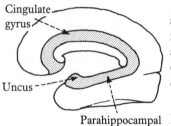

Cingulate gyrus

Uncus

Limbic system

Parahippocampal gyrus

Pathology:
The encephalitic process selectively affects the limbic system – with neuronal loss, astrocytic proliferation and perivascular inflammatory changes.

Clinical features:
Disturbance in behaviour precedes the development of complex partial (temporal lobe) seizures and memory impairment.
The course is progressive.

CEREBELLAR DEGENERATION Usually associated with bronchial or ovarian carcinoma.

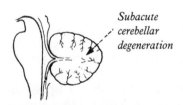

Subacute cerebellar degeneration

Pathology:
Purkinje cell loss with some involvement of the dentate nucleus. Brain stem changes also occur.

Clinical features:
The patient presents with a rapidly developing ataxia.
Brain stem involvement results in nystagmus, ophthalmoplegia and facial weakness.
The course is one of rapid progression.

MYELITIS

Subacute necrotising myelopathy ——

Selective posterolateral column degeneration
A rapidly evolving syndrome which mimics subacute combined degeneration due to B12 deficiency.

Pathology:
Axonal and myelin destruction with microglial proliferation.

Clinical features:
Back pain with ascending paraesthesia, weakness and loss of sphincter control. Upper limb involvement is followed by respiratory paralysis and death.

527

Non-Metastatic Manifestations of Malignant Disease

NEUROPATHY (see page 428)

Sensory neuropathy: Destruction of posterior root ganglion with progressive sensory symptomatology. The neuropathy is subacute or chronic in evolution. Combined axonal and demyelinative peripheral nerve damage. Steroids may evoke a period of remission.

Sensorimotor neuropathy: A mixed neuropathy with weakness and sensory loss. The syndrome may predate the recognition of the underlying neoplasm.

MYOPATHY

Establishing a causal relationship may be difficult.
– Muscle weakness can develop long before evidence of neoplasia.
– In patients with unexplained myopathy, malignancy may be detected only at autopsy.

Proximal Myopathy: A slowly progressive syndrome with weakness of proximal limb muscles. In myopathy occurring in middle/late life, underlying neoplasm is a likely explanation.

Inflammatory Myopathy   (Polymyositis dermatomyositis)   (See page 458):

The overall incidence of associated neoplasm in inflammatory myopathy is 15%. The typical patient is in middle age with a proximal weakness, elevated ESR and muscle enzymes with or without the skin features of dermatomyositis.

Myopathy with Endocrine disturbance: Ectopic hormone production (by malignant cells) may induce a myopathy characterised by chronic progressive proximal weakness, e.g. ectopic ACTH production from oat cell carcinoma of lung.

NEUROMUSCULAR JUNCTION DISTURBANCE

The Myasthenic syndrome   (Eaton-Lambert syndrome)
A disorder of the neuromuscular junction.
Acetylcholine release following nerve stimulation is deficient.

Clinical features:

The patient develops weakness of lower then upper limbs with a tendency to fatigue. Following brief exercise, power may paradoxically suddenly improve – second wind phenomenon. Examination reveals a proximal pattern of weakness and wasting with diminished tendon reflexes.

Diagnosis:

Confirmed electrophysiologically; the 'second wind phenomenon' is shown up as an incrementing response to repetitive nerve stimulation (as opposed to the decrementing response in myasthenia gravis, page 58).

Treatment:

Treatment attempts to increase the presynaptic release of acetylcholine using drugs such as guanidine HCl with some success.
Side effects – paraesthesia, ataxia and confusion may limit usage.
The myasthenic syndrome may develop in the absence of neoplasia, especially so in women.
Patients may present following an abnormal reaction to muscle relaxants during anaesthesia.

These syndromes may respond to the removal of the underlying neoplasm. A totally resectible primary tumour is rarely encountered and the response to resection is unpredictable.

Degenerative Disorders

INTRODUCTION

This heterogeneous group of neurological diseases is grouped together by the lack of known aetiology. As causes of such diseases are identified (e.g. metabolic, viral) they have been reclassified in their appropriate category. Of the remaining conditions many are familial.

Characteristically these disorders
- are gradually progressive.
- are symmetrical (bilateral symptoms and signs).
- may affect one or several specific levels of the nervous system.
- may demonstrate a specific pathology or just show neuronal atrophy and eventual loss without other features.

Classification:

Degenerative disorders are classified according to the specific part or parts of the central/peripheral nervous system affected and according to the ensuing clinical manifestations. The degenerative disorders may be alternatively termed the *system degenerations* because of their propensity to affect only part of the nervous system.

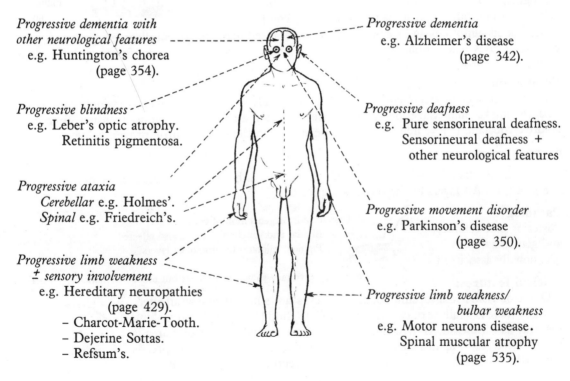

Progressive dementia with other neurological features
      e.g. Huntington's chorea
           (page 354).

Progressive blindness
      e.g. Leber's optic atrophy.
          Retinitis pigmentosa.

Progressive ataxia
      Cerebellar e.g. Holmes'.
      Spinal e.g. Friedreich's.

Progressive limb weakness ± sensory involvement
      e.g. Hereditary neuropathies
           (page 429).
        – Charcot-Marie-Tooth.
        – Dejerine Sottas.
        – Refsum's.

Progressive dementia
      e.g. Alzheimer's disease
           (page 342).

Progressive deafness
      e.g. Pure sensorineural deafness.
          Sensorineural deafness +
           other neurological features

Progressive movement disorder
      e.g. Parkinson's disease
           (page 350).

Progressive limb weakness/ bulbar weakness
      e.g. Motor neurons disease.
         Spinal muscular atrophy
           (page 535).

Most of these conditions are discussed in other chapters.

Progressive Blindness

LEBER's OPTIC ATROPHY

Leber's optic atrophy is a familial disorder of variable inheritance with a tendency to affect males significantly more than females.

Pathology: 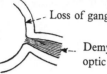 -- Loss of ganglion cells in the retina.

-- Demyelination and axonal loss in the optic nerve (papillomacular bundle).

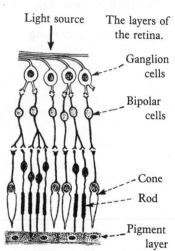

The layers of the retina.

- Ganglion cells
- Bipolar cells
- Cone
- Rod
- Pigment layer

Clinical features:

Onset of visual loss in late teens/early twenties.
- This is usually slow and insidious.
- Both eyes are simulatneously affected (rarely one eye months before the other).
- Central vision is lost with large bilateral scotomata.

Characteristically, blue/yellow colour discrimination is affected before red/green. The optic disc, initially blurred, eventually becomes pale and atrophic.

Progressive loss advances with peripheral constriction of the fields of vision, but visual impairment is rarely complete.

Associated symptoms and signs of a more generalised nervous system disorder occur in a proportion of cases – dementia, ataxia, progressive spastic paraplegia – and confusion with multiple sclerosis may arise.

Treatment:

There is no specific treatment. Patients should be advised to stop smoking – cyanide content of tobacco smoke may have deleterious effect on an already compromised visual function. Hydroxycobalamine (cyanide binder) has been used but appears of little proven value.

RETINITIS PIGMENTOSA

A hereditary disorder of the retina which may be inherited as an autosomal dominant or recessive trait. All layers of the retina are affected.

Pathology:

Posterior pale cataracts and glaucoma are occasionally associated.

-- Loss of rods, degeneration of cones.
Bipolar and ganglion cells are also affected.
Pigment migrates to superficial layers.

The optic nerve may show some gliosis but often is remarkably normal.

Clicical features:

Onset of visual loss in childhood. Both eyes are simultaneously affected. Initially there is a failure of twilight vision. The child has difficulty in making his way as darkness falls (nyctalopia). The retina around the macular area is first affected resulting in a characteristic ring scotoma. This gradually spreads outwards; eventually only a small 'tunnel' of central vision is left. Finally, complete blindness occurs. The majority of patients are completely blind by 50 years of age.

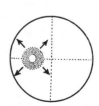

Progressive Blindness

RETINITIS PIGMENTOSA *(continued)*

The fundal appearance is diagnostic as a result of the superficial migration of pigment.

The electroretinogram – recording the electrical activity of the retina – is abnormal.

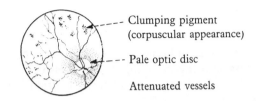

- - - Clumping pigment (corpuscular appearance)

- - - Pale optic disc

Attenuated vessels

Treatment:

None. Vitamins and steroids have been tried unsuccessfully.

Associated Conditions in Retinitis Pigmentosa

Several conditions are associated with retinitis pigmentosa:

- Hypogonadism/obesity/mental deficiency
- Spinocerebellar degeneration
- Polyneuropathy/ sensorineural deafness
- Myopathy/ophthalmoplegia/heart block

- Laurence Moon syndrome.
- Friedreich's ataxia.
- Refsum's syndrome.
- Kearns-Sayre syndrome.

Progressive Ataxia

The degenerative disorders manifested by progressive ataxia are termed *spinocerebellar degenerations*. Further classification is difficult in view of the many descriptions of familial cases in the literature, often bearing the eponymous title of the original author. The clinical overlap in these various forms is such that a broad concept of the disorders is the only pragmatic approach to them.

Familial cerebellar degeneration of *childhood* – Ataxia telangiectasia.

Familial spinocerebellar degeneratiof of *adults*:

1. *Spinal form*
   - Friedreich's ataxia.
   - Roussy-Levy syndrome.
   - Marie's spastic ataxia.

2. *Cerebellar form*
   - Cortical cerebellar degeneration of Holmes.
   - Dyssynergia cerebellaris myoclonica (Ramsay Hunt syndrome).
   - Olivopontocerebellar degeneration.

ATAXIA TELANGIECTASIA

An autosomal recessive disorder with onset in childhood.

Pathologically, widespread cerebellar neuronal loss occurs.

This is associated with ocular and cutaneous telangiectasia, which become more widespread with age.

Neurological features are those of mild mental retardation, progressive ataxia of stance/gait/limbs with dysarthria and nystagmus.

Patients are eventually confined to a wheelchair and, because of associated low serum levels of IgA and Ige, are susceptible to repetitive infections and the development of neoplasia.

Treatment is symptomatic.

Progressive Ataxia

SPINAL FORM

FRIEDREICH's ATAXIA

This is an inherited disorder with autosomal recessive and autosomal dominant forms; the recessive being more rapidly progressive.

The underlying cause of this condition is probably metabolic.

Pathology:

1. *Spinal:* The spinal cord is shrunken, especially in the thoracic region.
There is degeneration and gliosis of:

1.. Posterior columns.
2.. Corticospinal tracts.
3.. Dorsal spinocerebellar tracts.
4.. Ventral spinocerebellar tracts.

Dorsal roots and peripheral nerves are also shrunken when cases are. advanced.

2. *Cerebellar:* Changes in the cerebellum are less marked, There is Purkinje cell loss and atrophy of the dentate nucleus.

The corticobulbar tract and cerebrum are spared.

Clinical features:

Onset in 1st or 2nd decade. Sexes are equally affected.

Disturbance of gait is the initial symptom, progressing to lower limb ataxia   upper limb ataxia   truncal ataxia.

Involuntary movements of a myoclonic nature (see page 177) occur.

Corticospinal tract involvement results in limb weakness with absent abdominal reflexes and extensor plantar responses.

Posterior column involvement results in loss of vibration and joint position appreciation in the extremities.

Dorsal root involvement results in absent lower limb reflexes.

Involvement of myocardial muscle (cardiomyopathy) is common and results in cardiac failure or dysrhythmias.

Musculoskeletal abnormalities occur in 80% of cases.

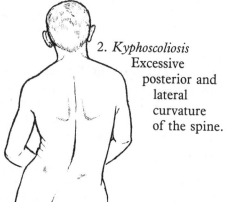

1. *Pes cavus* (club foot) with extension of metatarsophalangeal and flexion of interphalangeal joints.

2. *Kyphoscoliosis* Excessive posterior and lateral curvature of the spine.

Optic atrophy, retinitis pigmentosa, nystagmus, peroneal muscular atrophy and convulsions may all occur . occasionally in Friedreich's ataxia.

Progressive Ataxia

Friedreich's Ataxia *(continued)*

The disease is progressive. Patients are usually unable to walk within 5 years of onset, and death from cardiac (cardiomyopathy) or pulmonary (kyphoscoliosis) complications occurs within 10–20 years. Arrested cases without progression do occur but are rare.

Diagnosis:

Considered when midline and limb ataxia develops in childhood. As the disease progresses into a 'typical' case diagnosis is obvious, but initially exclusion of the many inborn errors of metabolism producing ataxia in childhood is necessary.

Aetiology:

A probable 'inborn' metabolic disorder; abnormal glucose tolerance and deficiency of enzyme *pyruvate dehydrogenase* have been identified in some patients.

Treatment:

Usually supportive. Choline and lecithin have been used for ataxia but without dramatic results. High fat diet to by-pass pyruvate dehydrogenase deficiency has had a limited success.

ROUSSY-LEVY SYNDROME

A probable variant of Friedreich's ataxia, associated with features of peroneal muscular atrophy (Charcot Marie Tooth disease).

The clinical course is more benign. Autosomal dominant and sex linked recessive inheritance is described. Nystagmus and dysarthria are infrequent findings.

The peripheral nerve component is evident clinically:
- wasting,
- sensory loss,
- hypertrophic nerves,

and can be confirmed by electromyography and nerve conduction studies.

MARIE'S SPASTIC ATAXIA

A probable variant of Friedreich's ataxia, associated with features of a progressive spastic paraplegia (more marked than that found in pure Friedreich's ataxia).

The onset is in adult life, much later than Friedreich's. The legs are noticeably 'stiff' when the patient walks. Dysarthria is rare.

Pes cavus and kyphoscoliosis are less common.

Progressive Ataxia

CEREBELLAR FORM

CORTICAL CEREBELLAR DEGENERATION OF HOLMES

A mendelian disorder.

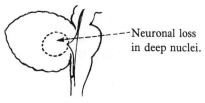

Neuronal loss
in deep nuclei.

Progressive degeneration of the cerebellar cortex
with Purkinje cell loss and reactive gliosis.

Clinical features:

Onset in middle age, with lower limb involvement, then
dysarthria and upper limb spread.

Seizures and myoclonus may ensue.

The disorder is progressive over 12–15 years.

Distinction should be made from acquired cerebellar degeneration e.g.

      alcohol/nutritional,

      hypothyroidism,

      drugs e.g. phenytoin.

DYSSYNERGIA CEREBELLARIS MYOCLONICA

(Ramsay Hunt syndrome)

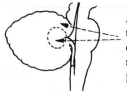

Myoclonus reflects
the damage to the
dentate nucleus and
superior cerebellar
peduncle.

Characterised by the presence of myoclonus in an early
onset cerebellar degeneration.

Mendelian dominant disorder with onset in childhood.
The disorder progresses with age. Myoclonic jerks of limbs
and trunk are associated with nystagmus, dysarthria, ataxia
of gait and stance and limb incoordination.

OLIVOPONTOCEREBELLAR DEGENERATION

A sporadically occurring disorder.

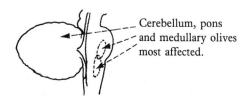

Cerebellum, pons
and medullary olives
most affected.

Diffuse cerebral atrophy and ventricular dilatation also occurs.

Variable age of onset.

Initial features are purely cerebellar then involvement of
bulbar musculature and extrapyramidal features become
evident.

The patient becomes immobile and develops progressive
speech and swallowing difficulties.

Autonomic features may be associated.

Survival ranges from 25–30 years from onset.

Motor Neurone Disease

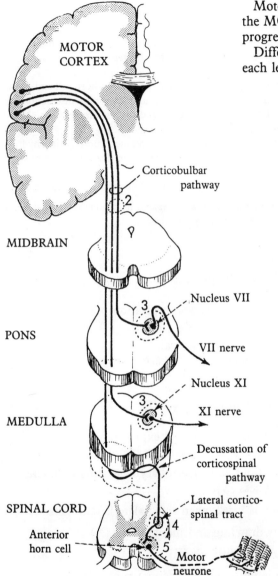

MOTOR CORTEX

Corticobulbar pathway

MIDBRAIN

2

PONS

3

Nucleus VII

VII nerve

Nucleus XI

MEDULLA

3

XI nerve

Decussation of corticospinal pathway

SPINAL CORD

Lateral cortico-spinal tract

Anterior horn cell

4

5

Motor neurone

Motor neurone disease is a degenerative disorder of the MOTOR SYSTEM affecting several levels. It is a progressive disorder with no specific treatment.

Different terms are used to describe involvement at each level:

1. The motor cortex.
2. The corticobulbar pathway:
   PSEUDOBULBAR PALSY.
3. The cranial nerve nuclei:
   PROGRESSIVE BULBAR PALSY.
4. The corticospinal tract:
   PRIMARY LATERAL SCLEROSIS.
5. The anterior horn cell:
   PROGRESSIVE MUSCULAR
   ATROPHY.

The clinical picture is always a mixture of the above.

When 4 and 5 predominate, the term AMYOTROPHIC LATERAL
SCLEROSIS is used.

Epidemiology:

Male : Female = 1.5 : 1.
Prevalence — 4 in 100,000.
Annual mortality — 1 in 100,000.
Age at onset — 35–50 years.
Geographical distribution — world wide.
Island of Guam, prevalence — 100 in
100,000.

Pathology

Naked eye: Thinning of anterior roots
of spinal cord.

Microscopic: Loss of neurones in motor cortex.
Loss of neurones in cranial nerve
nuclei and anterior horns.
Section of brain stem: reduction of corticobulbar and
corticospinal fibres.

No evidence of inflammatory response is seen in involved structures.

535

Motor Neurone Disease

Aetiology

The cause of motor neurone disease is unknown. Several possibilities have been suggested:

–Ageing: Premature ageing in certain motor cells may result in increasing metabolic demand upon survivors. As a consequence the survivors also suffer premature loss. This process could be 'triggered' by genetic and environmental factors.

–Viruses: Slow virus infection has been suggested. Polio virus will acutely damage the anterior horn cell and 'slow' polio infection could theoretically produce motor neurone disease. Some claim that motor neurone disease follows acute poliomyelitis; however, when this occurs the clinical picture is not typical and may resemble more closely Spinal Muscular Atrophy (see later).

–Disordered carbohydrate metabolism: Variable findings such as diabetic glucose tolerance curves, carbohydrate intolerance and insulin resistance, have been described in patients with motor neurone disease. No consistent abnormality has been found.

–Toxins: Certain metals, lead, selenium and manganese have been incriminated, but again evidence is inconclusive.

An increased incidence of *gastric surgery* in sufferers, the presence of *immune complexes* in small bowel biopsies and disordered *cellular immunity* have been noted but causative relationships are unclear.

CLINICAL FEATURES

The following features always occur in combination.

When bulbar or pseudobulbar features predominate the prognosis is:

> 2 – 3 years survival.
>
> Death from inanition and aspiration pneumonia.

When progressive muscular atrophy predominates the prognosis is:

> As long as 15 years survival.
>
> Periods of apparent disease arrest may occur.

Pseudobulbar Palsy

Features are due to degeneration of corticobulbar pathways to V, VII, X, XI and XII cranial nerve motor nuclei.

There is an apparent weakness of the muscles of mastication and expression, the patient has difficulty in chewing and the face is expressionless. The jaw jerk is exaggerated.

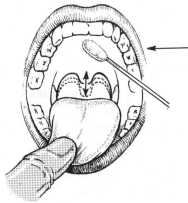

Food and fluid enter nasopharynx when swallowing – palatal weakness (X).

Gag reflex is brisk when soft palate is stimulated.

Speech is drawling and monotonous (X).

Swallowing is difficult (X).

Tongue is immobile and cannot protrude (XII).

Often spontaneous outbursts of laughing and crying occur – EMOTIONAL LABILITY.

Motor Neurone Disease

Progressive Bulbar Palsy

The symptoms and signs are due to a disturbance of the motor cranial nuclei rather than corticobulbar tracts. The condition is distinguished from pseudobulbar palsy by the presence of lower neurone (nuclear) signs.

Atrophy and *fasciculation* are present.

Fasciculations are visible muscle twitches which occur spontaneously and represent a discharging motor unit.

The tongue is best examined for these features.

At rest in the mouth, the tongue is wasted and folded, and fasciculation is evident giving a writhing appearance.

Jaw jerk and gag reflex are absent: fasciculation and atrophy may be present in other cranial nerve innervated muscles.

Primary Lateral Sclerosis

Signs of corticospinal tract disturbance with:
- –Increased tone.
- –Brisk reflexes.
- –Extensor plantar responses.
- –Distinctive distribution of weakness
  (extensors in upper limbs; flexors in lower limbs).

Spasticity is rarely severe (Intact extrapyramidal inhibition).

Progressive Muscular Atrophy

Signs and symptoms are due to anterior horn cell involvement.

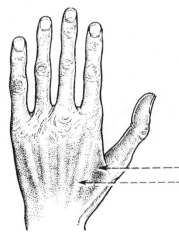

Atrophy,
weakness and
fasciculations are the cardinal features.

The patient is often aware of fasciculation.

Muscle cramps are common.

Weakness is not as severe as the degree of wasting suggests.

In the hand: wasting is evident.
1st dorsal interosseous muscle and tendons become prominent as hand muscles waste, giving 'guttered' appearance –
SKELETON HAND.

Gradual spread into all four limbs and trunk occurs as the disease progresses.

Motor Neurone Disease

Amyotrophic Lateral Sclerosis

Characterised by the unusual, almost diagnostic appearance of wasted, fasciculating muscles (anterior horn cell) with brisk reflexes (corticospinal tract). This is described as TONIC ATROPHY.

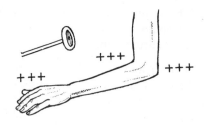

> *N.B.*   SENSORY SIGNS DO NOT OCCUR.
> BLADDER IS NEVER INVOLVED.
> OCULAR MUSCLES ARE NEVER AFFECTED.

Relentless progression of symptoms and signs is inevitable.

Diagnosis

The clinical findings are quite characteristic. These are supported by electromyography which reveals denervation with fibrillations widespread in different muscle groups (see EMG).

Differential Diagnosis includes disorders which produce combined upper and lower motor neurone signs e.g.
Cervical spondylosis.

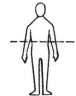

Segmental (LMN signs) weakness

Corticospinal muscle weakness

Pseudobulbar palsy may result also from cerebrovascular disease or multiple sclerosis.

Progressive muscular atrophy may be confused with a spinal muscular atrophy or limb girdle dystrophy.

Treatment

Specific: No effective treatment.
Antiviral drugs such as amantadine remain unproven.
Guanidine HCl – anecdotal reports of success.

Symptomatic:

Supportive – appliances to aid increasing weakness.
When dysphagia is the result of pseudobulbar palsy
- cricopharyngeal myotomy may greatly aid swallowing.
- section of the chorda tympani is helpful when swallowing saliva is difficult.

538

Chronic Spinal Muscular Atrophies

Chronic spinal muscular atrophies are hereditary disorders which are characterised by degeneration of cranial nerve nuclei and anterior horn cells of the spinal cord. As with motor neurone disease these disorders solely affect the motor system.

Werdnig Hoffman Disease

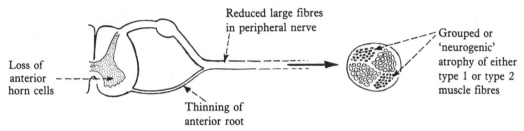

Clinical Features

An autosomal recessive disorder.
Reduced fetal movements are noted in late pregnancy with weakness and hypotonia at birth.
The child lies with arms and legs abducted and externally rotated.
Contractures, wasting and fasciculation become more evident.

Clinical Progress

May progress rapidly to death in 2–3 months.
In survivors, all motor milestones are delayed and 95 per cent of all cases are dead by 18 months.

Kugelberg Welander Disease

Pathological features similar to Werdnig Hoffman disease. Both autosomal dominant and sex-linked recessive inheritances have been described. Onset is in childhood, adolescence or early adult life.

Clinical Features

The disorder is characterised by weakness and wasting of proximal limb muscles. It is slowly progressive with great variability even within the same family. Survival into old age without serious disability can occur.

This disorder may easily be confused with *limb girdle dystrophy* and separated from it only by:
        1. The presence of fasciculation (50% of patients).
        2. EMG pattern (neurogenic).
        3. Muscle biopsy showing the grouped 'neurogenic' atrophy of muscle fibres.

There is no treatment for these conditions.
Genetic counselling is important.

Hereditary Spastic Paraplegia

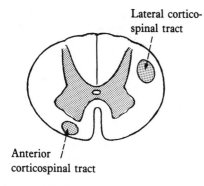

Lateral cortico-spinal tract

Anterior corticospinal tract

This is a mendelian dominant disorder in which there is progressive disturbance of motor function due to selective degeneration of the corticospinal tracts.

Clinical Features

Progressive spastic weakness involving initially the legs and then the arms.

High arched feet with flexion at knees and scissors-like gait are characteristic.

Reflexes are exaggerated, plantar responses extensor.

Bulbar and bladder function may eventually be disturbed.

Differential Diagnosis

When family history is present – consider familial multiple sclerosis.

When 'sporadic' (no family history) – diagnosis is by exclusion of all other inflammatory/vascular/compressive cord syndromes.

With negative investigation and a very slow pure motor clinical course – the diagnosis of *sporadic spastic paraplegia* may be made.

There is no treatment for this condition other than supportive.

Hereditary spastic paraplegia may be associated with degeneration in other neurological systems:

with spinocerebellar ataxia   with extrapyramidal involvement   with retinal degeneration   with optic atrophy

Here there are many syndromes described with eponymous titles. Their memorisation serves little purpose in view of the great rarity with which they are encountered.

The Phakomatoses

The phakomatoses are hereditary disorders characterised by multiorgan malformations and tumours. The tendency towards neurological and cutaneous involvement accounts for the alternative title of NEUROCUTANEOUS SYNDROMES.

These are: Neurofibromatosis,   Sturge-Weber disease,   Ataxia telangiectasia.
              Tuberose sclerosis,   Von Hippel-Lindau disease,

NEUROFIBROMATOSIS – Von Recklinghausen's disease

Incidence: / 1:2000.

Autosomal dominant inheritance.

Characterised by tumours of the skin, peripheral nervous system, central nervous system, viscera and vascular system as well as by a disturbance of cutaneous pigmentation.

Pathology:

An embryological disorder in which localised overgrowth of *mesodermal* or *ectodermal* tissue occurs.

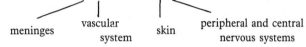

| meninges | vascular system | skin | peripheral and central nervous systems |

Clinical features:

Skin manifestations: —— Café au lait spots: light brown patches on the trunk with well demarcated edges.

Subcutaneous neurofibromata lying along peripheral nerves and enlarging with age.

Mollusca fibrosa: cutaneous fibromas – large, pedunculated and pink in colour.

Plexiform neuroma: diffuse neurofibromatosis associated with skin and subcutaneous overgrowth and occasional underlying bony abnormality.

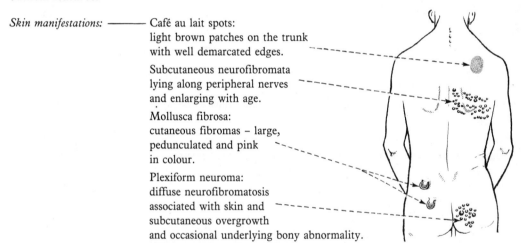

Skeletal manifestations: —— 50% of patients exhibit scoliosis.
Subperiosteal neurofibromas may give rise to bone hypertrophy or rarification with pathological fractures.

Hypertension: —— May result from intimal hyperplasia or coexistent phaeochromocytoma.

Neurological manifestations: – Mental retardation and epilepsy occur in 10–15% of patients without intracranial neoplasm.
Cerebrovascular accidents as a consequence of intimal hyperplasia are not uncommon.
Three patterns of neurological neoplasia are recognised:

1. *Intracranial neoplasms:*
   Optic nerve glioma.
   Acoustic nerve neuroma.
   Multiple meningioma.

2. *Intraspinal neoplasms:*
   Meningioma.
   Neurofibroma.
   Glioma.

3. *Peripheral nerve neoplasms:*
   Neurofibroma – a small
   proportion of which
   become sarcomatous.

541

The Phakomatoses

NEUROFIBROMATOSIS *(continued)*

Diagnosis:

A family history is obtained in over 50% of patients. The cutaneous manifestations are characteristic though they may be extremely mild with only café au lait spots (more than 6 in an individual is diagnostic). As a rule, the more florid the cutaneous manifestations the less likely is there nervous system involvement. CT scanning, caloric testing, X-rays of internal auditory meati and myelography may be necessary when nervous system involvement is suspected.

Treatment:

Surgical removal of symptomatic lesions.

TUBEROSE SCLEROSIS

Incidence: 1:30,000.

Autosomal dominant inheritance.

Characterised by skin lesions, epilepsy and occasionally mental retardation.

Pathology:

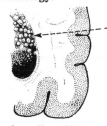

An embryological disorder.

Hard gliotic 'tubers' arise anywhere within the hemispheres but commonly around the ventricles. Projection into the ventricles produces a typical appearance like 'dripping candle wax'.

Tubers in the brain result from astrocytic overgrowth with large vacuolated cells and loss of surrounding myelin. ⟶ Transition may occur from gliosis to a subependymal astrocytoma.

As well as skin lesions, primitive renal tumours and cystic lung hamartomas occur.

Clinical features:

Skin manifestations:

The cutaneous lesions are characteristic – adenoma sebaceum appearing towards the end of the 1st year, though occasionally as late as the 5th year.

Red papular rash over the face and nose.

Depigmented areas on the trunk resembling vitiligo are common.

Fibromas and café au lait spots occur occasionally.

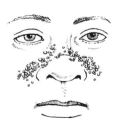

Neurological manifestations: — Mental retardation is present in 60% of cases, though the onset and its recognition may be delayed.

Seizures occur in almost all cases, often as early as the 1st week of life. Attacks are initially focal motor and eventually become generalised. The response to anticonvulsants is variable.

Intracranial neoplasms – astrocytomas – arise from tubers usually close to the ventricles and may result in an obstructive hydrocephalus.

Diagnosis:

The presence of epilepsy and adenoma sebaceum is diagnostic.

CT scan may show periventricular areas of calcium deposition.

Treatment:

Anticonvulsant therapy for epilepsy. Surgical removal of symptomatic lesions.

542

The Phakomatoses

STURGE-WEBER SYNDROME

Angiomatosis affecting the facial skin, eyes and leptomeninges produces the characteristic features of the Sturge-Weber syndrome:

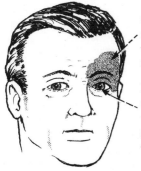

CAPILLARY NAEVUS or 'port wine stain' usually involving forehead and eyelid.

EYE DISORDERS are common –buphthalmos (congenital glaucoma), choroidal angioma.

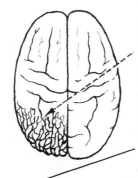

Thickened leptomeninges ipsilateral to the facial naevus and full of abnormal vessels overly an **ATROPHIC HEMISPHERE** with degenerative changes and calcification usually most marked in the parieto-occipital cortex.

↓

EPILEPSY occurs in 90%, usually presenting in infancy.

HEMIPARESIS, HOMONYMOUS HEMIANOPIA, BEHAVIOURAL DISORDER and MENTAL RETARDATION

Skull X-ray shows calcification and CT scan, in addition, shows the associated atrophic change.

Treatment:

Intractable epilepsy may require lobectomy or even hemispherectomy. Some recommend early excision of the surface lesion, but the rarity of the condition prevents thorough treatment evaluation.

VON HIPPEL-LINDAU DISEASE

An autosomal dominant disorder in which haemangioblastomas are found in the cerebellum, spinal canal and retina, and are associated with a number of visceral pathologies:

> Renal angioma,
> Renal cell carcinoma,
> Phaeochromocytoma,
> Pancreatic adenoma/cyst,
> Erythrocytosis.

Any of the above may produce signs and symptoms.

Retinal haemangioblastoma is seen in fundoscopy and may produce sudden blindness.

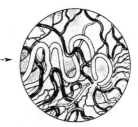

Cerebellar haemangioblastoma presents with progressive ataxia. Compression of the fourth ventricle may cause hydrocephalus with a subsequent rise in intracranial pressure.

Spinal canal haemangioblastoma – intradural lesion presenting with signs and symptoms of cord or root compression.

In long term survivors, renal carcinoma and phaeochromocytoma are the principle causes of death.

Treatment: depends on symptomatology.

ATAXIA TELANGIECTASIA   See page 531.

543

FURTHER READING

Adams R D, Victor M 1985 Principles of neurology, 3rd edn. McGraw-Hill, New York

Bickerstaff E R 1977 Neurological examination in clinical practice, 4th edn. Arnold, London

Brodal A 1981 Neurological anatomy, 3rd edn. Oxford University Press

Jennett W B, Teasdale G 1981 Management of head injuries. Davis, Philadelphia

Northfield D W C 1973 The surgery of the central nervous system. Blackwell, Oxford.

Ross Russell R W 1983 Vascular diseases of the central nervous system, 2nd edn. Churchill Livingstone, Edinburgh

Russell D S, Rubinstein LJ 1977 Pathology of tumours of the nervous system, 4th edn. Arnold, London

Walton J N 1985 Brain's diseases of the nervous system, 9th edn. Oxford University Press, Oxford

Wilkins R H, Rengachary S S (eds) 1985 Neurosurgery. McGraw-Hill, New York

INDEX

548